Barbara Fowble • Sue S. Yom
Florence Yuen • Sarah Arron
Editors

Keith Sharee • Abhishek Jairam
Associate Editors

Skin Care in Radiation Oncology

A Practical Guide

Springer

Editors
Barbara Fowble, MD, FACR, FASTRO
Department of Radiation Oncology
University of California San Francisco
San Francisco, CA, USA

Sue S. Yom, MD, PhD
Department of Radiation Oncology
University of California San Francisco
San Francisco, CA, USA

Florence Yuen, RN, MSN, AOCNP
Department of Radiation Oncology
University of California San Francisco
San Francisco, CA, USA

Sarah Arron, MD, PhD
Department of Dermatology
University of California San Francisco
San Francisco, CA, USA

Associate Editors
Keith Sharee, BA
Department of Radiation Oncology
University of California San Francisco
San Francisco, CA, USA

Abhishek Jairam, BA
Department of Radiation Oncology
University of California San Francisco
San Francisco, CA, USA

ISBN 978-3-319-31458-7 ISBN 978-3-319-31460-0 (eBook)
DOI 10.1007/978-3-319-31460-0

Library of Congress Control Number: 2016947072

This Springer imprint is published by Springer Nature
The registered company is Springer International Publishing AG Switzerland

Skin Care in Radiation Oncology

Preface

On any given day, thousands of patients will receive radiation for cancer or other conditions. Most of these patients will experience some degree of skin reaction that may affect quality of life and, if severe enough, result in treatment interruptions. Minimizing the frequency and severity of these reactions is important not only for improving quality of life but to avoid interruptions that could compromise local-regional control. Intervention strategies are divided into those with the goal of preventing a skin reaction and those with the goal of managing a skin reaction. Ideally these strategies are evidence based. However, despite many systematic reviews and meta-analyses, no single best practice has been identified and practice guidelines are lacking. While the armamentarium of available products is rapidly expanding, their use and acceptance in radiation oncology has been slow. For many radiation oncologists, skin care is limited to the use of aloe or an aqueous cream and Domeboro's solution.

This guide documents our clinical experience and observations with radiation skin changes at the University of California, San Francisco. We present the range and frequency of expected reactions, the factors that influence the reactions, and the interventions we employ. We provide evidence where it exists for the intervention. We have included photographs to illustrate the various reactions and their response to our intervention(s). The photographs facilitate identification of the skin changes in the clinic or inpatient unit. Our goal is to provide a framework for patient care in an era of advancing technology and systemic and targeted therapies and to highlight the importance of preventing and managing the side effects of our treatment.

San Francisco, CA, USA

Editors
Barbara Fowble
Sue S. Yom
Florence Yuen
Sarah Arron

Associate Editors
Keith Sharee
Abhishek Jairam

Acknowledgments

We would like to acknowledge the significant contributions of Patrick Martin-Tuite in the preparation and organization of all the chapters. His assistance has been paramount to the completion of this project. We would also like to acknowledge the incredible cooperation of our patients who have allowed us to photograph them on multiple occasions during and after their treatment and document their experience. Many individuals have participated in the care of our patients, and we would like to thank them for their meticulous and compassionate care.

Contents

Contributors

Mekhail Anwar, MD, PhD Department of Radiation Oncology, University of California San Francisco, San Francisco, CA, USA

Sarah Arron, MD, PhD Department of Dermatology, University of California San Francisco, San Francisco, CA, USA

Jennifer Bohm, RN, BSN Department of Radiation Oncology, University of California San Francisco, San Francisco, CA, USA

Steve E. Braunstein, MD, PhD UCSF Ron Conway Family, Gateway Medical Building, San Francisco, CA, USA

Department of Radiation Oncology, University of California San Francisco, San Francisco, CA, USA

Barbara Fowble, MD, FACR, FASTRO Department of Radiation Oncology, University of California San Francisco, San Francisco, CA, USA

Alex Gottschalk, MD, PhD Department of Radiation Oncology, University of California San Francisco, San Francisco, CA, USA

Daphne Adele Haas-Kogan, MD Harvard Medical School, Boston, MA, USA

Department of Radiation Oncology, Harvard Medical School, Brigham and Women's Hospital, Dana-Farber Cancer Institute, Boston Children's Hospital, Boston, MA, USA

Abhishek Jairam, BA Department of Radiation Oncology, University of California San Francisco, San Francisco, CA, USA

Kaveh Maghsoudi, MD, PhD Department of Radiation Oncology, University of California San Francisco, San Francisco, CA, USA

Catherine Park, MD Department of Radiation Oncology, University of California San Francisco, San Francisco, CA, USA

Anna K. Paulsson, MD Department of Radiation Oncology, University of California San Francisco, San Francisco, CA, USA

Diane Sandman, RN, CWOCN, MSN, FNP Department of Nursing, University of California San Francisco Medical Center, San Francisco, CA, USA

Keith Sharee, BA Department of Radiation Oncology, University of California San Francisco, San Francisco, CA, USA

Tracy Sherertz, MD Department of Radiation Oncology, University of California San Francisco, San Francisco, CA, USA

Joyce Tang, RN, MN Department of Radiation Oncology, University of California San Francisco Medical Center, San Francisco, CA, USA

Lisa Tsang, RN, MN Departments of Pediatric Hematology, Oncology, and Bone Marrow Transplant, UCSF Benioff Children's Hospital, San Francisco, CA, USA

Sue S. Yom, MD, PhD Department of Radiation Oncology, University of California San Francisco, San Francisco, CA, USA

Florence Yuen, RN, MSN, AOCNP Department of Radiation Oncology, University of California San Francisco, San Francisco, CA, USA

1 Scope of the Problem

Barbara Fowble

In 2015 it is estimated that 1,658,370 individuals in the United States will be given a new diagnosis of cancer [1]. Radiation will play a role in the treatment of at least 50 % of these patients [2, 3]. Acute radiation dermatitis is a common side effect, especially in disease sites where there are skin folds or the skin is the target of treatment. These sites include the breast, chest wall, head and neck, perineum, anal canal, vulva, groin, axilla, skin, and soft tissues. A recent study of head and neck, lung, and breast cancer patients treated in 2012–2013 reported significant skin toxicity in more than 50 % of the patients [4]. Typical acute reactions include erythema (redness caused by flushing with dilatation of dermal capillaries), dry desquamation with shedding of the outer layers of the skin, and moist desquamation where the desquamated skin begins to weep. Macmillan et al. [5] reported moist desquamation in 36 % of anal cancer patients, 29 % of head and neck cancer patients, and 27 % of breast cancer patients. Symptoms include pruritus, dryness, a burning sensation, swelling, increased warmth, tightness, tenderness, discomfort, and pain. The usual course of acute radiation dermatitis is the appearance of distinct erythema during the second and third week of treatment, dry desquamation during the later weeks of treatment, and moist desquamation at the end of treatment or within 1 week of treatment completion. Acute reactions peak the first 1–3 weeks after treatment is completed. Most acute reactions are reversible. Late reactions include changes in pigmentation (hyperpigmentation or hypopigmentation), telangiectasia, fibrosis, edema, atrophy, and ulceration. The frequency and severity of the reactions vary.

Factors which contribute to acute skin reactions are divided into patient related and treatment related. Patient-related factors include the anatomic site, sex, body mass index, age, ethnicity, sun-reactive skin type, bra or breast size, comorbidities including collagen vascular disease and HIV, smoking, and genetic mutations [5–20]. Treatment-related factors include the expanse of the skin within the treatment field, the beam energy, total dose and fractionation, the use of bolus and its frequency, the use of tangential beams, intensity-modulated radiation, the use of radiosensitizers, chemotherapy, and targeted agents [5, 8, 15, 18, 19, 21–29]. Minimizing the frequency and severity of acute radiation dermatitis is important. Significant toxicities can result in the interruption of treatment which may compromise local-regional control [30], and late reactions have been correlated with the severity of acute reactions [19, 31–33]. Intervention strategies for acute radiation dermatitis are divided into prevention or prophylaxis and management of the acute reaction. Ideally these strategies

B. Fowble, MD, FACR, FASTRO (✉)
Department of Radiation Oncology, University of California San Francisco, 1600 Divisadero St. H1031, San Francisco, CA 94115, USA
e-mail: barbara.fowble@ucsf.edu

B. Fowble et al. (eds.), *Skin Care in Radiation Oncology*, DOI 10.1007/978-3-319-31460-0_1

should be evidence based. However, there are many obstacles to this approach. Multiple systematic reviews and meta-analyses have failed to identify a single best practice [34–43]. The largest meta-analysis to date of 5688 patients reviewed 47 studies published prior to November 2012 [34]. Chan et al. [44] reported significant variability in the quality and scope of six systematic reviews and suggested that methodological flaws may have resulted in bias in the results and practice recommendations. Additional limitations of meta-analyses are the inclusion of older studies with small numbers of patients and with different disease sites, as well as failure to document or control for differences in radiation technique and dose, and systemic therapy. The majority of studies have focused on breast cancer patients with an emphasis on prevention. Placebo creams have varied among studies making comparisons difficult and often indirect. The use of different end points and scoring systems as well as different times at which reactions are assessed contributes to the lack of a consensus. Failure to assess reactions at their peak will underestimate their frequency and severity. In addition, the impact of interventions on patient symptoms has received less attention. An intervention may ameliorate patient symptoms without diminishing the appearance of the acute skin reaction [45].

Therefore, it is not surprising that recommendations for the prevention and/or management of acute radiation dermatitis have been driven by anecdotal evidence, physician or patient preference, experience, tradition, testimonials, word of mouth, or information obtained from internet searches [46]. Practice guidelines for the use of specific products/agents are lacking. Guidelines developed by the Oncology Nursing Society [47] included only the use of intensity-modulated radiation and allowing patients to wash their skin and to use nonaluminum-based deodorants during treatment. Similar guidelines were recommended by Dendaas et al. [48] from the University of Wisconsin. An international panel from the Multinational Association of Supportive Care in Cancer (MASCC) Skin Toxicity Study Group developed clinical practice guidelines based on a literature review of randomized clinical trials, meta-analyses, systematic reviews, and practice guidelines published prior to July 2012 [49]. The panel supported the recommendation for skin washing with or without a mild soap, the use of antiperspirants, and the use of topical prophylactic corticosteroids to decrease discomfort and itching. The panel concluded that silver sulfadiazine decreased the dermatitis score and is strongly recommended against the use of trolamine and aloe vera for prophylaxis. No recommendation was made for the use of topical sucralfate, hyaluronic acid, ascorbic acid, silver leaf dressing, Theta-Cream, dexpanthenol, and calendula for prophylaxis, given what was considered insufficient or weak evidence. Pulsed dye laser was recommended for the treatment of telangiectasia.

Despite the lack of consensus regarding best practice, there are some general principles of skin care management [27, 50, 51] given that it is unlikely that acute radiation dermatitis can be completely prevented. Exposure to irritants such as perfume or aftershave lotions should be avoided. Tape should not be used in the treatment area. Loose or soft fitting clothing is preferable to diminish friction and trauma to the skin surface. Shaving, if necessary, should be with an electric razor. Nutrition and hydration should be maintained to promote healing. Sun exposure of the treated area is not recommended. Extremes of temperature (extremely hot or cold) should be avoided. Topical efforts to maintain clean, hydrated skin are important. Appropriate dressings should be used for moist desquamation. Mild analgesics may diminish discomfort. Cornstarch should be avoided for skin chafing since it has been associated with bacterial proliferation and an exaggerated inflammatory response [52]. Topical steroids should not be used on an open wound, and gentian violet should be avoided due to its potential carcinogenic effect [53].

Numerous products and agents are available for the prevention and treatment of acute radiation dermatitis. A practice survey from the United Kingdom [54] noted that the most commonly used product for prophylaxis was an aqueous cream. Erythema and dry desquamation were commonly treated with hydrocortisone and moist desquamation with a hydrogel dressing. A separate online practice survey of 181 institutions from the United States and Europe (89 % Europe, United Kingdom excluded) reported similar findings [55]. An aqueous cream and aloe were the two most commonly used products for prophylaxis. However, the most common product used for erythema was an aqueous cream followed by hydrocortisone. Silicone dressing was the most common dressing used for moist desquamation. Hydrogel dressing was the second most common.

In light of the above findings, we recognized the need for a practical guide for the prevention and treatment of radiation dermatitis. The guide is based on our clinical experience and observations as well as evidence where it exists. It is not meant to be an exhaustive review of the literature. Nor is it meant to endorse a particular product or agent. We have documented the typical and not so typical reactions seen and the results of our interventions. Each chapter is devoted to a specific disease site. We have included separate chapters for pediatrics and wound care for locally advanced cancers. For each disease site, we present the range and frequency of the observed reactions, factors influencing these reactions, the typical course of each reaction and its resolution, and the interventions used. Our objective is to provide a framework on which to build strategies that will mitigate radiation dermatitis in an era of advancing and evolving technology and the increasing complexity of combining radiation with new systemic and targeted therapies.

References

1. Cancer Facts and Figures 2015. American Cancer Society. 2015. http://www.cancer.org/acs/groups/content/@editorial/documents/document/acspc-044552.pdf. Accessed 29 Apr 2015.
2. Delaney G, Jacob S, Featherstone C, Barton M. The role of radiotherapy in cancer treatment: estimating optimal utilization from a review of evidence-based clinical guidelines. Cancer. 2005;104:1129–37. doi:10.1002/cncr.21324.
3. Tyldesley S, Delaney G, Foroudi F, Barbera L, Kerba M, Mackillop W. Estimating the need for radiotherapy for patients with prostate, breast, and lung cancers: verification of model estimates of need with radiotherapy utilization data from British Columbia. Int J Radiat Oncol Biol Phys. 2011;79:1507–15. doi:10.1016/j.ijrobp.2009.12.070.
4. Chan RJ, Mann J, Tripcony L, Keller J, Cheuk R, Blades R, et al. Natural oil-based emulsion containing allantoin versus aqueous cream for managing radiation-induced skin reactions in patients with cancer: a phase 3, double-blind, randomized, controlled trial. Int J Radiat Oncol Biol Phys. 2014;90:756–64. doi:10.1016/j.ijrobp.2014.06.034.
5. Macmillan MS, Wells M, MacBride S, Raab GM, Munro A, MacDougall H. Randomized comparison of dry dressings versus hydrogel in management of radiation-induced moist desquamation. Int J Radiat Oncol Biol Phys. 2007;68:864–72. doi:10.1016/j.ijrobp.2006.12.049.
6. Smith KJ, Skelton HG, Tuur S, Yeager J, Decker C, Wagner KF. Increased cutaneous toxicity to ionizing radiation in HIV-positive patients. Military Medical Consortium for the Advancement of Retroviral Research (MMCARR). Int J Dermatol. 1997;36:779–82.
7. Fitzpatrick TB. The validity and practicality of sun-reactive skin types I through VI. Arch Dermatol. 1988;124:869–71.
8. Pignol JP, Vu TT, Mitera G, Bosnic S, Verkooijen HM, Truong P. Prospective evaluation of severe skin toxicity and pain during postmastectomy radiation therapy. Int J Radiat Oncol Biol Phys. 2015;91:157–64. doi:10.1016/j.ijrobp.2014.09.022.
9. Sharp L, Johansson H, Hatschek T, Bergenmar M. Smoking as an independent risk factor for severe skin reactions due to adjuvant radiotherapy for breast cancer. Breast. 2013;22:634–8. doi:10.1016/j.breast.2013.07.047.
10. Wells M, Macmillan M, Raab G, MacBride S, Bell N, MacKinnon K, et al. Does aqueous or sucralfate cream affect the severity of erythematous radiation skin reactions? A randomised controlled trial. Radiother Oncol. 2004;73:153–62. doi:10.1016/j.radonc.2004.07.032.
11. Hoopfer D, Holloway C, Gabos Z, Alidrisi M, Chafe S, Krause B, et al. Three-arm randomized phase III trial: quality aloe and placebo cream versus powder as skin treatment during breast cancer radiation therapy. Clin Breast Cancer. 2014;15(3):181–90. doi:10.1016/j.clbc.2014.12.006.
12. Wright JL, Takita C, Reis IM, Zhao W, Lee E, Hu JJ. Racial variations in radiation-induced skin toxicity severity: data from a prospective cohort receiving post-mastectomy radiation. Int J Radiat Oncol Biol Phys. 2014;90:335–43. doi:10.1016/j.ijrobp.2014.06.042.
13. Ryan JL. Ionizing radiation: the good, the bad, and the ugly. J Invest Dermatol. 2012;132:985–93. doi:10.1038/jid.2011.411.
14. De Ruyck K, Van Eijkeren M, Claes K, Morthier R, De Paepe A, Vral A, et al. Radiation-induced damage to normal tissues after radiotherapy in patients treated for gynecologic tumors: association with single nucleotide polymorphisms in XRCC1, XRCC3, and OGG1 genes and in vitro chromosomal radiosensitivity in lymphocytes. Int J Radiat Oncol Biol Phys. 2005;62:1140–9. doi:10.1016/j.ijrobp.2004.12.027.

15. Freedman GM, Li T, Nicolaou N, Chen Y, Ma CC, Anderson PR. Breast intensity-modulated radiation therapy reduces time spent with acute dermatitis for women of all breast sizes during radiation. Int J Radiat Oncol Biol Phys. 2009;74:689–94. doi:10.1016/j.ijrobp.2008.08.071.
16. Twardella D, Popanda O, Helmbold I, Ebbeler R, Benner A, von Fournier D, et al. Personal characteristics, therapy modalities and individual DNA repair capacity as predictive factors of acute skin toxicity in an unselected cohort of breast cancer patients receiving radiotherapy. Radiother Oncol. 2003;69:145–53.
17. Ho AY, Fan G, Atencio DP, Green S, Formenti SC, Haffty BG, et al. Possession of ATM sequence variants as predictor for late normal tissue responses in breast cancer patients treated with radiotherapy. Int J Radiat Oncol Biol Phys. 2007;69:677–84. doi:10.1016/j.ijrobp.2007.04.012.
18. De Langhe S, Mulliez T, Veldeman L, Remouchamps V, van Greveling A, Gilsoul M, et al. Factors modifying the risk for developing acute skin toxicity after whole-breast intensity modulated radiotherapy. BMC Cancer. 2014;14:711. doi:10.1186/1471-2407-14-711.
19. Pignol JP, Olivotto I, Rakovitch E, Gardner S, Sixel K, Beckham W, et al. A multicenter randomized trial of breast intensity-modulated radiation therapy to reduce acute radiation dermatitis. J Clin Oncol. 2008;26:2085–92. doi:10.1200/JCO.2007.15.2488.
20. Meyer F, Fortin A, Wang CS, Liu G, Bairati I. Predictors of severe acute and late toxicities in patients with localized head-and-neck cancer treated with radiation therapy. Int J Radiat Oncol Biol Phys. 2012;82:1454–62. doi:10.1016/j.ijrobp.2011.04.022.
21. Tieu MT, Graham P, Browne L, Chin YS. The effect of adjuvant postmastectomy radiotherapy bolus technique on local recurrence. Int J Radiat Oncol Biol Phys. 2011;81:e165–71. doi:10.1016/j.ijrobp.2011.01.002.
22. Back M, Guerrieri M, Wratten C, Steigler A. Impact of radiation therapy on acute toxicity in breast conservation therapy for early breast cancer. Clin Oncol (R Coll Radiol). 2004;16:12–6.
23. Hannan R, Thompson RF, Chen Y, Bernstein K, Kabarriti R, Skinner W, et al. Hypofractionated whole-breast radiation therapy: does breast size matter? Int J Radiat Oncol Biol Phys. 2012;84:894–901. doi:10.1016/j.ijrobp.2012.01.093.
24. Satzger I, Degen A, Asper H, Kapp A, Hauschild A, Gutzmer R. Serious skin toxicity with the combination of BRAF inhibitors and radiotherapy. J Clin Oncol. 2013;31:e220–2. doi:10.1200/JCO.2012.44.4265.
25. Churilla TM, Chowdhry VK, Pan D, de la Roza G, Damron T, Lacombe MA. Radiation-induced dermatitis with vemurafenib therapy. Pract Radiat Oncol. 2013;3:e195–8. doi:10.1016/j.prro.2012.11.012.
26. Pulvirenti T, Hong A, Clements A, Forstner D, Suchowersky A, Guminski A, et al. Acute radiation skin toxicity associated with BRAF inhibitors. J Clin Oncol. 2014;34:e17–9. doi:10.1200/JCO.2013.49.0565.
27. Bernier J, Bonner J, Vermorken JB, Bensadoun RJ, Dummer R, Giralt J, et al. Consensus guidelines for the management of radiation dermatitis and coexisting acne-like rash in patients receiving radiotherapy plus EGFR inhibitors for the treatment of squamous cell carcinoma of the head and neck. Ann Oncol. 2008;19:142–9. doi:10.1093/annonc/mdm400.
28. Tejwani A, Wu S, Jia Y, Agulnik M, Millender L, Lacouture ME. Increased risk of high-grade dermatologic toxicities with radiation plus epidermal growth factor receptor inhibitor therapy. Cancer. 2009;115:1286–99. doi:10.1002/cncr.24120.
29. Levy A, Hollebecque A, Bourgier C, Loriot Y, Guigay J, Robert C, et al. Targeted therapy-induced radiation recall. Eur J Cancer. 2013;49:1662–8. doi:10.1016/j.ejca.2012.12.009.
30. Robertson C, Robertson AG, Hendry JH, Roberts SA, Slevin NJ, Duncan WB, et al. Similar decreases in local tumor control are calculated for treatment protraction and for interruptions in the radiotherapy of carcinoma of the larynx in four centers. Int J Radiat Oncol Biol Phys. 1998;40:319–29.
31. Fernando IN, Ford HT, Powles TJ, Ashley S, Glees JP, Torr M, et al. Factors affecting acute skin toxicity in patients having breast irradiation after conservative surgery: a prospective study of treatment practice at the Royal Marsden Hospital. Clin Oncol (R Coll Radiol). 1996;8:226–33.
32. Bentzen SM, Overgaard M. Relationship between early and late normal-tissue injury after postmastectomy radiotherapy. Radiother Oncol. 1991;20:159–65.
33. Lilla C, Ambrosone CB, Kropp S, Helmbold I, Schmezer P, von Fournier D, et al. Predictive factors for late normal tissue complications following radiotherapy for breast cancer. Breast Cancer Res Treat. 2007;106:143–50. doi:10.1007/s10549-006-9480-9.
34. Chan RJ, Webster J, Chung B, Marquart L, Ahmed M, Garantziotis S. Prevention and treatment of acute radiation-induced skin reactions: a systematic review and meta-analysis of randomized controlled trials. BMC Cancer. 2014;14:53. doi:10.1186/1471-2407-14-53.
35. Bolderston A, Lloyd NS, Wong RK, Holden L, Robb-Blenderman L, Supportive Care Guidelines Group of Cancer Care Ontario Program in Evidence-Based C. The prevention and management of acute skin reactions related to radiation therapy: a systematic review and practice guideline. Support Care Cancer. 2006;14:802–17. doi:10.1007/s00520-006-0063-4.
36. Butcher K, Williamson K. Management of erythema and skin preservation; advice for patients receiving radical radiotherapy to the breast: a systematic literature review. J Radiother Pract. 2012;11:44–54. doi:10.1017/S1460396910000488.
37. Kedge E. A systematic review to investigate the effectiveness and acceptability of interventions for moist desquamation in radiotherapy patients. Radiography. 2009;15:247–57.
38. Koukourakis GV, Kelekis N, Kouvaris J, Beli IK, Kouloulias VE. Therapeutics interventions with anti-inflammatory creams in post radiation acute skin reac-

tions: a systematic review of most important clinical trials. Recent Pat Inflamm Allergy Drug Discov. 2010;4:149–58.
39. Richardson J, Smith JE, McIntyre M, Thomas R, Pilkington K. Aloe vera for preventing radiation-induced skin reactions: a systematic literature review. Clin Oncol. 2005;17:478–84.
40. Salvo N, Barnes E, van Draanen J, Stacey E, Mitera G, Breen D, et al. Prophylaxis and management of acute radiation-induced skin reactions: a systematic review of the literature. Curr Oncol. 2010;17:94–112.
41. Zhang Y, Zhang S, Shao X. Topical agent therapy for prevention and treatment of radiodermatitis: a meta-analysis. Support Care Cancer. 2013;21:1025–31. doi:10.1007/s00520-012-1622-5.
42. Hardefeldt PJ, Edirimanne S, Eslick GD. Deodorant use and the risk of skin toxicity in patients undergoing radiation therapy for breast cancer: a meta-analysis. Radiother Oncol. 2012;105:378–9. doi:10.1016/j.radonc.2012.08.020.
43. Meghrajani CF, Co HC, Ang-Tiu CM, Roa FC. Topical corticosteroid therapy for the prevention of acute radiation dermatitis: a systematic review of randomized controlled trials. Expert Rev Clin Pharmacol. 2013;6:641–9. doi:10.1586/17512433.2013.841079.
44. Chan RJ, Larsen E, Chan P. Re-examining the evidence in radiation dermatitis management literature: an overview and a critical appraisal of systematic reviews. Int J Radiat Oncol Biol Phys. 2012;84:e357–62. doi:10.1016/j.ijrobp.2012.05.009.
45. Miller RC, Schwartz DJ, Sloan JA, Griffin PC, Deming RL, Anders JC, et al. Mometasone furoate effect on acute skin toxicity in breast cancer patients receiving radiotherapy: a phase III double-blind, randomized trial from the North Central Cancer Treatment Group N06C4. Int J Radiat Oncol Biol Phys. 2011;79:1460–6. doi:10.1016/j.ijrobp.2010.01.031.
46. Freedman GM. Topical agents for radiation dermatitis in breast cancer: 50 shades of red or same old, same old? Int J Radiat Oncol Biol Phys. 2014;90:736–8. doi:10.1016/j.ijrobp.2014.07.001.
47. Feight D, Baney T, Bruce S, McQuestion M. Putting evidence into practice. Clin J Oncol Nurs. 2011;15:481–92. doi:10.1188/11.CJON.481-492.
48. Dendaas N. Toward evidence and theory-based skin care in radiation oncology. Clin J Oncol Nurs. 2012;16:520–5. doi:10.1188/12.CJON.520-525.
49. Wong RK, Bensadoun RJ, Boers-Doets CB, Bryce J, Chan A, Epstein JB, et al. Clinical practice guidelines for the prevention and treatment of acute and late radiation reactions from the MASCC Skin Toxicity Study Group. Support Care Cancer. 2013;21:2933–48. doi:10.1007/s00520-013-1896-2.
50. Glover D, Harmer V. Radiotherapy-induced skin reactions: assessment and management. Br J Nurs. 2014;23:S28–5.
51. Bauer C, Laszewski P, Magnan M. Promoting adherence to skin care practices among patients receiving radiation therapy. Clin J Oncol Nurs. 2015;19:196–203. doi:10.1188/15.CJON.196-203.
52. Odum BC, O'Keefe JS, Lara W, Rodeheaver GT, Edlich RF. Influence of absorbable dusting powders on wound infection. J Emerg Med. 1998;16:875–9.
53. Naylor W, Mallett J. Management of acute radiotherapy induced skin reactions: a literature review. Eur J Oncol Nurs. 2001;5:221–33. doi:10.1054/ejon.2001.0145.
54. Harris R, Probst H, Beardmore C, James S, Dumbleton C, Bolderston A, et al. Radiotherapy skin care: a survey of practice in the UK. Radiography. 2012;18:21–7.
55. O'Donovan A, Coleman M, Harris R, Herst P. Prophylaxis and management of acute radiation-induced skin toxicity: a survey of practice across Europe and the USA. Eur J Cancer Care. 2015;24:425–35.

Part I

Background

Anatomy of the Skin and Pathophysiology of Radiation Dermatitis

2

Sarah Arron

2.1 Anatomy of the Skin

2.1.1 The Epidermis

The outermost layer of the skin is the epidermis, which is primarily made up of keratinocytes (Fig. 2.1). Keratinocytes produce the keratin protein that serves as the major structural component of the epidermal barrier.

2.1.1.1 The Stratum Basale

The deepest layer of the epidermis is the basal layer, which contains rounded keratinocytes that continually divide to replenish the epidermis. As the cells divide, some retain their replicative potential and others become transit amplifying cells that mature into squamous keratinocytes. These push older cells up toward the surface of the skin, where they are shed. Malignant transformation of basal keratinocytes leads to basal cell carcinoma.

Embedded among the basal keratinocytes are melanocytes, the cells that produce the pigment of the skin. Melanin functions to protect the skin from ultraviolet radiation. Production of melanin is stimulated by UV or other injury to the skin, leading to tanning, freckling, or age spots. Malignant transformation of melanocytes leads to melanoma.

The basal layer also contains Merkel cells, which are tactile sensory cells of neuroectodermal origin. Malignant transformation of these cells leads to Merkel cell carcinoma.

2.1.1.2 The Stratum Spinosum

Just superior to the basal layer is the spinous layer or squamous layer, the thickest layer of the epidermis. This layer is characterized by polygonal keratinocytes, interspersed with Langerhans cells. These are cells of the immune system that detect foreign antigen.

2.1.1.3 The Stratum Granulosum and Stratum Lucidum

As keratinocytes continue to mature and progress toward the outer surface of the skin, they become larger and flatter. The stratum granulosum or granular layer is characterized by basophilic keratohyalin granules that bind keratin together, resulting in a dense barrier layer. These cells also contain lamellar bodies containing lipids and proteins that are secreted into the extracellular space to provide the hydrophobic lipid envelope of the skin. Clearing of these keratinocytes forms the stratum lucidum. These cells ultimately fuse together and die, transitioning into the stratum corneum.

S. Arron, MD, PhD (✉)
Department of Dermatology, University of California, San Francisco, 1701 Divisadero Street, Box 0316, San Francisco, CA 94115, USA
e-mail: Sarah.Arron@ucsf.edu

B. Fowble et al. (eds.), *Skin Care in Radiation Oncology*, DOI 10.1007/978-3-319-31460-0_2

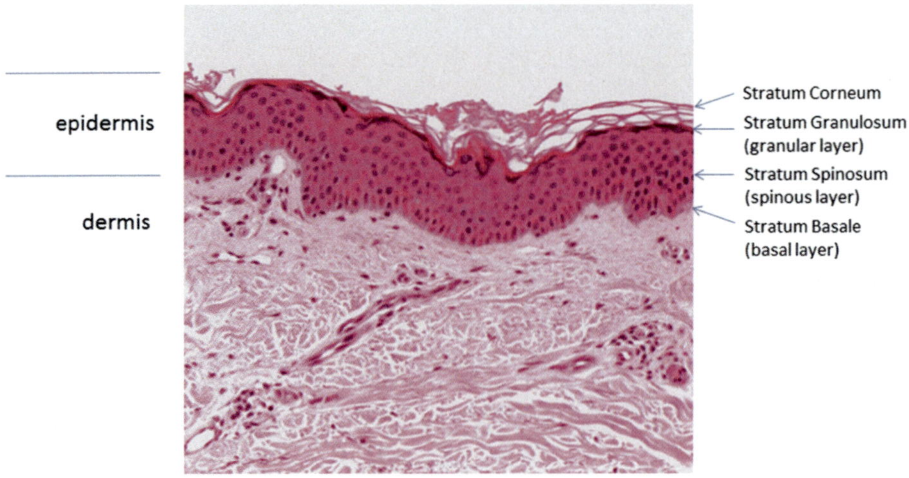

Fig. 2.1 Diagram of the skin. Photo shows normal arm skin, 100×. Photo courtesy of John Geisse, MD

2.1.1.4 The Stratum Corneum

The outermost later of the epidermis is made up of multiple layers of dead keratinocytes. The stratum corneum is continuously sloughed off as underlying keratinocytes mature and take their place. The entire epidermal turnover takes approximately 4 weeks in younger people and 5–7 weeks in older people.

2.1.2 The Dermis

The dermis lies beneath the epidermis and is the thickest layer of the skin. Its main function is to regulate body temperature and supply the epidermis with blood. The dermis is primarily made up of collagen and elastin produced by fibroblasts. Collagen supports the skin with structural durability, while elastin provides skin flexibility and elasticity. The dermis contains a papillary outer layer and a reticular inner layer, which are primarily distinguished by the density of collagen and the specialized structures within. Specialized structures include blood vessels, lymphatics, pain and touch receptors, hair follicles, and sebaceous glands.

2.2 Radiation Skin Reactions

2.2.1 Acute Radiation Dermatitis

Ionizing radiation exposure results in non-visible or prodromal erythema of the skin within 24 h of exposure. It is followed by a second visible phase of erythema beginning 10–14 days after exposure and lasting for up to 1 month [1, 2]. Acute radiation dermatitis is characterized by erythema, edema, blistering, and erosion of the skin. There is often tanning or darkening of the skin preceding desquamation and slough. This reaction usually resolves, but the skin that receives large doses of radiation will typically lose adnexae including hair follicles and eccrine and sebaceous glands. The skin may have permanent telangiectasia, mottled pigmentation, dry texture, and alopecia. Less common presentations of acute radiation dermatitis include morbilliform rash, annular or ring-shaped lesions, and bullae or blisters.

The erythema results from an increased blood supply via the dermal vascular plexus, while dry desquamation results from the inability of basal keratinocyte replication to proliferate fast enough to replenish the damaged squamous epithelium. Injury to sebaceous glands causes skin dryness and injury to follicles results in hair loss. Moderate to severe erythema is most common in skin folds or areas of friction and moist occlusion. Focal loss of the epidermis with a serious drainage and fibrinous exudate are characteristic of moist desquamation. Moist desquamation may be limited to skin folds (groin, axilla, or inframammary fold region) or appear confluent in locations other than skin folds. Bullae may develop. Areas of moist desquamation or ruptured bullae are susceptible to infection, especially with *Staphylococcus aureus*.

2.2.2 Histological Features of Acute Radiation Dermatitis

Acute radiation dermatitis is rarely biopsied, as the clinical presentation is typically sufficient to render the diagnosis. The histopathologic features include keratinocyte necrosis with spongiosis. There may be subepidermal vesiculation progressing to bullae or epidermal slough. Edema is present in the dermis and endothelial cells. Vasodilatation and erythrocyte extravasation may be present. Fibrin thrombin may obstruct arterioles [3]. The inflammatory infiltrate in the dermis includes lymphocytes, eosinophils, macrophages, and plasma cells. Hair follicles may shift into the catagen phase, resulting in synchronized but reversible hair loss. Hyperkeratosis is associated with dry desquamation.

2.2.3 Chronic Radiation Dermatitis

Radiation dermatitis is deemed chronic if the resulting changes appear after a latent period of months to years [4] or if they appear as an extension or progression of the acute process. An example of the latter is breast edema which may persist for several years after breast-conserving surgery and radiation and typically resolves after 2–3 years [5]. The most common chronic changes are hypopigmentation and telangiectasia, which can occur in over 80 % of patients who received moderate doses in the range of 40–50 Gy [6]. Hyperpigmentation, depressed scarring, induration, and keratosis (growths of keratin on the skin) are seen less commonly. Chronic changes typically continue to evolve over a period of about 4 years following treatment [7].

Changes in pigmentation (hypopigmentation or hyperpigmentation) which appear with acute radiation dermatitis may persist or gradually normalize. Textural changes in the skin include atrophic plaques, hyperkeratosis, and xerosis. Loss of hair follicles results in alopecia. If hair follicles have not been destroyed, the hair may be brittle. Telangiectasias are dilated superficial blood vessels. Their appearance has been correlated with the extent and severity of acute reactions with an increased incidence in areas of prior moist desquamation [8, 9]. They are permanent and tend to increase with time [5, 10]. Atrophy of the skin results in fragility and a predisposition to delayed or non-healing of ulcerations or insults to the skin and infection. Fibrosis and contraction result from injury to the fibroblasts. Radiation necrosis results from dermal ischemia and impairment of the reparative process. In this most severe process, superinfection is not uncommon and skin grafts may be required.

2.2.4 Histological Features of Chronic Radiation Dermatitis

Histopathologic examination of chronic radiation dermatitis demonstrates dermal sclerosis and elastosis (Fig. 2.2). The epidermal histology is variable, with hyperkeratosis, focal parakeratosis, atypia, and dyskeratosis. There may be basal vacuolar change and liquefactive degeneration.

Chronic radiation dermatitis is characterized by "radiation fibroblasts," bizarre dermal fibroblasts with large atypical nuclei and basophilic cytoplasm. These may raise concern for malignant transformation, but they do not appear to have malignant potential. Radiation fibroblasts typically express factor XIIIa and may express CD34 [11]. Dermal blood vessels may dilate and become tortuous, particularly in high-grade dermatitis. This correlates with the telangiectasia

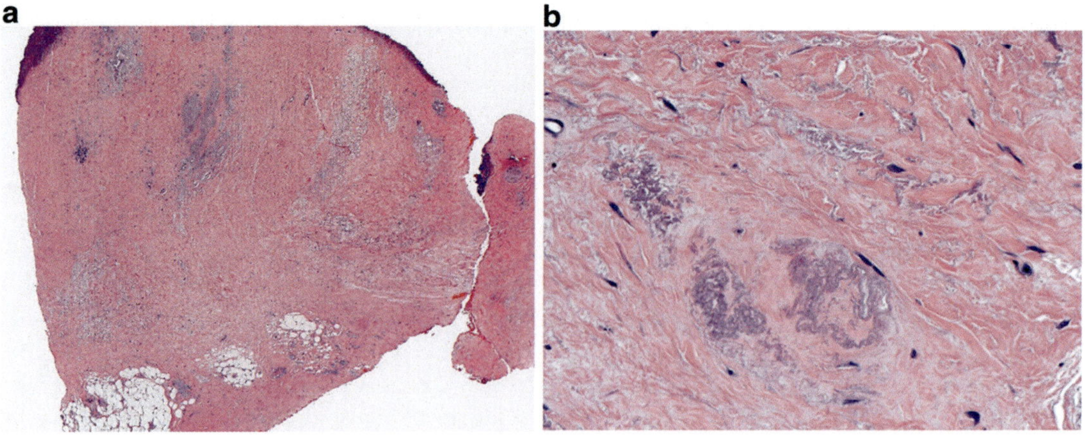

Fig. 2.2 Chronic radiation dermatitis. (**a**) 40×, (**b**) 400×. Photos courtesy of Jeffrey North, MD

and poikiloderma seen on clinical examination. Vessels are reduced in number and may have hyaline change and narrowing of the lumen. Ablation of the pilosebaceous unit results in irreversible alopecia, and there may be eccrine atrophy which results in loss of sweat formation. In contrast to thermal burns, the arrector pili muscles remain and are often surrounded by sclerotic collagen.

2.3 Pathophysiology of Radiation Dermatitis

Radiation dermatitis is the result of injury to multiple skin structures including epidermal keratinocytes, dermal fibroblasts, cutaneous vasculature, and hair follicles. It interferes with the maturation, reproduction, and repopulation of these cells [12]. It is the result of direct tissue injury as well as the inflammation recruited to the injured skin [13, 14]. DNA damage is mediated by the production of free radicals. Leukocytes and other immune cells migrate from the circulation to the skin [15, 16]. Increased formation of cytokines and chemokines (IL-1 alpha, IL-1 beta, TNF-alpha, IL-6, IL-8, CL4, CXCL10, and CCL2) has been associated with acute radiation dermatitis [15, 17, 18]. Radiation causes immediate direct injury to keratinocytes, which results in oxidative stress. Production of free radicals such as reactive oxygen species superoxides, hydrogen peroxides, and hydroxyl radicals cause damage to the tissue [19]. This triggers vasodilation, vascular permeability, and recruitment of inflammatory cells. These immune cells secrete pro-inflammatory cytokines that drive fibroblast differentiation into myofibroblasts, which produce collagen and smooth muscle actin [20]. Extracellular matrix deposition by activated myofibroblasts results in wound healing, but persistent activation from repeated radiation injury can lead to fibrosis [21, 22]. Acute injury results from reduced and impaired stem cells, changes in endothelial cells, inflammation, and epidermal cell apoptosis and necrosis [13].

Fibrosis is primarily driven by transforming growth factor beta (TGFβ), which is upregulated in response to ionizing radiation [23, 24]. TGFβ plays a key role in tissue fibrosis by stimulating fibroblasts to secrete extracellular matrix proteins (connective tissue growth factor) [25]. TGFβ-induced fibrosis appears to be mediated via Smad3, as Smad3 knockout mice exhibit accelerated healing and decreased damage after irradiation [26].

Macrophages play a major role in radiation dermatitis and fibrosis. Macrophages may be activated by tumor necrosis factor alpha (TNFα) and interferon gamma (IFNγ) to polarize into an M1 pro-inflammatory phenotype producing IL1β, TNFα, IL-6, and IL-12 or may be activated by IL-4 and IL-13 to polarize into an anti-inflammatory phenotype marked by production of TGFβ [27]. The complex balance of these macrophage populations during radiation injury and tissue repair are not well understood and likely shift over time to promote resolution of inflammation and myofibroblast activity.

2.4 Radiosensitizers and Radiation Recall

Radiation recall skin reactions are precipitated by the administration of systemic agents. They occur in areas of acute skin reactions that had previously returned to normal and should not be confused with delayed healing. They are unpredictable and uncommon. The onset is typically within days to weeks after exposure to the inciting agent. It may appear as erythema, dry desquamation, vesicles, maculopapular lesions, and in severe cases ulceration and skin necrosis. Some of the agents which have been associated with radiation recall dermatitis include bleomycin, capecitabine, docetaxel, paclitaxel, cisplatin, cyclophosphamide, epirubicin, doxorubicin, actinomycin D, etoposide, 5-fluorouracil, gemcitabine, methotrexate, tamoxifen, and vinblastine [28].

In addition, numerous systemic agents can be used to augment the effect of radiation therapy (radiation sensitizers), including chemotherapeutic agents such as 5-fluorouracil, gemcitabine, capecitabine, and platinum analogs and targeted molecular inhibitors such as EGFR inhibitors [29, 30].

2.5 Other Skin Eruptions Associated with Radiation Therapy

A less common presentation of radiation dermatitis is the eosinophilic, polymorphous, pruritic eruption, often associated with radiation therapy for breast cancer. This eruption favors the extremities and may arise outside of the radiation field. There is a lymphohistiocytic infiltrate with eosinophils.

Other skin conditions that have been reported as arising within radiation fields include lichen planus, lichen sclerosus, morphea, graft vs. host disease, and pseudosclerodermatous panniculitis. Conditions that can be induced by radiation therapy and extend beyond the radiation field include erythema multiforme, bullous and cicatricial pemphigoid, herpes zoster, pemphigus vulgaris and pemphigus foliaceus.

References

1. Simonen P, Hamilton C, Ferguson S, Ostwald P, O'Brien M, O'Brien P, et al. Do inflammatory processes contribute to radiation induced erythema observed in the skin of humans? Radiother Oncol. 1998;46:73–82.
2. Schmuth M, Sztankay A, Weinlich G, Linder DM, Wimmer MA, Fritsch PO, et al. Permeability barrier function of skin exposed to ionizing radiation. Arch Dermatol. 2001;137:1019–23.
3. Archambeau JO, Pezner R, Wasserman T. Pathophysiology of irradiated skin and breast. Int J Radiat Oncol Biol Phys. 1995;31:1171–85. doi:10.1016/0360-3016(94)00423-I.
4. Salvo N, Barnes E, van Draanen J, Stacey E, Mitera G, Breen D, et al. Prophylaxis and management of acute radiation-induced skin reactions: a systematic review of the literature. Curr Oncol. 2010;17:94–112.
5. Freedman GM, Anderson PR, Bleicher RJ, Litwin S, Li T, Swaby RF, et al. Five-year local control in a phase II study of hypofractionated intensity modulated radiation therapy with an incorporated boost for early stage breast cancer. Int J Radiat Oncol Biol Phys. 2012;84:888–93. doi:10.1016/j.ijrobp.2012.01.091.
6. Turesson I, Notter G. The influence of fraction size in radiotherapy on the late normal tissue reaction—II: comparison of the effects of daily and twice-A-week fractionation on human skin. Int J Radiat Oncol Biol Phys. 1984;10:599–606.
7. Rupprecht R, Lippold A, Auras C, Bramkamp G, Breitkopf C, Elsmann HJ, et al. Late side-effects with cosmetic relevance following soft X-ray therapy of cutaneous neoplasias. J Eur Acad Dermatol Venereol. 2007;21:178–85. doi:10.1111/j.1468-3083.2006.01886.x.
8. Bentzen SM, Overgaard M. Relationship between early and late normal-tissue injury after postmastectomy radiotherapy. Radiother Oncol. 1991;20:159–65.
9. Lilla C, Ambrosone CB, Kropp S, Helmbold I, Schmezer P, von Fournier D, et al. Predictive factors for late normal tissue complications following radiotherapy for breast cancer. Breast Cancer Res Treat. 2007;106:143–50. doi:10.1007/s10549-006-9480-9.
10. Toledano A, Garaud P, Serin D, Fourquet A, Bosset JF, Breteau N, et al. Concurrent administration of adjuvant chemotherapy and radiotherapy after breast-conserving surgery enhances late toxicities: long-term results of the ARCOSEIN multicenter randomized study. Int J Radiat Oncol Biol Phys. 2006;65:324–32. doi:10.1016/j.ijrobp.2005.12.020.

11. Meehan SA, LeBoit PE. An immunohistochemical analysis of radiation fibroblasts. J Cutan Pathol. 1997;24:309–13.
12. Malkinson FD, Hanson WR. Physiology, biochemistry, and molecular biology of the skin. Oxford: Oxford University Press; 1991.
13. Hymes SR, Strom EA, Fife C. Radiation dermatitis: clinical presentation, pathophysiology, and treatment 2006. J Am Acad Dermatol. 2006;54:28–46. doi:10.1016/j.jaad.2005.08.054.
14. Mancini ML, Sonis ST. Mechanisms of cellular fibrosis associated with cancer regimen-related toxicities. Front Pharmacol. 2014;5:51. doi:10.3389/fphar.2014.00051.
15. Holler V, Buard V, Gaugler MH, Guipaud O, Baudelin C, Sache A, et al. Pravastatin limits radiation-induced vascular dysfunction in the skin. J Invest Dermatol. 2009;129:1280–91. doi:10.1038/jid.2008.360.
16. Muller K, Meineke V. Radiation-induced alterations in cytokine production by skin cells. Exp Hematol. 2007;35:96–104. doi:10.1016/j.exphem.2007.01.017.
17. Okunieff P, Xu J, Hu D, Liu W, Zhang L, Morrow G, et al. Curcumin protects against radiation-induced acute and chronic cutaneous toxicity in mice and decreases mRNA expression of inflammatory and fibrogenic cytokines. Int J Radiat Oncol Biol Phys. 2006;65:890–8. doi:10.1016/j.ijrobp.2006.03.025.
18. Xiao Z, Su Y, Yang S, Yin L, Wang W, Yi Y, et al. Protective effect of esculentoside A on radiation-induced dermatitis and fibrosis. Int J Radiat Oncol Biol Phys. 2006;65:882–9. doi:10.1016/j.ijrobp.2006.01.031.
19. Pan J, Su Y, Hou X, He H, Liu S, Wu J, et al. Protective effect of recombinant protein SOD-TAT on radiation-induced lung injury in mice. Life Sci. 2012;91:89–93. doi:10.1016/j.lfs.2012.06.003.
20. Eckes B, Zigrino P, Kessler D, Holtkotter O, Shephard P, Mauch C, et al. Fibroblast-matrix interactions in wound healing and fibrosis. Matrix Biol. 2000;19:325–32.
21. Wynn TA, Ramalingam TR. Mechanisms of fibrosis: therapeutic translation for fibrotic disease. Nat Med. 2012;18:1028–40. doi:10.1038/nm.2807.
22. Ueha S, Shand FH, Matsushima K. Cellular and molecular mechanisms of chronic inflammation-associated organ fibrosis. Front Immunol. 2012;3:71. doi:10.3389/fimmu.2012.00071.
23. Canney PA, Dean S. Transforming growth factor beta: a promotor of late connective tissue injury following radiotherapy? Br J Radiol. 1990;63:620–3. doi:10.1259/0007-1285-63-752-620.
24. Schultze-Mosgau S, Wehrhan F, Grabenbauer G, Amann K, Radespiel-Troger M, Neukam FW, et al. Transforming growth factor beta1 and beta2 (TGFbeta2 / TGFbeta2) profile changes in previously irradiated free flap beds. Head Neck. 2002;24:33–41.
25. Leask A, Abraham DJ. TGF-beta signaling and the fibrotic response. FASEB J. 2004;18:816–27. doi:10.1096/fj.03-1273rev.
26. Flanders KC, Major CD, Arabshahi A, Aburime EE, Okada MH, Fujii M, et al. Interference with transforming growth factor-beta/ Smad3 signaling results in accelerated healing of wounds in previously irradiated skin. Am J Pathol. 2003;163:2247–57.
27. Novak ML, Koh TJ. Macrophage phenotypes during tissue repair. J Leukoc Biol. 2013;93:875–81. doi:10.1189/jlb.1012512.
28. Burris 3rd HA, Hurtig J. Radiation recall with anti-cancer agents. Oncologist. 2010;15:1227–37. doi:10.1634/theoncologist.2009-0090.
29. Lawrence TS, Blackstock AW, McGinn C. The mechanism of action of radiosensitization of conventional chemotherapeutic agents. Semin Radiat Oncol. 2003;13:13–21. doi:10.1053/srao.2003.50002.
30. Lacouture ME, Maitland ML, Segaert S, Setser A, Baran R, Fox LP, et al. A proposed EGFR inhibitor dermatologic adverse event-specific grading scale from the MASCC skin toxicity study group. Support Care Cancer. 2010;18:509–22. doi:10.1007/s00520-009-0744-x.

Types of Radiation-Related Skin Reactions

3

Barbara Fowble, Sue S. Yom, and Florence Yuen

Radiation-related skin reactions can be divided into acute and late reactions. Acute reactions are those that occur during treatment or within several weeks after the completion of treatment. Late reactions are those that occur more than 90 days after treatment is completed.

3.1 Scoring Systems for Radiation-Induced Skin Reactions

Various scoring systems have been used to assess acute and late skin toxicity from radiation. The three most common systems are the RTOG (Radiation Therapy Oncology Group)/EORTC (European Organization for Research and Treatment of Cancer) [1], the LENT (Late Effect on Normal Tissue)/SOMA (Symptom Objective Measures, Management, Assessment) [2], and the CTCAE (Common Terminology Criteria for Adverse Events) [3]. The RTOG/EORTC system grades acute and late effects, the LENT/SOMA grades only late effects, and the National Cancer Institute's CTCAE system grades only acute effects. A comparison of these three systems is presented in Table 3.1. In surveys of radiation oncology departments in the United Kingdom, Europe, and the United States, the most commonly used system was the RTOG/EORTC [4, 5]. Modifications of the systems have been proposed to more accurately reflect the acute reactions for breast cancer [6, 7]. Lacouture et al. [8], in recognizing the limitations of the CTCAE scoring system in characterizing the very specific types of adverse events associated with targeted therapies such as the epidermal growth factor receptor (EGFR) inhibitors, also proposed a new dermatologic grading scale. This scale includes more detailed descriptions of the adverse dermatologic events which correlate with a specific grade.

An issue with clinician-based professional assessments is the lack of consideration of the impact on the patient's experience. Additional grading scales that incorporate patient-reported outcomes include the RISRAS (radiation-induced skin reaction assessment scale) [9], the Catterall Skin Scoring Profile [10], the Skindex-16, the Skin Cancer Index, and the Dermatology Life Quality Index [11–14]. The RISRAS scale includes both a professional assessment and patient-rated symptom scale. The Skindex-16 measures quality of life in patients with skin conditions and does not include a professional assessment. The Skin Cancer Index is a 15-item instrument with three components (emotion, social, and appearance) developed to assess quality of life in patients with nonmelanoma skin cancers. The DLQI is a widely validated

B. Fowble, MD, FACR, FASTRO (✉) • S.S. Yom, MD, PhD • F. Yuen, RN, MSN, AOCNP
Department of Radiation Oncology, University of California, San Francisco, 1600 Divisadero, H1031, Box 1708, San Francisco, CA 94115, USA
e-mail: BFowble@radonc.ucsf.edu

B. Fowble et al. (eds.), *Skin Care in Radiation Oncology*, DOI 10.1007/978-3-319-31460-0_3

Table 3.1 Standard scoring systems for acute and late radiation skin toxicity

	CTCAE v4.0 [3]	RTOG [1]	LENT/SOMA [2]
Toxicity	Acute	Acute/late	Late
Score			
0	No change	No change	No change
1	Faint erythema Dry desquamation	Faint or dull erythema Dry desquamation Follicular reaction Epilation Decreased sweating	Minor symptoms No treatment
2	Moderate-brisk erythema Patchy moist desquamation in skin folds and creases Moderate edema	Tender or bright erythema Patchy moist desquamation Moderate edema	Moderate symptoms Conservative treatment
3	Moist desquamation other than skin folds Bleeding with minor trauma	Confluent moist desquamation other than skin folds Pitting edema	Severe symptoms Aggressive treatment
4	Skin necrosis or ulceration Spontaneous bleeding Skin graft needed	Ulceration, hemorrhage Necrosis	Irreversible damage Major intervention
5	Death	Death related to treatment	Death or loss organ

10-question survey applicable to a variety of different skin conditions and has been used in the context of evaluating the impact of dermatologic treatments and targeted therapies.

For quality of life impact of targeted therapies, major available patient-reported instruments include the FACT-EGFRI-18 [15], an 18-question survey that assesses the physical, emotional, social, and functional impact of the skin, nail, and hair toxicities from EGFR-inhibition therapy, and the hand-foot syndrome 14 (HFS-14), a 14-item questionnaire for patients experiencing chemotherapy-associated hand-foot syndrome and hand-foot skin reaction [16].

Radiation-related skin reactions vary in frequency, intensity, and severity. Factors which influence the observed reactions are divided into patient and treatment related. Patient-related factors include the anatomic site, sex, body mass index, age, ethnicity, sun-reactive skin type, bra or breast size, comorbidities including collagen vascular disease and HIV, smoking, and genetic mutations [6, 7, 17–30]. Treatment-related factors include the expanse of the skin within the treatment field, the beam energy, total dose and fractionation, the use of bolus and its frequency, the use of tangential beams, intensity-modulated radiation, the use of radiosensitizers, chemotherapy, and targeted agents [19, 25, 31–41].

The characterization of the skin reaction differs among the scoring systems as noted in Table 3.1. Interobserver variability is a common challenge. Below we provide descriptions and photographic examples of acute and late skin reactions. The examples highlight the spectrum of changes that may be seen.

3.2 Acute Reactions

3.2.1 Erythema

While the initial reaction to radiation therapy occurs as early as the first treatment, the earliest visible manifestation of a radiation-related skin reaction is erythema. It typically occurs in the second to third week of treatment and initially appears as a slight pink discoloration. It may progress to a bright red or reddish purple color as the cumulative dose increases. It can be described as mild, moderate (brisk), or marked. It is a result of the destruction of the basal cells with an inflammatory response characterized by erythrocyte extravasation and capillary dilatation in the dermis (Table 3.2).

3.2.2 Hyperpigmentation

Erythema may be accompanied by hyperpigmentation especially in African-American patients or patients of other ethnicities with darker skin pigment. The hyperpigmentation often involves the nipple/areolar complex in women with breast cancer and may persist for several months following completion of treatment (Table 3.3).

3.2.3 Dry Desquamation

Dry desquamation typically occurs at doses of 3000 cGy or higher. It is characterized by shedding of the outer layers of the skin as new cells migrate to replace the damaged cells (Table 3.4).

3.2.4 Moist Desquamation

Moist desquamation occurs when the epidermis sloughs and the underlying surface are moist and edematous. Epidermal loss may increase the risk of infection and moist desquamation may be associated with purulent exudate. Moist desquamation occurs at doses above 4000 cGy and is most likely to occur in skin folds where there is self-bolus. Reepithelialization should occur within 10–14 days of the onset of moist desquamation and is characterized by the appearance of islands of new skin cells which are white in color and should not be confused with infection (Table 3.5).

3.2.5 Folliculitis

Folliculitis is an infection of the hair follicles which is characterized by the appearance of multiple small erythematous lesions that are raised and pruritic. Purulent material (pustule) may be present in the center of the lesions. The infectious agent is usually *Staphylococcus aureus*. Management includes the use of topical agents (Table 3.6).

3.2.6 Cutaneous Candidiasis

Cutaneous candidiasis may develop in moist areas such as the groin, axilla, or inframammary fold region of the breast. It has a characteristic appearance of areas of erythema with plaque like lesions with peripheral scaling. Papules and pustules may be present. These changes should not be mistaken for erythema related to radiation. A topical antifungal should be added to the skin care regimen for areas of suspected candidiasis (Fig. 3.1)

3.3 Late Reactions

3.3.1 Pigmentation Changes

Reepithelialization in areas of moist desquamation may result in hypopigmentation or hyperpigmentation of the skin or a combination of the two. A change in pigmentation is most often seen in African-American patients. Hypopigmentation of the nipple/areolar complex is also seen in some Caucasian women. The acute hyperpigmentation seen in African-American patients may not resolve completely, leaving the treated area hyperpigmented for long periods or even permanently (Table 3.7).

3.3.2 Telangiectasia

Telangiectasias are dilated superficial blood vessels. Their incidence is increased in areas of prior moist desquamation. They are permanent and tend to increase with time. They can be removed with laser therapy but generally require multiple sessions and may reappear (Fig. 3.2).

3.3.3 Edema

Edema is characterized by persistent interstitial swelling of the tissues. It is more common in areas of dependency (extremities, pendulous breast) and may be chronic in nature. In breast cancer it has been reported to peak at 3–6 months with resolution by 3 years (Table 3.8) [7].

Table 3.2 Erythema

Mild erythema	Moderate erythema	Marked erythema
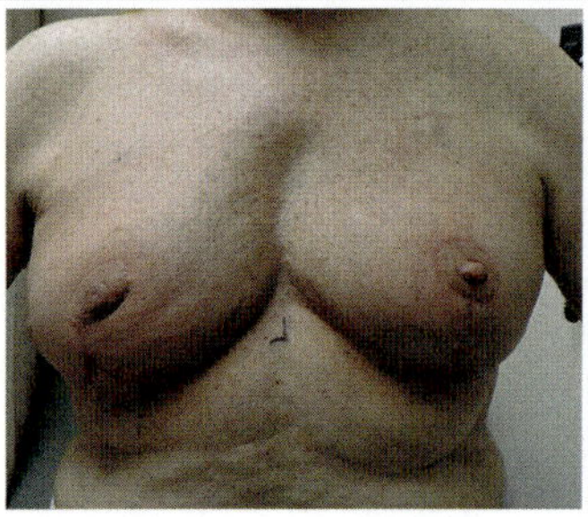 Week 2, bilateral breast cancer, reduction mammoplasty, beginning of mild erythema	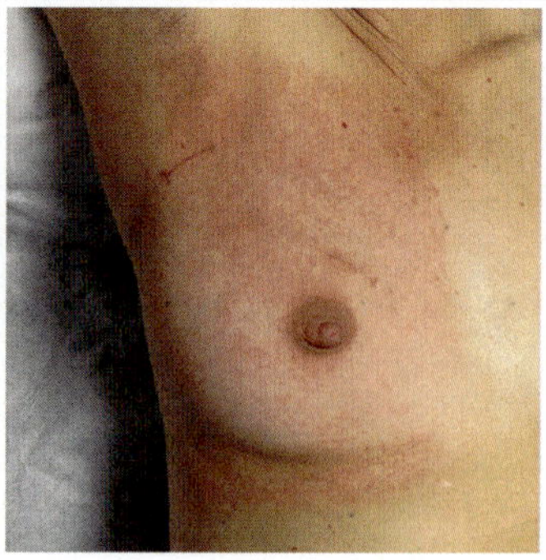 Week 4, moderate erythema, right breast whole breast radiation, breast-conserving surgery	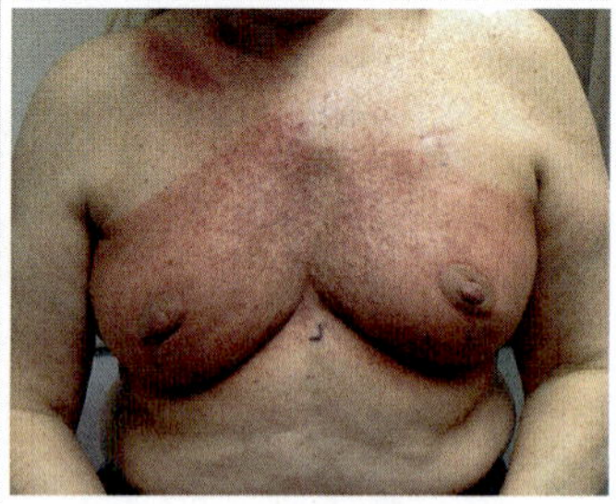 Week 5, bilateral breast cancer, reduction mammoplasty, marked erythema
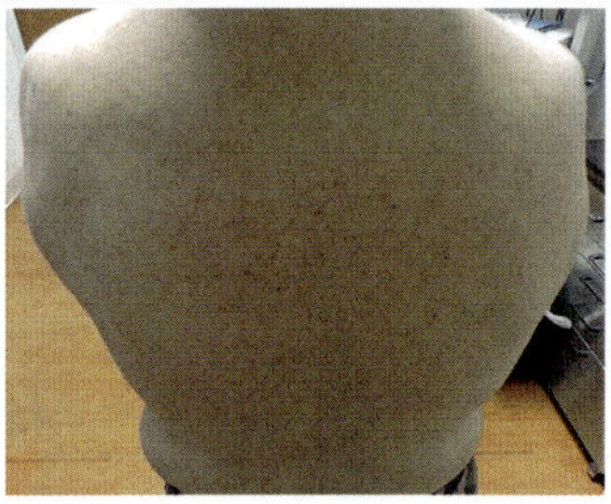 Week 4, IMRT, adenocarcinoma of the left lung, posterior thoracic region	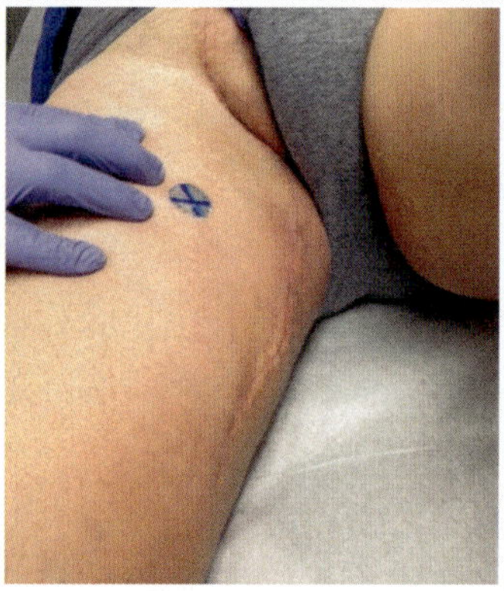 Week 4, sarcoma treated to right proximal medial thigh	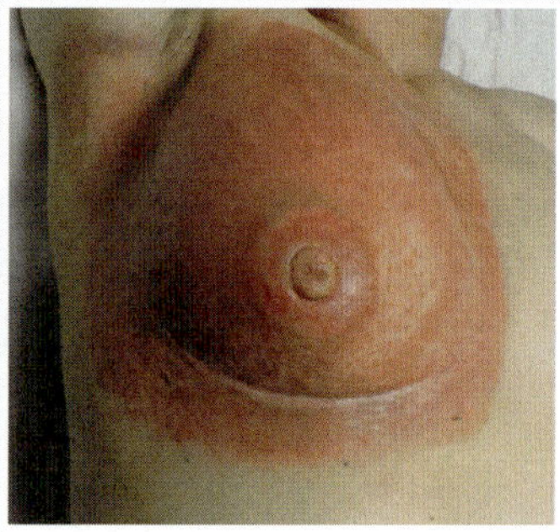 Week 5, reconstructed breast with transverse upper gracilis microvascular flap. Custom bolus every other day
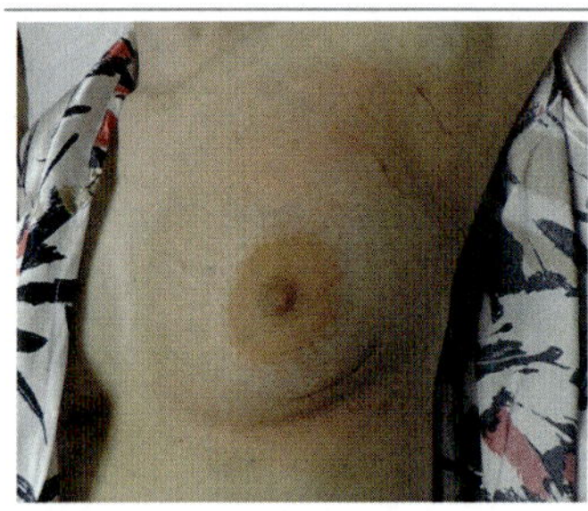 Week 3, breast-conserving surgery	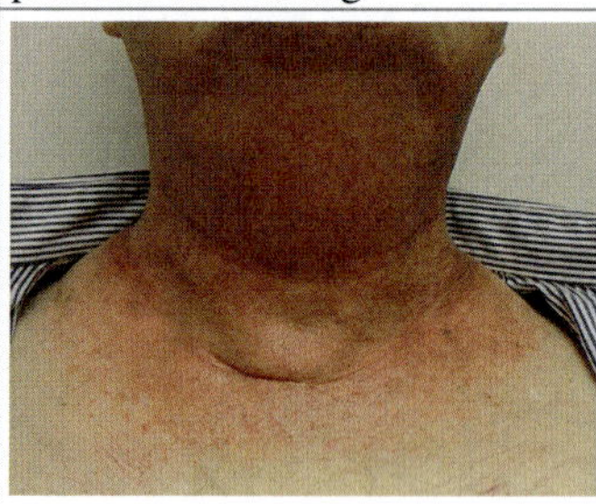 Week 6, cancer, base of tongue	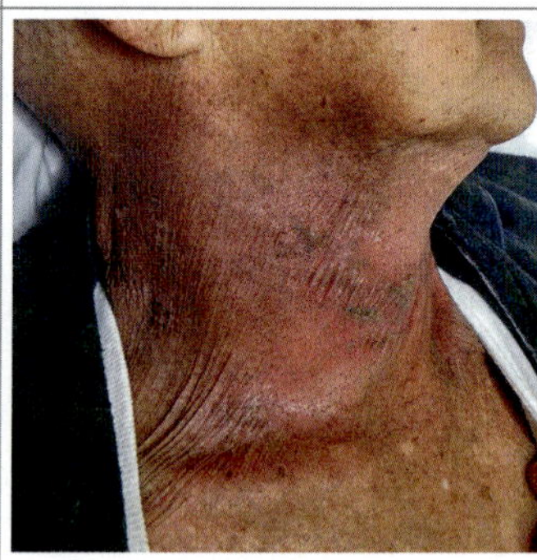 Week 5, cancer of the pyriform sinus

Table 3.3 Hyperpigmentation

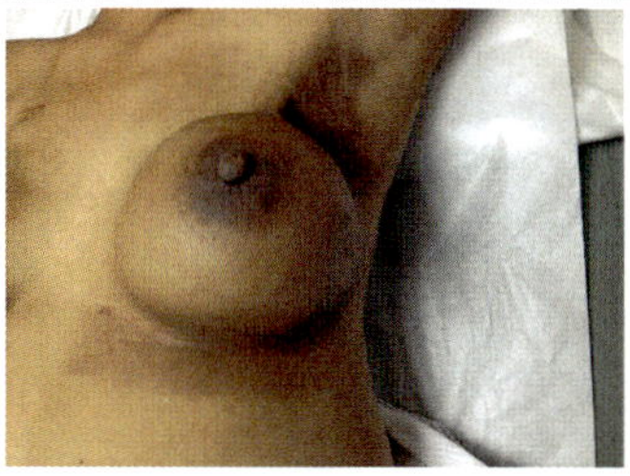 6 weeks postradiation. Filipino, total nipple skin sparing mastectomy, custom bolus every other day 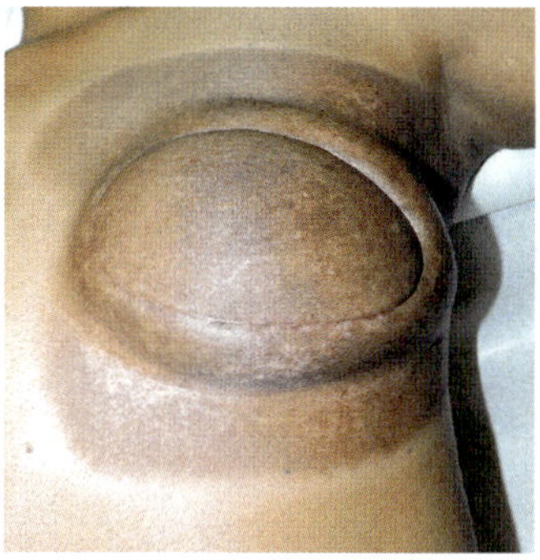 6 months postradiation, Indian female with locally recurrent inflammatory breast cancer, TRAM flap. Bolus daily with concurrent Xeloda and chest wall boost	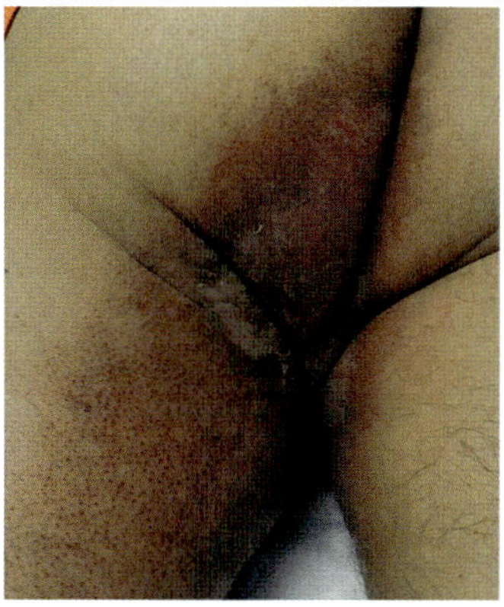 Week 6. Hispanic male, sarcoma, thigh	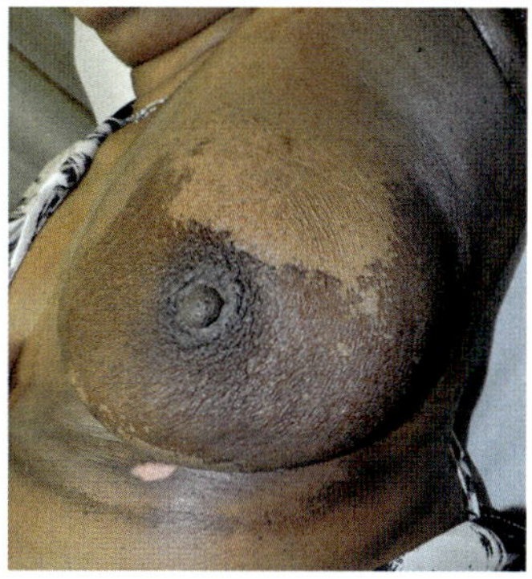 3 weeks postradiation. Resolving hyperpigmentation. Breast-conserving surgery, African-American female

Table 3.4 Dry desquamation

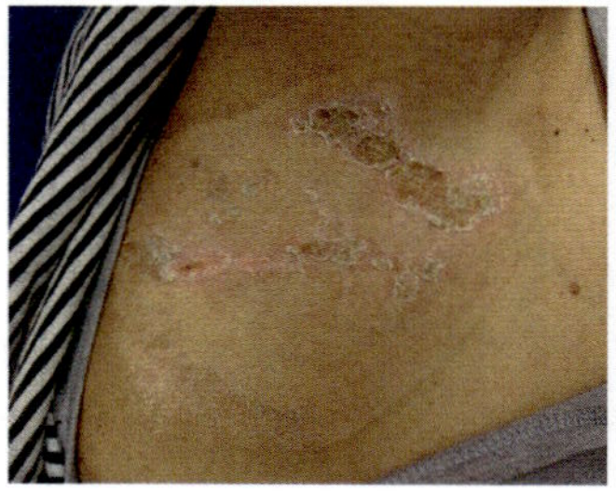 1 week postradiation, Ewing's sarcoma, dry desquamation in the clavicular region	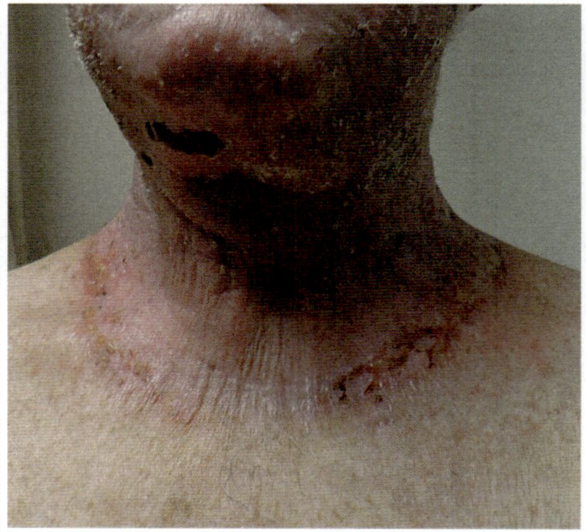 2 weeks postradiation, squamous cell carcinoma of the left lower lip, concurrent cetuximab. Exhibits dry desquamation in surrounding neck	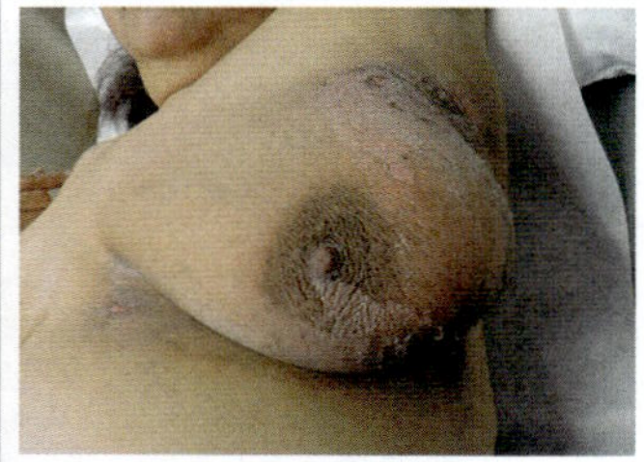 2 weeks postradiation, dry desquamation, intact breast

Table 3.5 Moist desquamation

Moist desquamation	Diffuse moist desquamation
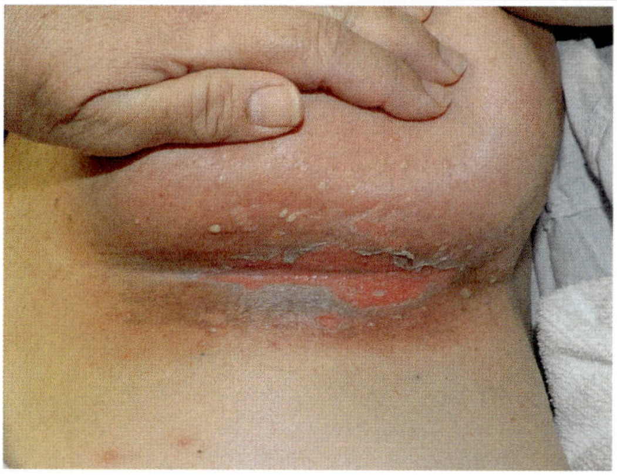 1 week postradiation, focal moist desquamation, inframammary fold, without exudate	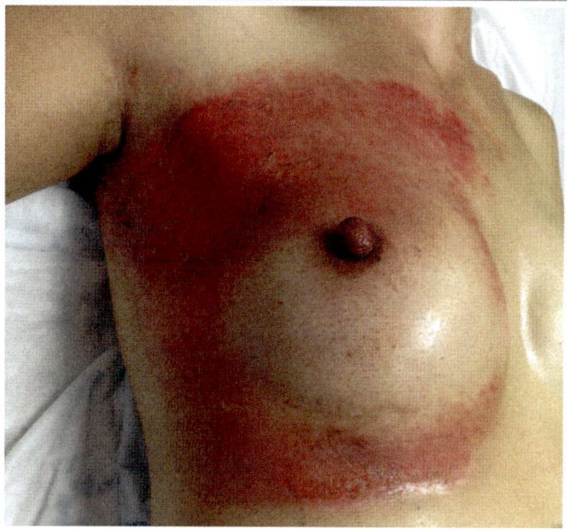 1 week postradiation, chest wall recurrence, implant-reconstructed breast
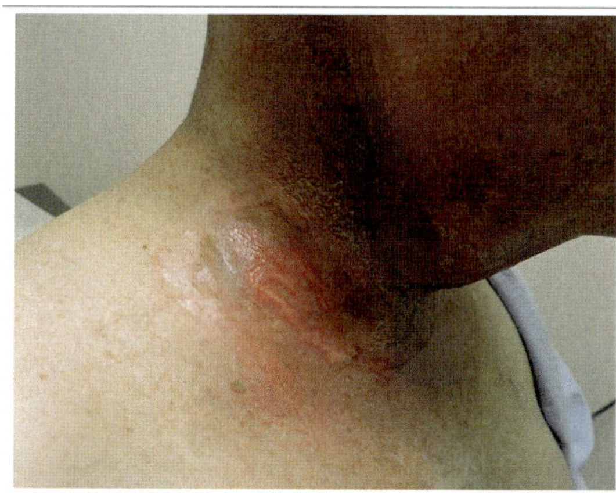 2 weeks postradiation, concurrent weekly cisplatin, focal moist desquamation; cancer, base of tongue	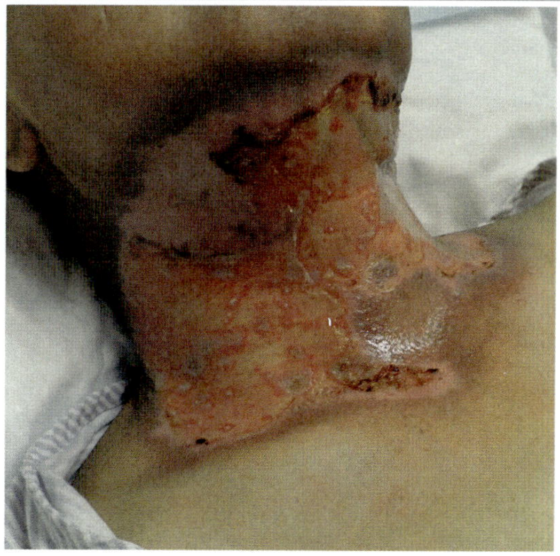 2 weeks postradiation; concurrent cisplatin, squamous cell carcinoma, left oral tongue; diffuse moist desquamation

(continued)

Table 3.5 (continued)

Moist desquamation	Diffuse moist desquamation
	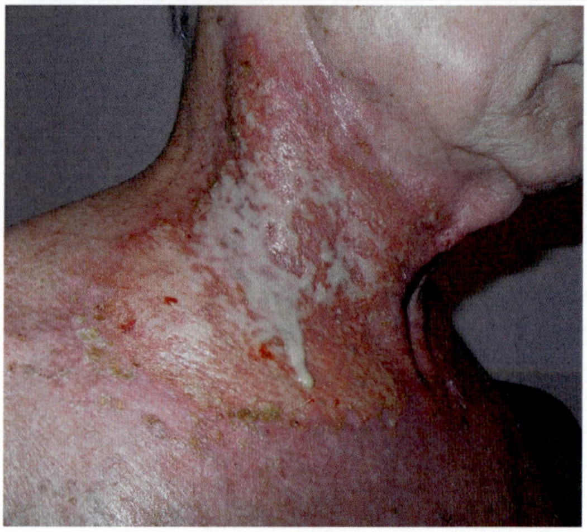 Week 4, post-squamous cell carcinoma of the upper esophagus, status post endoscopic mucosal resection and subsequent hiatal esophagectomy for multifocal dysplasia throughout esophagus. Recurrence in the right supraclavicular node, level 3 and paratracheal areas. Radiation with concurrent carboplatin and Taxol, moist desquamation with purulent exudate
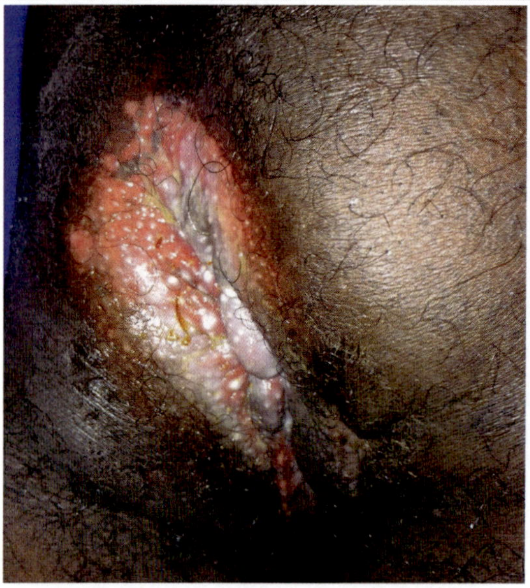 African-American male, anal cancer, IMRT with concurrent 5-FU, and mitomycin C. Perineum with moist desquamation and beginning reepithelialization (white patches)	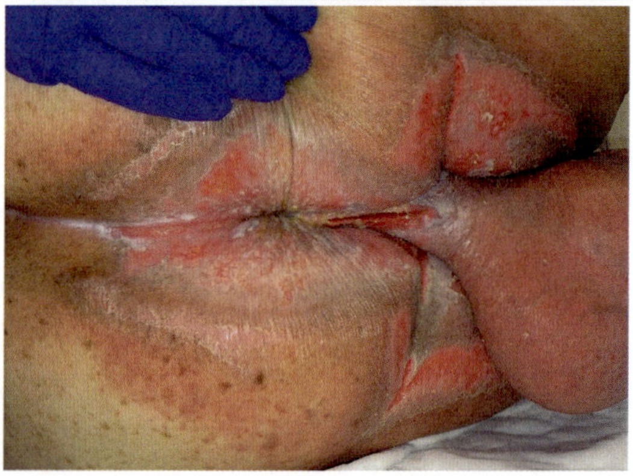 Week 6, squamous cell carcinoma of the perianal region, perineum with diffuse moist desquamation. Treated with IMRT and concurrent 5-FU and mitomycin C

Table 3.5 (continued)

<table>
<tr><th>Moist desquamation</th><th>Diffuse moist desquamation</th></tr>
<tr><td></td><td>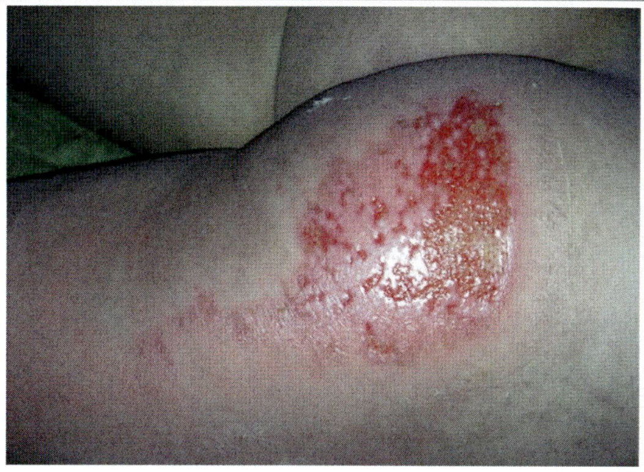
2.5 weeks postradiation; Ewing's sarcoma, desquamation, and beginning epithelization</td></tr>
</table>

Table 3.6 Folliculitis

<table>
<tr><td>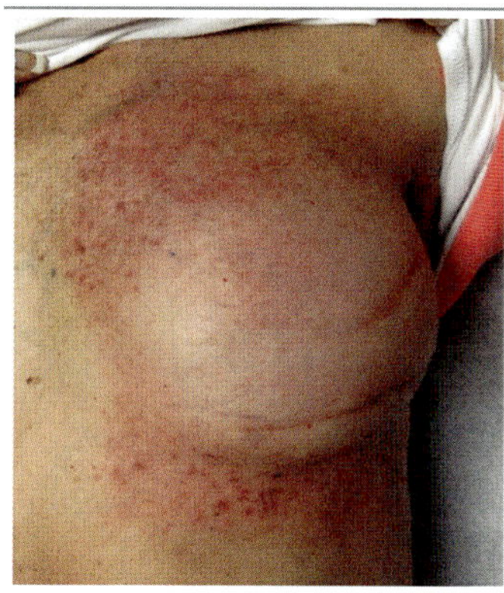
Week 6, reconstructed breast with areas of folliculitis, upper inner quadrant and inframammary fold</td><td>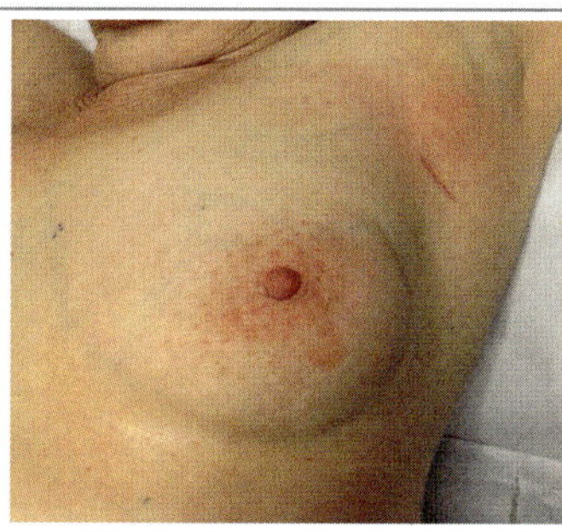
Week 4, intact breast with central area of folliculitis</td><td>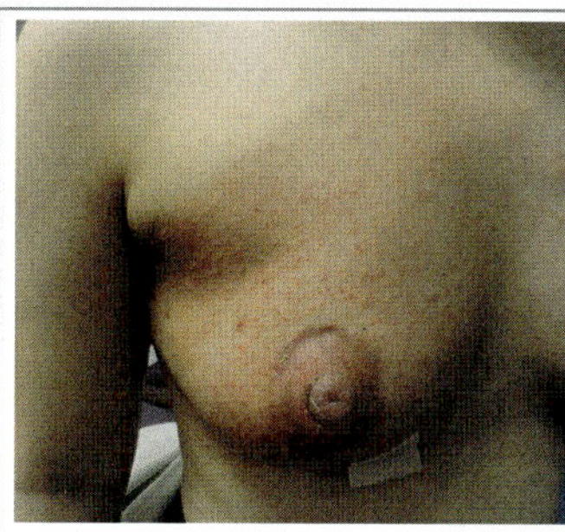
1 week postradiation, breast with wide area of folliculitis</td></tr>
</table>

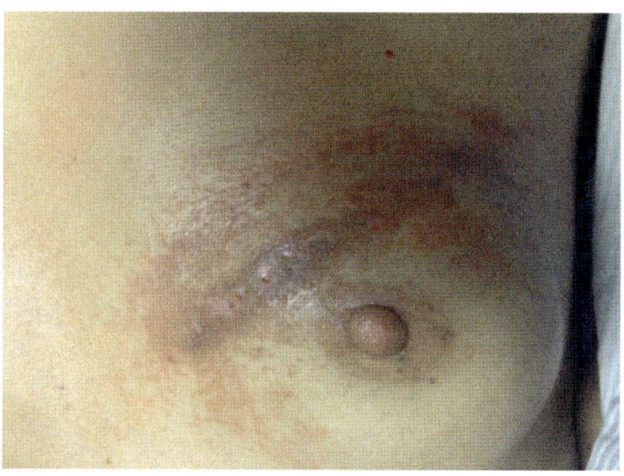

Fig. 3.1 Breast cancer; development of cutaneous candidiasis along incision site that had been sealed with glue

3.3.4 Fibrosis

Radiation fibrosis results in loss of parenchymal cells with the increased formation of fibrous tissue. In the skin and soft tissues, the affected area(s) becomes firmer and tighter and at times painful. It is correlated with total radiation dose, the volume(s) treated [42, 43], and overlapping fields [44]. The changes have been thought to be irreversible, but preclinical models and limited success with clinical interventions suggest some degree of reversibility (Fig. 3.3) [44–46].

Table 3.7 Pigmentation changes

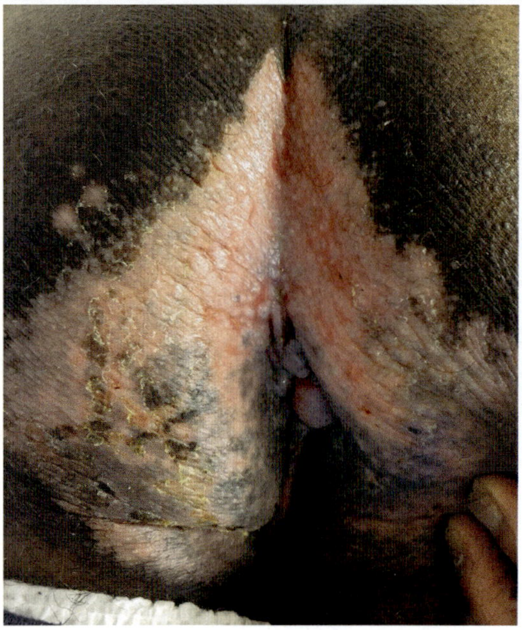 2 week break between weeks 5 and 6 of treatment. African-American male, anal cancer, hypopigmentation during second week of 2-week break	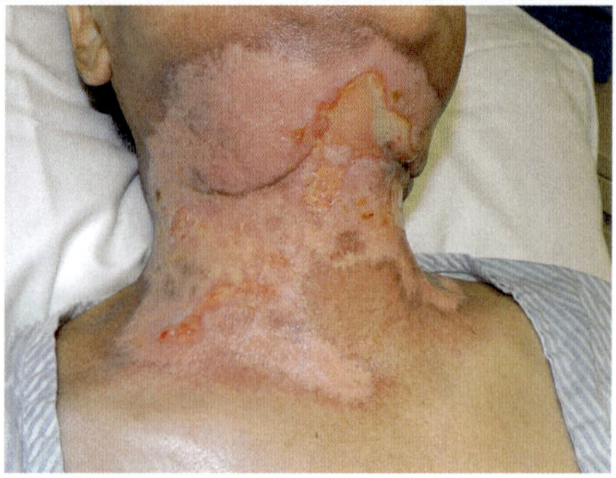 5 weeks postradiation, concurrent cisplatin, left oral tongue cancer

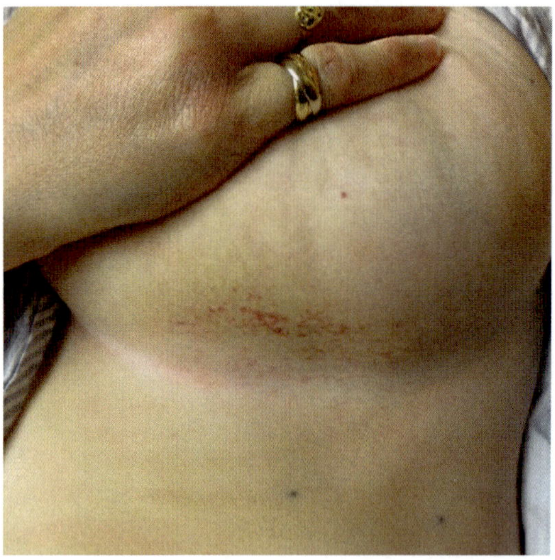

Fig. 3.2 5.5 years postradiation. Intact breast with telangiectasia inframammary fold. Status post-breast-conserving surgery

3.3.5 Morphea

Morphea is a localized form of scleroderma. It is characterized by circumscribed patches or plaques of sclerosis with induration. The areas may be erythematous or hypopigmented. Radiation-induced morphea has been reported in women with breast cancer treated with breast-conserving surgery and whole breast radiation [47–49] or partial breast radiation [50]. The changes may appear outside of the area of radiation [49]. It is reported to occur in 1/500 women treated for breast cancer [51, 52]. The interval from radiation to the appearance of morphea ranges from 1 month to 32 years [51, 53, 54]. It is not a precursor to systemic sclerosis. It should not be confused with a recall reaction (Table 3.9).

Table 3.8 Edema

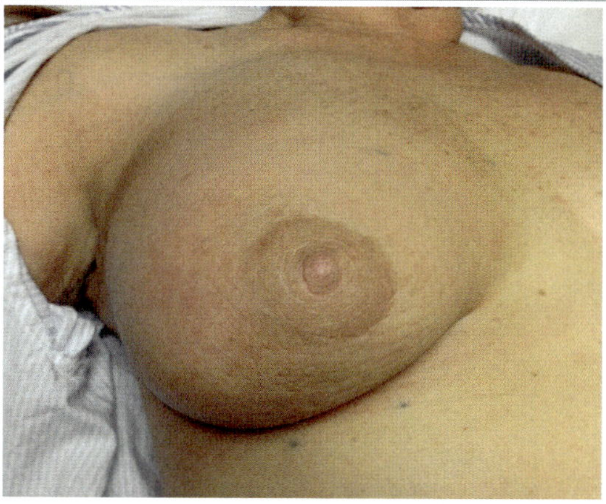 4 months postradiation. Breast edema	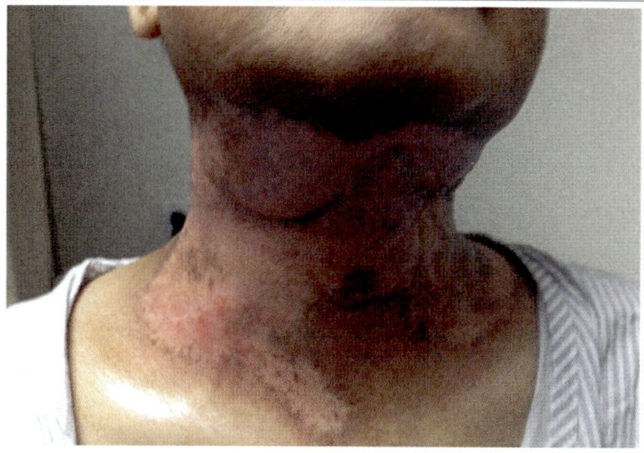 5 weeks postradiation, concurrent cisplatin upper neck edema related to surgery and radiation

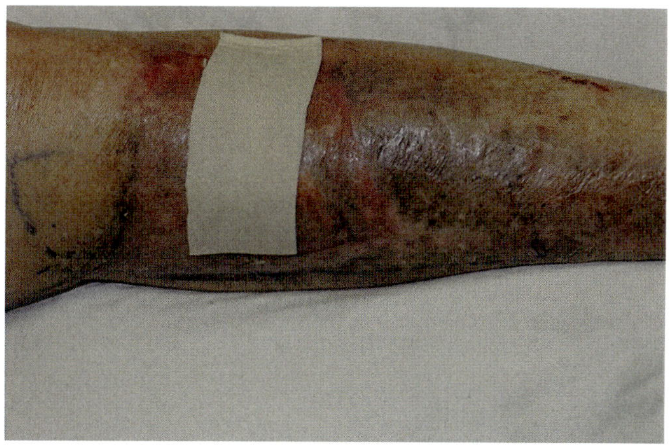

Fig. 3.3 Week 3, recurrent pleomorphic undifferentiated sarcoma with invasion into the tibia, fibrosis of the anterior tibia. Status post-resection and IORT 15 Gy

Table 3.9 Morphea

<table>
<tr><td>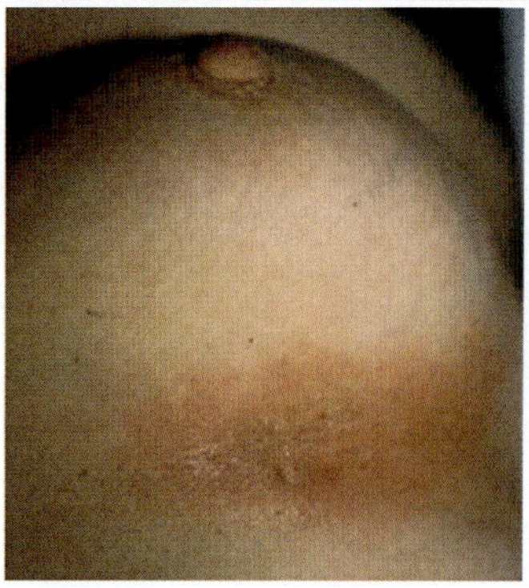
2 years postradiation. Breast cancer, radiation-induced morphea
Photo courtesy of M. Kari Connolly, MD</td><td>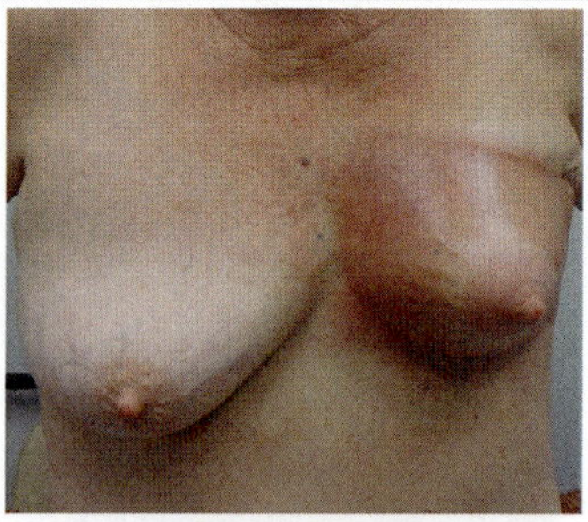
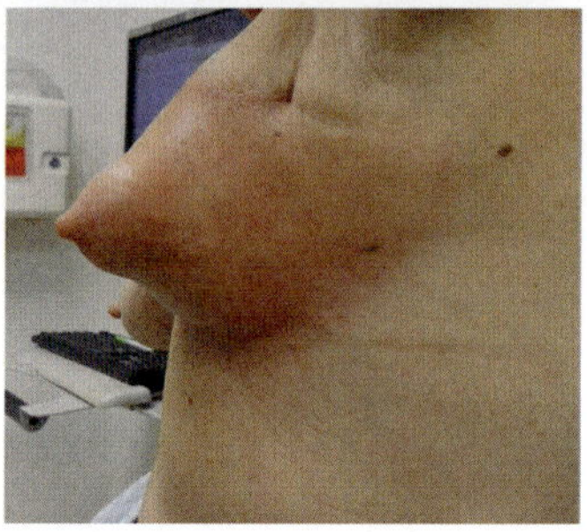
Radiation-induced morphea presenting 7 months posttreatment. 70-year-old female with pT2N0 luminal A cancer s/p lumpectomy and radiation
Photos courtesy of Jyoti Mayadev, MD</td></tr>
</table>

Table 3.10 Recall skin reactions

<table>
<tr><td>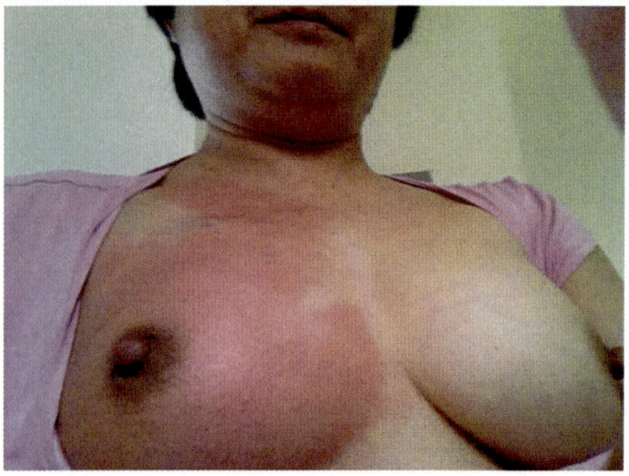
9 months postradiation; recall reaction related to doxorubicin, with erythema in breast and supraclavicular region</td><td>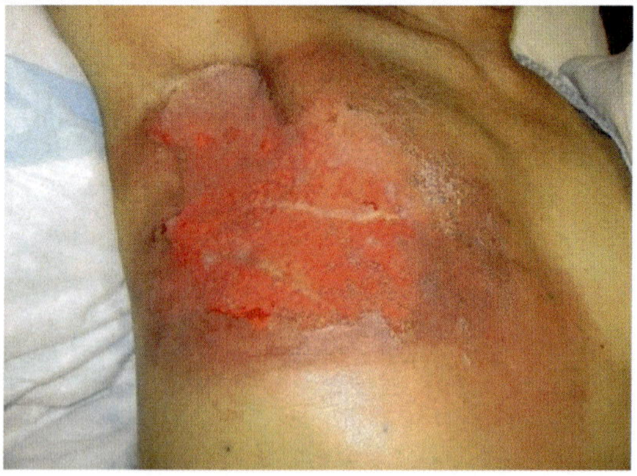
Postmastectomy radiation for chest wall recurrence with recall reaction; moist desquamation following liposomal doxorubicin transarterial chemoembolization for hepatocellular cancer</td></tr>
</table>

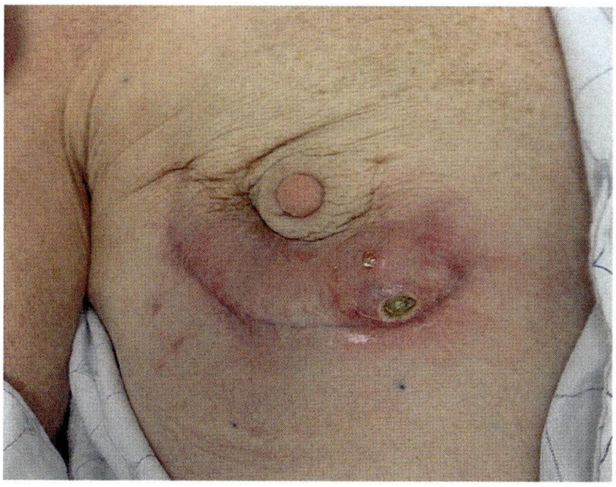

Fig. 3.4 Chronic cellulitis, postradiation necrosis; implant-reconstructed breast

3.3.6 Recall Skin Reactions

Radiation recall skin reactions are precipitated by the administration of systemic agents or targeted therapies. They occur in areas of acute skin reactions that had previously returned to normal and should not be confused with delayed healing. They are unpredictable and uncommon. The onset is typically within days to weeks after exposure to the inciting agent. It may appear as erythema, dry desquamation, vesicles, maculopapular lesions, and in severe cases ulceration and skin necrosis. Some of the agents which have been associated with radiation recall dermatitis include bleomycin, capecitabine, docetaxel, paclitaxel, cisplatin, cyclophosphamide, epirubicin, doxorubicin, actinomycin D, etoposide, 5-fluorouracil, gemcitabine, methotrexate, tamoxifen, and vinblastine (Table 3.10) [55]. One influential report indicated that a variety of targeted therapies such as those inhibiting MTOR, EGFR, HDAC, and BRAF pathways, for example, as well as other experimental systemic agents, may produce radiation recall [37].

3.3.7 Ulceration

Ulceration of the skin is an uncommon event after conventional radiation. It has been reported to occur in less than 5 % of patients receiving radiation for squamous cell cancer of the head and neck [35]. Management requires multimodality therapy. Full-thickness graft may be indicated for healing (Fig. 3.4).

References

1. Cox JD, Stetz J, Pajak TF. Toxicity criteria of the Radiation Therapy Oncology Group (RTOG) and the European Organization for Research and Treatment of Cancer (EORTC). Int J Radiat Oncol Biol Phys. 1995;31:1341–6. doi:10.1016/0360-3016(95)00060-C.
2. LENT SOMA scales for all anatomic sites. Int J Radiat Oncol Biol Phys. 1995;31:1049–91.
3. Common Terminology Criteria for Adverse Events (CTCAE) Version 4.0. In: Cancer Therapy Evaluation Program. National Cancer Institute, National Institutes of Health, U.S. Department of Health and Human Services. 2010. http://evs.nci.nih.gov/ftp1/CTCAE/CTCAE_4.03_2010-06-14_QuickReference_8.5x11.pdf. Accessed 16 Apr 2015.
4. Harris R, Probst H, Beardmore C, James S, Dumbleton C, Bolderston A, et al. Radiotherapy skin care: a survey of practice in the UK. Radiography. 2012; 18:21–7.
5. O'Donovan A, Coleman M, Harris R, Herst P. Prophylaxis and management of acute radiation-induced skin toxicity: a survey of practice across Europe and the USA. Eur J Cancer Care. 2015;24:425–35. doi:10.1111/ecc.12213.
6. Wright JL, Takita C, Reis IM, Zhao W, Lee E, Hu JJ. Racial variations in radiation-induced skin toxicity severity: data from a prospective cohort receiving postmastectomy radiation. Int J Radiat Oncol Biol Phys. 2014;90:335–43. doi:10.1016/j.ijrobp.2014.06.042.
7. Freedman GM, Li T, Nicolaou N, Chen Y, Ma CC, Anderson PR. Breast intensity-modulated radiation therapy reduces time spent with acute dermatitis for women of all breast sizes during radiation. Int J Radiat Oncol Biol Phys. 2009;74:689–94. doi:10.1016/j.ijrobp.2008.08.071.
8. Lacouture ME, Maitland ML, Segaert S, Setser A, Baran R, Fox LP, et al. A proposed EGFR inhibitor dermatologic adverse event-specific grading scale from the MASCC skin toxicity study group. Support Care Cancer. 2010;18:509–22. doi:10.1007/s00520-009-0744-x.
9. Noble-Adams R. Radiation-induced skin reactions. 3: Evaluating the RISRAS. Br J Nurs. 1999;8:1305–12. doi:10.12968/bjon.1999.8.19.1305.
10. Catterall M, Rogers C, Thomlinson RH, Field SB. An investigation into the clinical effects of fast neutrons. Methods and early observations. Br J Radiol. 1971; 44:603–11. doi:10.1259/0007-1285-44-524-603.
11. Chren MM, Lasek RJ, Quinn LM, Mostow EN, Zyzanski SJ. Skindex, a quality-of-life measure for patients with skin disease: reliability, validity, and

responsiveness. J Invest Dermatol. 1996;107: 707–13.
12. Chren MM, Lasek RJ, Sahay AP, Sands LP. Measurement properties of Skindex-16: a brief quality-of-life measure for patients with skin diseases. J Cutan Med Surg. 2001;5:105–10. doi:10.1007/s102270000010.
13. Rhee JS, Matthews BA, Neuburg M, Logan BR, Burzynski M, Nattinger AB. The skin cancer index: clinical responsiveness and predictors of quality of life. Laryngoscope. 2007;117:399–405. doi:10.1097/MLG.0b013e31802e2d88.
14. Lewis V, Finlay AY. 10 years experience of the Dermatology Life Quality Index (DLQI). J Investig Dermatol Symp Proc. 2004;9:169–80. doi:10.1111/j.1087-0024.2004.09113.x.
15. Wagner LI, Berg SR, Gandhi M, Hlubocky FJ, Webster K, Aneja M, et al. The development of a Functional Assessment of Cancer Therapy (FACT) questionnaire to assess dermatologic symptoms associated with epidermal growth factor receptor inhibitors (FACT-EGFRI-18). Support Care Cancer. 2013;21:1033–41. doi:10.1007/s00520-012-1623-4.
16. Sibaud V, Dalenc F, Chevreau C, Roche H, Delord JP, Mourey L, et al. HFS-14, a specific quality of life scale developed for patients suffering from hand-foot syndrome. Oncologist. 2011;16:1469–78. doi:10.1634/theoncologist.2011-0033.
17. Macmillan MS, Wells M, MacBride S, Raab GM, Munro A, MacDougall H. Randomized comparison of dry dressings versus hydrogel in management of radiation-induced moist desquamation. Int J Radiat Oncol Biol Phys. 2007;68:864–72. doi:10.1016/j.ijrobp.2006.12.049.
18. Smith KJ, Skelton HG, Tuur S, Yeager J, Decker C, Wagner KF. Increased cutaneous toxicity to ionizing radiation in HIV-positive patients. Military Medical Consortium for the Advancement of Retroviral Research (MMCARR). Int J Dermatol. 1997;36: 779–82.
19. Fitzpatrick TB. The validity and practicality of sun-reactive skin types I through VI. Arch Dermatol. 1988;124:869–71.
20. Pignol JP, Vu TT, Mitera G, Bosnic S, Verkooijen HM, Truong P. Prospective evaluation of severe skin toxicity and pain during postmastectomy radiation therapy. Int J Radiat Oncol Biol Phys. 2015;91:157–64. doi:10.1016/j.ijrobp.2014.09.022.
21. Sharp L, Johansson H, Hatschek T, Bergenmar M. Smoking as an independent risk factor for severe skin reactions due to adjuvant radiotherapy for breast cancer. Breast. 2013;22:634–8. doi:10.1016/j.breast.2013.07.047.
22. Wells M, Macmillan M, Raab G, MacBride S, Bell N, MacKinnon K, et al. Does aqueous or sucralfate cream affect the severity of erythematous radiation skin reactions? A randomised controlled trial. Radiother Oncol. 2004;73:153–62. doi:10.1016/j.radonc.2004.07.032.
23. Hoopfer D, Holloway C, Gabos Z, Alidrisi M, Chafe S, Krause B, et al. Three-Arm randomized phase III trial: quality aloe and placebo cream versus powder as skin treatment during breast cancer radiation therapy. Clin Breast Cancer. 2014;15(3):181–90. doi:10.1016/j.clbc.2014.12.006.
24. Ryan JL. Ionizing radiation: the good, the bad, and the ugly. J Invest Dermatol. 2012;132:985–93. doi:10.1038/jid.2011.411.
25. De Ruyck K, Van Eijkeren M, Claes K, Morthier R, De Paepe A, Vral A, et al. Radiation-induced damage to normal tissues after radiotherapy in patients treated for gynecologic tumors: association with single nucleotide polymorphisms in XRCC1, XRCC3, and OGG1 genes and in vitro chromosomal radiosensitivity in lymphocytes. Int J Radiat Oncol Biol Phys. 2005;62:1140–9. doi:10.1016/j.ijrobp.2004.12.027.
26. Twardella D, Popanda O, Helmbold I, Ebbeler R, Benner A, von Fournier D, et al. Personal characteristics, therapy modalities and individual DNA repair capacity as predictive factors of acute skin toxicity in an unselected cohort of breast cancer patients receiving radiotherapy. Radiother Oncol. 2003;69:145–53.
27. Ho AY, Fan G, Atencio DP, Green S, Formenti SC, Haffty BG, et al. Possession of ATM sequence variants as predictor for late normal tissue responses in breast cancer patients treated with radiotherapy. Int J Radiat Oncol Biol Phys. 2007;69:677–84. doi:10.1016/j.ijrobp.2007.04.012.
28. De Langhe S, Mulliez T, Veldeman L, Remouchamps V, van Greveling A, Gilsoul M, et al. Factors modifying the risk for developing acute skin toxicity after whole-breast intensity modulated radiotherapy. BMC Cancer. 2014;14:711. doi:10.1186/1471-2407-14-711.
29. Pignol JP, Olivotto I, Rakovitch E, Gardner S, Sixel K, Beckham W, et al. A multicenter randomized trial of breast intensity-modulated radiation therapy to reduce acute radiation dermatitis. J Clin Oncol. 2008;26:2085–92. doi:10.1200/JCO.2007.15.2488.
30. Meyer F, Fortin A, Wang CS, Liu G, Bairati I. Predictors of severe acute and late toxicities in patients with localized head-and-neck cancer treated with radiation therapy. Int J Radiat Oncol Biol Phys. 2012;82:1454–62. doi:10.1016/j.ijrobp.2011.04.022.
31. Tieu MT, Graham P, Browne L, Chin YS. The effect of adjuvant postmastectomy radiotherapy bolus technique on local recurrence. Int J Radiat Oncol Biol Phys. 2011;81:e165–71. doi:10.1016/j.ijrobp.2011.01.002.
32. Hannan R, Thompson RF, Chen Y, Bernstein K, Kabarriti R, Skinner W, et al. Hypofractionated whole-breast radiation therapy: does breast size matter? Int J Radiat Oncol Biol Phys. 2012;84:894–901. doi:10.1016/j.ijrobp.2012.01.093.
33. Satzger I, Degen A, Asper H, Kapp A, Hauschild A, Gutzmer R. Serious skin toxicity with the combination of BRAF inhibitors and radiotherapy. J Clin Oncol. 2013;31:e220–2. doi:10.1200/JCO.2012.44.4265.

34. Pulvirenti T, Hong A, Clements A, Forstner D, Suchowersky A, Guminski A, et al. Acute radiation skin toxicity associated with BRAF inhibitors. J Clin Oncol. 2014. doi:10.1200/JCO.2013.49.0565.
35. Bernier J, Bonner J, Vermorken JB, Bensadoun RJ, Dummer R, Giralt J, et al. Consensus guidelines for the management of radiation dermatitis and coexisting acne-like rash in patients receiving radiotherapy plus EGFR inhibitors for the treatment of squamous cell carcinoma of the head and neck. Ann Oncol. 2008;19:142–9. doi:10.1093/annonc/mdm400.
36. Tejwani A, Wu S, Jia Y, Agulnik M, Millender L, Lacouture ME. Increased risk of high-grade dermatologic toxicities with radiation plus epidermal growth factor receptor inhibitor therapy. Cancer. 2009; 115:1286–99. doi:10.1002/cncr.24120.
37. Levy A, Hollebecque A, Bourgier C, Loriot Y, Guigay J, Robert C, et al. Targeted therapy-induced radiation recall. Eur J Cancer. 2013;49:1662–8. doi:10.1016/j.ejca.2012.12.009.
38. Robertson C, Robertson AG, Hendry JH, Roberts SA, Slevin NJ, Duncan WB, et al. Similar decreases in local tumor control are calculated for treatment protraction and for interruptions in the radiotherapy of carcinoma of the larynx in four centers. Int J Radiat Oncol Biol Phys. 1998;40:319–29.
39. Fernando IN, Ford HT, Powles TJ, Ashley S, Glees JP, Torr M, et al. Factors affecting acute skin toxicity in patients having breast irradiation after conservative surgery: a prospective study of treatment practice at the Royal Marsden Hospital. Clin Oncol (R Coll Radiol). 1996;8:226–33.
40. Bentzen SM, Overgaard M. Relationship between early and late normal-tissue injury after postmastectomy radiotherapy. Radiother Oncol. 1991;20: 159–65.
41. Lilla C, Ambrosone CB, Kropp S, Helmbold I, Schmezer P, von Fournier D, et al. Predictive factors for late normal tissue complications following radiotherapy for breast cancer. Breast Cancer Res Treat. 2007;106:143–50. doi:10.1007/s10549-006-9480-9.
42. Collette S, Collette L, Budiharto T, Horiot JC, Poortmans PM, Struikmans H, et al. Predictors of the risk of fibrosis at 10 years after breast conserving therapy for early breast cancer: a study based on the EORTC Trial 22881–10882 'boost versus no boost'. Eur J Cancer. 2008;44:2587–99. doi:10.1016/j.ejca.2008.07.032.
43. Davis AM, O'Sullivan B, Turcotte R, Bell R, Catton C, Chabot P, et al. Late radiation morbidity following randomization to preoperative versus postoperative radiotherapy in extremity soft tissue sarcoma. Radiother Oncol. 2005;75:48–53.
44. Delanian S, Porcher R, Balla-Mekias S, Lefaix JL. Randomized, placebo-controlled trial of combined pentoxifylline and tocopherol for regression of superficial radiation-induced fibrosis. J Clin Oncol. 2003;21:2545–50. doi:10.1200/JCO.2003.06.064.
45. Westbury CB, Yarnold JR. Radiation fibrosis—current clinical and therapeutic perspectives. Clin Oncol (R Coll Radiol). 2012;24:657–72. doi:10.1016/j.clon.2012.04.001.
46. Delanian S, Balla-Mekias S, Lefaix JL. Striking regression of chronic radiotherapy damage in a clinical trial of combined pentoxifylline and tocopherol. J Clin Oncol. 1999;17:3283–90.
47. Dancey AL, Waters RA. Morphea of the breast. Two case reports and discussion of the literature. J Plast Reconstr Aesthet Surg. 2006;59:1114–7. doi:10.1016/j.bjps.2006.01.018.
48. Cheah NL, Wong DW, Chetiyawardana AD. Radiation-induced morphea of the breast: a case report. J Med Case Rep. 2008;2:136. doi:10.1186/1752-1947-2-136.
49. Ardern-Jones MR, Black MM. Widespread morphoea following radiotherapy for carcinoma of the breast. Clin Exp Dermatol. 2003;28:160–2.
50. Wernicke AG, Goltser Y, Trichter S, Sabbas A, Gaan J, Swistel AJ, et al. Morphea as a consequence of accelerated partial breast irradiation. Clin Breast Cancer. 2011;11:67–70. doi:10.3816/CBC.2011.n.012.
51. Bleasel NR, Stapleton KM, Commens C, Ahern VA. Radiation-induced localized scleroderma in breast cancer patients. Australas J Dermatol. 1999; 40:99–102.
52. Davis DA, Cohen PR, McNeese MD, Duvic M. Localized scleroderma in breast cancer patients treated with supervoltage external beam radiation: radiation port scleroderma. J Am Acad Dermatol. 1996;35:923–7.
53. Walsh N, Rheaume D, Barnes P, Tremaine R, Reardon M. Postirradiation morphea: an underrecognized complication of treatment for breast cancer. Hum Pathol. 2008;39:1680–8. doi:10.1016/j.humpath.2008.04.010.
54. Schaffer JV, Carroll C, Dvoretsky I, Huether MJ, Girardi M. Postirradiation morphea of the breast presentation of two cases and review of the literature. Dermatology. 2000;200:67–71.
55. Burris 3rd HA, Hurtig J. Radiation recall with anticancer agents. Oncologist. 2010;15:1227–37. doi:10.1634/theoncologist.2009-0090.

4 Skin Care Products Used During Radiation Therapy

Florence Yuen and Sarah Arron

Skin care during radiation therapy is an essential component of the radiation oncology treatment plan. Skin reactions and their complications affect a majority of patients who undergo external beam radiotherapy [1–4]. If not addressed effectively, the ramifications can influence multiple aspects of patient care and patient well-being. These include pain, infection, decreased activity, altered sleep patterns, decreased quality of life, and potential treatment interruptions which may adversely affect cure rates.

The development of radiation-induced skin changes begins with the onset of radiotherapy and continues over a period of weeks beyond the completion of treatment. The initial skin changes may not be noticeable to the patient, as individual tolerance to treatment is variable. There are certain skin types that appear to be more at risk of breakdown. These include patients who are African American, have darker skin in general, have increased skinfolds, have fragile skin such as the elderly, and have sites of prior treatment or sites with uncontrolled tumor [4].

Currently there is no standard of care for the prevention and management of skin reactions in the radiation oncology patient population. There is a multitude of prescription and nonprescription skin care products currently on the market for patients undergoing radiation therapy. These products can range in out-of-pocket cost from a few dollars to more than a hundred dollars. A 2012 retrospective study by Schnur et al. [5], looking at out-of-pocket expenses for women undergoing external beam radiation for breast cancer, reported that 94 % of women incurred an average $131.00 out-of-pocket expense for products related to skin care toxicity.

At present, there is limited and insufficient evidence, with the exception of prophylactic topical steroid creams [1], to support the use of any specific topical agent over another for the prevention of radiation dermatitis. Trials focused on the effectiveness of products are beginning to address the need and desire for more evidence-based practice in this population.

The following are some of the more commonly used skin care products available for patients undergoing radiation therapy. Some of these products have been investigated and have or have not been shown to significantly benefit patients by decreasing radiation reactions. However, some products have not been evaluated in a controlled setting but have demonstrated utility and are commonly used by consensus opinion.

F. Yuen, RN, MSN, AOCNP (✉)
Department of Radiation Oncology, University of California, San Francisco, 1600 Divisadero, Cancer Cntr Room 1031, Box 1708, San Francisco, CA 94143, USA
e-mail: Florence.Yuen@ucsf.edu

S. Arron, MD, PhD
Department of Dermatology, University of California San Francisco, San Francisco, CA, USA

B. Fowble et al. (eds.), *Skin Care in Radiation Oncology*, DOI 10.1007/978-3-319-31460-0_4

4.1 Moisturizers and Emollients

The efficacy of moisturizers for the prevention and management of radiation skin reactions has been evaluated in several studies [1, 2, 6–11]. DiFranco et al. [6] demonstrated that skin hydration prior to, during, and following radiation therapy could have a positive effect on the skin.

Moisturizers have a safe treatment profile [12]. They may be useful in the prevention and management of the acute skin reactions associated with radiation dermatitis. Moisturizing and emollient agents come in various vehicles of delivery such as ointments (least irritation), creams, pastes, foams, lotions, and gels (drying with potential for irritation). The delivery vehicle of a topical formulation may help enhance penetration of the active agent. From a dermatological perspective, ointments are generally preferred over creams and lotions as they are more penetrating and hydrating. However, patients may find ointments too greasy, and, from a radiation oncology perspective, an ointment may be too occlusive at the start of treatment. Care should also be taken to avoid application of any agent immediately prior to the radiation treatment visit as it may create an undesired bolus effect.

As there is no strong evidence in radiation oncology to suggest one preparation over the other, consideration should be given to the effect desired and to patient preference. It is also prudent to consider the vehicle of delivery in evaluating and comparing the efficacy of agents in clinical trials. In order to have an optimum effect, moisturizers should be selected and tailored to address the needs of the individual patient along the continuum and site of radiation treatment [12].

At the start of treatment, moisturizers that are easily absorbed are preferred, leaving minimum residue that could serve as a bolus effect. Moisturizers that are comedogenic and that contain chemical components that may cause a sensitivity reaction which could further irritate radiated skin should be avoided. Our institution recommends that no skin care product be applied within 3 h prior to radiation.

Moisturizers do not add moisture to the skin but rather help the skin maintain its moisture. They are most effective when applied directly to the skin after bathing, to lock in moisture. They may consist of a combination of natural oils, ceramides, humectants, emollients, lubricants, etc. Moisturizers protect the skin's moisture by three means: replacement of deficient agents (present in the product), occlusion, and humectant action [12, 13]. Occlusive agents work by forming a thin film on the surface of the skin which prevents moisture loss. Examples are A&D Ointment, white petroleum, etc. Humectants, such as urea, sorbitol, sodium lactate, ammonium lactate, propylene glycol, panthenol, hyaluronic acid, honey, glycerin, and gelatin, promote moisture by two means. Humectants enhance water absorption from the dermis into the epidermis, or they can attract water vapor from the air to moisturize the skin [12, 13]. When used alone, a humectant can increase water loss from the skin by pulling water from the dermis and allowing it to evaporate. Therefore, in many products, humectants are combined with an occlusive agent or emollient to prevent moisture loss due to evaporation (e.g., Aveeno moisturizing cream, Cetaphil cream, Eucerin original).

4.1.1 Various Moisturizers

Lotion Soft: Lotion Soft™ is an easily absorbed light lotion that contains emollients and moisturizers. Lotion Soft Skin Conditioner is petroleum and mineral oil-free [14].

Remedy Lotion: Remedy Lotions are manufactured by Medline, which provides a variety of moisturizing lotions. Commonly used products include Remedy Basics Moisturizing Body Lotion, which is an unscented light moisturizer that is easily absorbed [15]. Remedy Phytoplex Nourishing Skin Cream is a blend of emollients, containing lipids such as safflower and carrageenan, essential fatty acids, oat kernel, licorice root extract, and plant botanicals [16].

Calendula: Calendula has been used in alternative medicine practice and various cultures for many years. It has purported anti-inflammatory and healing properties. *Calendula officinalis* is an herbaceous plant [17]. A (2004) randomized study compared calendula ointment with trolamine in 254 women undergoing breast irradiation [18]. The study showed that calendula cream was statistically better at reducing the occurrence of Radiation Therapy Oncology Group (RTOG) grade 2 or higher skin reaction, pain associated with the skin reaction, and treatment interruption. Many of the patients were satisfied with the calendula, but one third of the participants reported that the cream was difficult to apply. A 2009 Cochrane review [19] reported preliminary data indicating that calendula may be beneficial for management of acute radiation-induced erythema. The MASCC (2013) skin toxicity group felt there was insufficient evidence to support or refute a recommendation for use of calendula [1]. A 2015 double-blind study by Schneider et.al [20], comparing calendula against essential fatty acids in head and neck cancer patients undergoing radiotherapy, found that calendula was significantly more effective. The authors felt calendula provided protection in patients undergoing radiation and concomitant chemotherapy.

At our institution, we use calendula cream as a moisturizing agent for the management of dermatitis. It is applied topically twice daily, during, and following radiation treatment, to moisturize the skin, reduce irritation, and soothe irritated tissue. Patients find the cream formulation easy to apply. It is readily absorbed, leaving minimal to no residue on the skin. Calendula is also available in cream, ointment, gel, and tincture.

Petroleum-based bland emollients: These heavier emollients are more occlusive. Petrolatum has been noted to have a barrier-repairing effect in delipidized stratum corneum [12]. Bland petrolatum-based emollients are the preferred products, as emollients containing lanolin, beeswax, or fragrances may cause a sensitivity reaction and may block pores. Petrolatum-based products are widely available and inexpensive. Examples of these are A&D Ointment, Aquaphor, and white petroleum jelly. We defer the use of petroleum-based emollients until the patient begins to develop erythema or dry desquamation as we have found them to be too occlusive at the start of treatment.

Biafine (trolamine): This is an oil-in-water emulsion humectant-like moisturizer. It is reported to heal by recruiting macrophages to the wound and promoting the production of granulation tissue [1, 3]. This product has been used for many years and is frequently requested by patients and used in the radiation oncology setting. However, clinical trials have not found this cream to be either superior or effective in decreasing radiation-induced dermatitis. Two randomized non-blinded studies in women with breast cancer compared trolamine with best supportive care (Aquaphor, aloe vera, Lipiderm) [21, 22]. These studies concluded that trolamine did not provide a radioprotective benefit. Another study, conducted by Laffin et al. [23], comparing trolamine cream against Cavilon No Sting Barrier creams used by patients in humid climates, also showed no benefit in the trolamine arm. In that study, patients reported that the trolamine cream was thick, not well absorbed, and difficult to use. Based on the available evidence, the Multinational Association for Supportive Care in Cancer (MASCC) skin toxicity group does not recommend trolamine for prevention of radiation dermatitis [1].

EpiCeram: This is a replenishing emulsion containing ceramide (key ingredient), cholesterol, and free fatty acids. Ceramides are the major lipid components present in the stratum corneum. They are thought to play an essential role in maintaining the barrier function and water permeability of the skin. It is thought that ceramide content may be deficient in many skin disorders with a diminished barrier function [24]. The emulsion is designed to replenish the lipids within the stratum corneum and has been used effectively in the management of atopic dermatitis. The manufacturer's indications for use include the management of radiation dermatitis [25]. It is available by prescription only.

Hyaluronic acid cream: Hyaluronic acid is a naturally occurring polymer that is widely distributed in connective tissues. It is a key component of the dermal extracellular matrix. It has been shown to stimulate fibroblasts and fibrin development and assist in tissue granulation and healing [2]. However, in a study that compared topical hyaluronic acid-based gels to the bland emollient Aquaphor, no benefit was seen in reduction of grade 2 or greater dermatitis in the hyaluronic acid arm [26]. However, a study of patients with breast, head, neck, and pelvic malignancies reported a benefit of hyaluronic acid in delaying and diminishing the intensity and duration of the reactions [27].

Sucralfate: Sucralfate, a nonabsorbable substance, is thought to act directly on prostaglandin synthesis, promote angiogenesis, and bind epidermal growth factor to tissues [3, 7]. It is also thought to produce an anti-inflammatory effect by inhibiting gamma interferon and interleukin-2 [7].

There have been conflicting results in trials using different patient cohorts, treatment doses, and formulations of sucralfate cream. Although many patients report that the cream is soothing, no evidence to date has shown that sucralfate is effective in decreasing or preventing radiation dermatitis [2]. A study by Wells et al. [7] randomized 357 patients with head and neck, breast, or anorectal cancer to receive either aqueous cream, sucralfate cream, or no cream, from the start of treatment. The authors concluded that there was no benefit from a prophylactic application of a cream to the treatment area. The authors went on to identify several risk factors related to severe skin reactions, suggesting the need for further study in patients at higher risk.

Oils: Oils such as long-chain saturated fatty acids, medium-chain triglycerides, essential fatty acids, and fatty alcohols are thought to exert their benefits on the skin partially through improved repair by supplying lipids and improved permeability. There is limited evidence on the use of natural oils and its benefit in radiation oncology. We generally do not recommend the use of oils on the skin while the patient is on treatment. If oils are used, we recommend that they be thoroughly removed prior to treatment as they may leave a residue which could cause a bolus effect. Some examples of commonly used complementary oils are the following:

Emu oil: The emu is a large bird that originated in Australia. Emu oil is derived from the bird's subcutaneous and retroperitoneal fat. The oil contains high amounts of polyunsaturated fatty acids and antioxidants. Emu oil is gaining increased popularity among patients. It has been used both topically and orally. Emu oil is purported to have anti-inflammatory properties, as well as enhance skin permeation and moisture. Ultra emu oil has been processed to remove impurities [28].
In the oncology setting, emu oil has been used for the management of mucositis and to prevent osteopenia as a result of chemotherapy. Its mechanism of action is unclear at this time but is being investigated for additional uses [29]. Most recently ultra emu oil was utilized in a study on the prevention of radiation dermatitis, by Rollmann et al. [28]. The study concluded that the use of oil-based treatments may be safe for use with radiation treatments and that the use of ultra emu oil was not associated with any increased adverse effects.

Coconut oil: Coconut oil has been widely used in complementary medicine, cooking, cosmetics, and skin care products for many years. It is derived from the meat or flesh of the coconut. It is a highly saturated fat containing medium-chain triglycerides and polyphenols. Medium-chain triglycerides are thought to work differently than other types of saturated fat in the body. Research on the effects of medium-chain triglycerides found in coconut oil on the body is very preliminary. Coconut oil has been noted to be safe for ingestion and topical application [30–32].

Olive oil: The oil, extracted from ripe olives, is composed of mainly monounsaturated fatty acids. It also contains linoleic acid and numerous other chemical compounds including tocopherols, beta-carotene, and phytosterols [33]. The oil has been used as an emollient for management of eczema and psoriasis as well as in neonatal skin care [34]. A small study, by Danby et al. [34], compared olive oil application twice daily to sunflower seed oil over a

5-week period. The olive oil arm showed a significant reduction in the integrity of the stratum corneum layer of the skin and induced mild erythema at 4 weeks of use. This effect was not seen in the sunflower seed oil arm. Sunflower seed oil improved hydration, did not induce erythema, and preserved stratum corneum integrity. The study authors felt that the use of topical olive oil in atopic dermatitis could potentially exacerbate the dermatitis and challenged its use in infant massage [34]. Although not tested in patients undergoing radiation, the findings highlight the need for additional evidence-based research with regard to the benefits of natural oils that are widely accepted for use.

Avocado oil: Avocado oil has been noted to be rich in proteins, minerals, and vitamins A, D, and E [35]. It has been used for eczema and is purported to reduce itching and inflammation of the skin. People who suffer from very dry skin or from eczema often find avocado oil to have soothing properties.

Tea tree oil: Also known as melaleuca oil, this is an essential oil from the leaves of the *Melaleuca alternifolia* plant [36]. It has been used for many years in skin washes and shampoos for its antimicrobial effects (against acne, skin infections, as well as foot and toenail fungus) [37]. Tea tree oil should not be used in or around the mouth, as it is toxic if ingested. It is not recommended for use with pediatric patients due to its limited testing in this population [38]. Although tea tree oil continues to be widely used in alternative medicine, there is no clinical evidence to support the effectiveness of tea tree oil for treating radiation dermatitis.

4.2 Topical Steroids

Topical steroids have long been used to reduce the inflammatory response in the skin. Topical steroids are available in many different preparations. There are numerous topical steroids, available as ointments, creams, and lotions. They are categorized by their strengths and range from super-high potency to low potency.

MASCC (2013) guidelines [1] support the use of prophylactic topical steroids for the prevention and management of radiation dermatitis. A systematic review by Meghrajani et al. [8]. and a recent study by Hindley et al. [9] further support the evidence for topical steroid use during radiation therapy. Hindley et al. [9] concluded that the use of mometasone furoate 0.1 %, a mid-potency steroid cream, during and for 2 weeks postradiation was effective in reducing radiation dermatitis.

There is no standard for the type of topical steroid to be used in the radiation oncology population. The concentration, frequency, and duration of steroid application vary by institution. The long-term use of high-potency corticosteroids is contraindicated in order to prevent complications such as thinning of the skin, stretch marks (striae), or topical steroid addiction. Topical steroid addiction is a rebound effect that results in worsening skin inflammation requiring a stronger topical steroid to get the same result. The side effects of topical steroids capable of reducing inflammation can be mitigated by limiting their use to the lowest potency, by limiting their use to no more than twice daily, and by discontinuing their use with resolution of inflammation.

Topical steroids are ranked by class, from super potent (Class 1) to weakest (Class 7). Cutaneous side effects are rare with low-potency topical corticosteroids. In the adult population, high-potency and medium-strength preparations, used in areas other than the face and intertriginous and genital areas, are unlikely to cause cutaneous side effects if used for 6 weeks or less. In general, occluded areas such as the anogenital region and axilla should be treated with Class 6 or 7. Topical steroids stronger than Class 6 should be used sparingly on the face.

Steroids should be discontinued once the skin condition has improved. Because of their potential for increased side effects, the concentration and duration of their use should be minimized with children and in thin-skinned sites such as the face, perineum, axillae, and reconstructed thin skin flaps and moist desquamation sites. The use of steroids under these conditions may result in increased absorption and increased cutaneous side effects.

At our institution we begin our patients on a very low-potency 1 % hydrocortisone cream which is available over the counter. It is used in combination with an emollient. The patient should apply the steroid first, then followed with an emollient approximately 30 min later. The patients apply the mixture twice daily. Patients are instructed to discontinue the steroid at the completion of treatment or if the skin becomes excoriated.

4.3 Miscellaneous Products

RadiaGel™: This is a water-soluble hydrogel. Its purported use is for skin conditioning and management of radiation skin reactions before and throughout radiation treatment. The active ingredient is acemannan, a polysaccharide found in aloe leaves. The manufacturer's recommendation is to apply a thin layer to the radiation site two to three times a day. Per its distributor (Medline), RadiaGel will not create a bolus effect. RadiaGel has been noted to change from a translucent to an amber color over time. This has no impact on product efficacy [39].

RadiaPlex™ gel: Product by MPM. This is a wound gel, advertised for use during radiation treatment. It contains glycerin, hyaluronic acid, and aloe vera polysaccharides [40].

My Girls Breast Cream™: My Girls™ Skin Care cream is plant based. Its primary ingredients are calendula and rosemary. The cream is made without parabens, fragrance, or dyes. It is a moisturizer intended for women undergoing breast radiation. The cream has a whipped cream like texture. This makes it easy to apply over irritated skin [41].

4.4 Cleansers/Antiseptics

Cleansers help remove contaminants such as dirt, perspiration, oil, and dead skin cells from the skin within the treatment area. Cleansing aids in decreasing potential bacterial and bio-burden on the treatment site. Cleansing or washing of the site should be performed daily as this has been shown to be more effective than rinsing with water alone [42]. Rinsing of the site each time the patient urinates or has a bowel movement, in addition to daily cleansing, may be advisable in cases involving the genitalia, anal canal, or rectum.

Soaps and synthetic detergents: The skin's surface pH is ~4.7 on average, while water has a neutral pH of 7. Soaps, such as Ivory or Castile soap, are made up of long-chain fatty acid alkali salts and have a pH of 9 or 10. The higher pH of soaps can change the pH balance of the skin and lead to increased irritation and bacterial overgrowth. Soaps may contain the humectant glycerine or additional lipids or oils to counteract the drying effect. Some soaps, such as Lever or Dial, contain antibacterial agents. These tend to be further irritating and are best reserved for patients with intact skin and a history of superficial bacterial infections such as folliculitis or abscesses. Synthetic detergent cleansers (Syndets) such as Dove or Cetaphil have nonsoap surfactants and free fatty acids and are typically neutral or slightly acidic. These maintain the lipid and proteins of the epidermal barrier and are less irritating to the skin. These are generally recommended for patients undergoing radiation.

Chlorhexidine gluconate (Hibiclens™): Chlorhexidine is the active ingredient in Hibiclens™. Chlorhexidine has activity against gram-positive and gram-negative organisms. Chlorhexidine body baths and impregnated washcloths have shown to be effective in decreasing the colonization of vancomycin-resistant enterococci (VRE) and methicillin-resistant *Staphylococcus aureus* (MRSA) in hospitalized patients [43]. It is also readily available in 2 and 4 % solutions. In lower concentrations (2 %), it is bacteriostatic. In the higher 4 % concentration, it is bactericidal. It is not recommended for wound care in the 4 % concentration but is more commonly used on intact skin, for surgical preparation or hand washing [44, 45]. In our practice, we dilute the 2 or 4 % solution to yield a 0.5 % solution or lower. It has been suggested that this low chlorhexidine concentration may reduce the bacterial bio-burden of the wound, allowing for tissue healing [46]. We use it as a gentle wash, on areas of moist desquamation and as a cleansing sitz bath for our anal cancer patients, followed by moisturization, as it can be drying. Hibiclens® can be purchased over the counter at many drug stores [47].

Skintegrity Wound Cleanser™: This product assists with gentle wound cleansing by loosening proteins and wound debris, thus helping prevent buildup of devitalized and necrotic tissue [48].

Manual debridement: Debridement removes loose, devitalized, and necrotic tissue. This helps to decrease the bio-burden that may promote infection. Debridement is typically performed using very gentle mechanical techniques, such as sterile tweezers or dry gauze, to gently pull off the necrotic tissue.

4.5 Drying Agents

Burow's solution (Domeboro, Domeboro Otic): The solution has astringent and antibacterial properties. Burow's solution has been shown to have antibacterial effects against *Staphylococcus aureus* and *Pseudomonas aeruginosa* [49]. The active ingredients in Burow's solution are aluminum sulfate tetradecahydrate and calcium acetate monohydrate. It is available as an over-the-counter powder preparation. The powder is diluted with water to make a solution. The solution is poured onto 4×4 gauze or a clean washcloth. The saturated cloth or gauze is applied to the skin as a compress, for 15 min, three to four times a day. The solution assists with the cleansing and drying of weeping dermatitis. Overuse will result in excessive drying [50].

Aloe vera: Aloe vera is a succulent plant species. The leaves contain various phytochemicals such as acetylated mannans, polymannans, anthraquinones, and various lectins [51]. Aloe vera is widely used in herbal and alternative medicine. The extract from the leaf is used on cuts and burns for its soothing and purported healing effects and is popular among patients. The scientific evidence for the therapeutic effectiveness of aloe vera is limited [51]. With regard to the use of aloe vera in radiation oncology, a study by Heggie et al. [10] compared aloe vera gel with a topical aqueous cream, each applied three times a day during radiation treatment and for 2 weeks following treatment. They found that the dry desquamation rate was higher in the aloe vera group (70 % vs. 41 %). Topical application of aloe vera is not an effective preventative for radiation-induced dermatitis, and the MASCC skin toxicity study group recommends against its use [1, 52, 53].

4.6 Topical Anti-infective Agents

Topical antibacterial and antifungal agents have been used with radiation treatment skin reactions because of their ability to treat a localized area with minimal systemic absorption. In the radiation oncology setting, antibiotics are not recommended for prophylactic antibacterial management but rather for management of minor secondary infections and moist desquamation that are at high risk of infection. If there is a clinical concern for cellulitis or a soft tissue infection, systemic antibiotics should be considered.

Antifungal agents: Antifungal medications are used to treat mycoses such as candidiasis that may develop due to radiation altering the skin's integrity, as well as increased moisture in the skinfolds and intertriginous areas. Antifungal agents such as clotrimazole, miconazole, and nystatin are effective topical therapies for dermatitis complicated by *Candida* infection. The medication is available in ointment, cream, or powder form and is available over the counter. Commonly used products include 1 % clotrimazole cream [54] with 1 % hydrocortisone cream, miconazole, or Zeasorb-AF powder [55].

Bacitracin: This is an inexpensive over-the-counter topical antibiotic ointment, used for the prevention or management of localized skin infections. Bacitracin is a broad spectrum antibiotic that targets gram-positive and gram-negative bacteria such as *Staphylococcus aureus*, *Staphylococcus epidermidis*, and *Streptococcus pyogenes* [56].

Mupirocin (Bactroban): This is a topical antibiotic available in ointment or cream form. It is used for secondary bacterial skin infections. Mupirocin is effective against gram-positive bacteria including *S. aureus*, strep, and MRSA. Its effectiveness against MRSA is a primary advantage over other topical antibiotics. Mupirocin may be associated with systemic allergic reactions, including anaphylaxis, urticarial reactions, angioedema, and generalized rash. Mupirocin ointment is the vehicle of choice. It is also available as a cream which is well absorbed and is easier to use than the ointment. To minimize antibiotic resistance, mupirocin should not be used prophylactically or for an extended period. It can be applied to the skin two times daily and followed with a light emollient. Discontinue the mupirocin in 3–5 days if no clinical response is seen.

Mānuka honey: Mānuka honey is a viscous, saturated sugar solution, produced by honeybees, from the nectar of *Leptospermum scoparium*, the Mānuka tree, originating in New Zealand and Australia [57, 58]. Honey has been shown to have anti-infective, healing, and soothing actions. Honey assists the healing of burns and wounds in various ways. Firstly, it is a humectant which draws fluid from the environment and underlying dermis by osmosis, which assists in maintaining a moist wound environment, as well as facilitating autolytic debridement [57, 58]. Secondly, the enzymes of honey and its hydrogen peroxide by-product have been shown to exert an antibacterial effect. However, all honey varieties are not equivalent in their antibacterial effects [57]. Mānuka or *Leptospermum scoparium* honey has a low pH level and high osmolarity due to its high sugar content. This combination is purported to hinder the growth of and dehydrate microbes. It is a non-peroxide-producing honey but instead has a high level of methylglyoxal (MG) which is responsible for the honey's antibacterial effect. Mānuka honey has been shown to display significant biofilm reduction and antibacterial effects against gram-positive, gram-negative, anaerobic, and antibiotic-resistant bacteria, such as MRSA [57, 59–62].

To date, no bacterial resistance to honey has been noted [63]. Understandably, there is an increased interest in the use of *Leptospermum scoparium* Mānuka honey in this era of rising bacterial resistance to antibiotics. Medical-grade *Leptospermum scoparium* Mānuka honey-impregnated dressings are available in many forms, such as gel, impregnated gauze, impregnated hydrogels, foams, and alginates [64].

Silver sulfadiazine cream: Silver sulfadiazine cream is a combined formulation made from silver nitrate and sodium sulfadiazine. It is a sulfa drug with action against many gram-positive and gram-negative bacteria, including *Pseudomonas aeruginosa*, *Staphylococcus aureus*, and *Staphylococcus epidermidis* [65]. It was initially used in the 1970s as a topical treatment for burns, ulcerations, and wounds [66, 67].

Silver sulfadiazine cream is recommended for application once or twice daily as a thick coating. The cream should completely cover the entire treatment area. A secondary cover dressing should be applied. Prior to each new application, the previously placed silver sulfadiazine cream should be cleaned away along with any tissue debris. Pain and discomfort have been reported during removal of the old dressing. The dressing change procedure may also disrupt the healing skin cells and delay the wound-healing process. A very small trial comparing silver sulfadiazine cream to a polyantimicrobial gel reported that four out of eight women found that removing the cream caused too much pain to continue and that significantly more time was required to perform the dressing change [68].

Systemic absorption of silver sulfadiazine cream may cause adverse reactions. Adverse reactions include leukopenia (when applied to large areas), as well as allergic skin and systemic reactions [69].

MASCC (2013) skin toxicity group [1] has made a weak recommendation for the use of silver sulfadiazine cream. However, a Cochrane review has not recommended its use, as the authors found tentative evidence that silver sulfadiazine may prolong healing time [70].

Our practice has discontinued the use of silver sulfadiazine cream due to its potential for systemic absorption and untoward reactions, discomfort with daily dressing change, disruption of the healing wound bed, and the availability of improved silver ion and alternative dressings.

4.7 Skin Barriers

There is an increasing body of evidence suggesting that the protection of the skin from mechanical friction caused by clothing or other body parts may also reduce skin reaction severity. The use of barrier films or creams has been hypothesized to reduce trauma and retain moisture in intact skin, thereby reducing potential friction and radiation skin reactions [3].

Cavilon No Sting Barrier Film: This is a cream or solution that can be applied, swabbed, or sprayed onto the skin. It is alcohol-free, therefore making it sting- and pain-free on application. Once applied, it dries and leaves a flexible, breathable terpolymer film on the skin. The film is protective and assists in preventing maceration and tissue breakdown from wound fluid and friction. It also provides a secure base for the application of dressings [71].

Two studies, Graham et al. [11] and Laffin et. Al [23], have looked at Cavilon No Sting Barrier Film in comparison to sorbolene. The patients were women undergoing external beam radiation therapy for breast cancer. The studies concluded that the Cavilon No Sting Barrier Film was more effective than sorbolene in reducing pruritus and moist desquamation. More studies are needed, but it has been suggested that the skin barrier could be beneficial for skin protection and friction reduction [2, 11, 71].

Mepitel Film: Mepitel Film is made up of adherent, transparent Safetac-based soft silicone. The film adheres to the skin but not to open wounds; therefore, it does not traumatize the skin or wound on removal. The film is transparent, thin, and water resistant and assists in maintaining moisture. The film is indicated for use on the skin with scant to no drainage. Herst et al. [72] conducted a study which found that Mepitel Film is effective in preventing moist desquamation. Mepitel Film was placed on the patients at the start of radiation. The film was left in place through radiation treatments and replaced when it lifted off. According to the patients in this trial, the film also provided them with a sense of comfort and protection. The authors of the study concluded that the prophylactic use of Mepitel Film is a viable option for institutions with high moist desquamation rates. Once applied, the film can remain in place and does not need to be removed for radiation treatments, as the bolus effect is negligible [72]. The film will stay in place for about 10–14 days before it begins to lift off on its own [62, 72]. Its use is promising but needs further evaluation with regard to long-term outcomes.

4.8 Dressings

Dressings are used for various purposes in radiation oncology, including minimizing skin friction, preventing irritation, decreasing pain, promoting comfort, absorbing drainage, and managing moist desquamation. There are numerous dressings available, and there is considerable variation among practices. Standard gauze and tape dressings are not recommended and are rare if ever used on radiated skin, as they will stick to wounds and damage layers of the dermis on removal. There is no consensus or evidence supporting the use of one type or brand of dressing in the management of dry or moist desquamation. When considering the type of dressing to use, one should take moisture management into account. It has been shown that a moist wound-healing environment can help wounds heal faster by promoting reepithelialization and the migration of epithelial cells across the wound bed [62, 73]. Other considerations, when selecting a dressing, are management of bio-burden, antimicrobial action, infection, minimization of adverse effects, cost, ease of application, patient compliance with dressing changes, and comfort and pain reduction [3, 19]. In general, all dressings should be removed prior to patients receiving radiation treatments.

4.8.1 Collagen Dressings/Gels

Collagen is a protein that assists in giving the skin its tensile strength and promotes wound healing and new tissue growth. Collagen is thought to attract fibroblasts and keratinocytes to wounds, assisting with debridement, angiogenesis, and reepithelialization [74, 75].

Collagen dressings provide alternative collagen to the wound. The alternative collagen source may be from bovine, porcine, or avian sources. This collagen binds with matrix metalloproteinases found in the extracellular fluid of wounds. This allows the wound to utilize its own natural collagen to assist with wound healing by stimulating granulation and new tissue growth [74, 75].

The dressings can be used on a variety of wounds with scant to heavy exudates, as well as skin grafts. They are not recommended for use in wounds with dry eschar or in those patients with bovine, porcine, or avian sensitivities. They are available in various forms such as gel, powder, lotion, and gel sheets [75]. Dressing changes range from daily up to 7 days depending on the manufacturer's recommendation, the wound, and the treatment schedule. Products include Stimulen™ Collagen Gel, Lotion, Powder, or Sheets; Triple Helix Collagen Dressing, BGC Matrix®; BIOSTEP Collagen Matrix; Catrix® Wound Dressing; CellerateRX® Gel or Powder; ColActive® Plus; Excellagen®; FIBRACOL® Plus; and Puracol® Plus [75].

4.8.2 Hydrophilic Dressings/Hydrogels

MASCC guidelines, based on prior studies, indicate that the evidence on hydrocolloid dressings for radiation-induced moist desquamation remains unconvincing [1]. With respect to hydrogels, the evidence was conflicting; Mak et al. [76], in a small study of 42, mainly nasopharyngeal patients, and Macmillan et al. [77] in a larger study ($n = 357$) of head and neck, breast, and anorectal patients showed that hydrogels increased skin reaction severity, although only the Macmillan study found statistical significance. Gollins et al. [78] reported a significant decrease in skin reaction severity in 14 of 30 patients with breast and head and neck cancers. These studies involved the use of dry dressings, gentian violet, and sucralfate, all of which are not recommended for the management of moist desquamation [1].

Hydrocolloids: A hydrocolloid is a substance that forms a gel when it comes in contact with water.

Hydrocolloid dressings are self-adhering and nontraumatic to wound beds. The dressings consist of a gel, foam, or alginate colloidal matrix, with an occlusive, water-resistant outer layer. The dressings are effective in providing autolytic debridement. The colloidal portion of the dressing gels when it comes in contact with wound exudate, trapping bacteria, and wound debris while maintaining a moist healing environment [62, 79].

Hydrocolloid dressings are useful for the protection of healing noninfected wounds that are dry or that exhibit little to moderate exudate. The dressings are designed for extended wear of 3–7 days depending on the amount of exudate or per the manufacturer's recommendation. Care should be taken when removing the dressing as removal could cause trauma to fragile skin [80].

Hydrogels: Hydrogels are a mix of various synthetic polymers in a gel base consisting of greater than 90 % water. They are effective in helping to maintain fluid exchange on the wound surface [62, 81]. Hydrogels can assist with autolytic debridement of wounds. The dressing donates moisture which promotes a moist healing environment, granulation, and epithelialization. The high water content in a hydrogel dressing is cooling and soothing to wounds and can assist in decreasing discomfort. Hydrogel dressings usually do not adhere to wound beds; therefore, dressing change discomfort is decreased. The length of time the dressing can stay in place, generally 1–4 days, varies according to the manufacturer's recommendation [81, 82]. We have found hydrogel dressings effective for use with dry or slightly moist wounds, such as dry desquamation, follicular type radiation skin reactions, or pruritus. They are also effective with wounds that have granulation tissue or slough, with light to no drainage, that need debridement. Hydrogels are not recommended for wounds with heavy exudates.

Hydrogel is available as an amorphous gel or dressing. The gel is available in tubes, packets, or spray and is applied directly to the wound. The dressings are available in different forms, such as an impregnated hydrogel dressing or a hydrogel sheet, with or without a border. The dressings are usually translucent or clear. They can vary in viscosity and thickness, depending on the manufacturer [81]. Examples of the available hydrogel products include but are not limited to Elastogel™, Intrasite Gel™, Vigilon™, and Carrington Gel™ [81].

4.8.3 Alginate Dressings

Alginate is a complex polysaccharide extracted from marine algae. The dressings are made up of entangled fibers containing alginate, calcium, and sodium. Alginate dressings are conformable, lightweight, and highly absorbent. The dressings may be used with infected or noninfected wounds that have moderate to heavy exudate. They are capable of absorbing many times their weight. The wound exudate stimulates the alginate complex to exchange its calcium ions for sodium ions. This forms an amorphous gel that covers the wound. The dressing assists in maintaining a moist wound environment and assists with autolytic debridement. Alginates come in various forms including ribbons, beads, and pads. Alginate dressings are also available, impregnated with *Leptospermum* honey and silver ions. The dry dressing should be applied directly to the moist wound and then covered with a secondary dressing. The secondary dressing holds the alginate in place and prevents it from drying out. Alginate dressing is not recommended for use on wounds with minimal exudate as the dressing can dry out and stick to the wound, possibly traumatizing the healing tissue on removal. In this circumstance, wetting the dressing with fluid such as saline, water, or wound cleanser will loosen it and allow it to be easily removed [83, 84]. We have found the alginate dressings with silver ions to be effective in the management of our patients with moist desquamation. Examples of alginate dressings include but are not limited to Aquacel® Ag, Silverlon Calcium Alginate™, Medihoney Alginate™, and Restore Calcium Alginate™.

4.8.4 Silicone Dressings

Mepilex Lite: Mepilex products are absorbent, Safetac-based soft silicone dressings that adhere to healthy skin but not to open wounds. Mepilex Lite dressings have been proposed to decrease skin reaction severity but not moist desquamation rates. The dressings do not stick well in the axilla or on damp areas such as moisturized skin. Mepilex Lite dressings should be removed during radiation treatments as they will cause a small bolus effect (0.5 mm) [72] They need to be replaced approximately two times a week as they lose their adherence over time [85]. Additional products include Mepilex Transfer and Mepitel with and without Ag.

4.8.5 Silver Ion Dressings

Silver ion dressings: Silver has been noted to have antiseptic, antimicrobial, and anti-inflammatory properties [86]. In its elemental or uncharged form Ag (silver) is unreactive. The silver (Ag+) ion, when positively charged (cation), takes on a potent antimicrobial and bactericidal effect. This ionic reaction can occur when the silver cation binds to and reacts with tissue proteins and wound exudates causing structural changes in the bacterial cell membranes which in turn cause cell death [86].

Silver ions have been noted to be effective against a broad range of bacteria, including *Staphylococcus aureus*, methicillin-resistant *Staphylococcus aureus*, and vancomycin-resistant enterococci (VRE) [87]. Although there is a growing concern that the increased use of silver products may promote antibacterial resistance, there is no evidence to support this concern. An expert working group on the appropriate use of silver dressings in wounds suggested that the dressings are appropriate for use on wounds to decrease bio-burden and act as an antimicrobial barrier for acute or chronic wounds with a high risk of infection or reinfection [87]. The silver components of a dressing may be dispersed as a coating, or within the structure of the dressing, or as a combination of both. There are various silver ion dressing containing products including hydrogel (Silvasorb™ Gel) that are available.

When making a selection, consideration should be given to the degree of wound exudate production, as this may impact your choice of carrier dressing, the duration of silver efficacy, the use of secondary dressings, and patient preferences. The manufacturer's recommendations should be followed with regard to application and length of time the dressing can be left in place [86–88].

Vuong et al. [89] looked at the effect of silver leaf nylon dressing in 15 patients receiving radiation to the perineum. The patients wore a dressing made with silver leaf nylon from the initiation of radiation until 2 weeks postradiation. The mean RTOG dermatitis grades were significantly lower in the dressing versus control group. The benefit was thought to be attributable to the antimicrobial properties of the silver leaf nylon. Muangman et al. [66] compared Aquacel Ag (an ionic silver-coated hydrofiber dressing) to silver sulfadiazine for management of partial thickness burns. Aquacel Ag is a moisture-retention hydrofiber dressing with sustained silver ion release. It has an antimicrobial effect against pseudomonas, methicillin-resistant *S. aureus* (MRSA), and vancomycin-resistant enterococcus (VRE). The group noted that the Aquacel Ag provided a faster healing time, decreased pain symptoms, increased patient convenience, and was cost effective when compared to silver sulfadiazine.

In 2015, Mepilex Ag, a silver-impregnated foam dressing, was found to be successful in the management of partial thickness pediatric burns in comparison to a foam dressing used in conjunction with silver sulfadiazine cream. The authors found that patients required fewer (than daily) dressing changes, resulting in decreased pain, few infections, and a shorter length of hospital stay [67, 90].

There is currently no evidence-based recommendation for the routine use of silver ion dressings. To the contrary, the MASCC panel (2013) [1] made a weak recommendation against the use of silver leaf dressing, and a Cochrane review of silver dressings concluded that silver dressings do not improve healing rates [91]. However, the use of silver dressings in the Cochrane review may not have been within the scope of recommendations of the various manufacturers. In some cases they were used for extended periods and sometimes on wounds that were infected or contained a heavy bio-burden [87].

In our experience we have found silver ion containing hydrogel, hydrofiber, and alginate dressings to be effective with wound healing, infection prevention, pain control, and ease of use in our patients experiencing moist desquamation.

Photographs of many of the products mentioned in this chapter may be found in Appendix A.

References

1. Wong RK, Bensadoun RJ, Boers-Doets CB, Bryce J, Chan A, Epstein JB, et al. Clinical practice guidelines for the prevention and treatment of acute and late radiation reactions from the MASCC Skin Toxicity Study Group. Support Care Cancer. 2013;21:2933–48. doi:10.1007/s00520-013-1896-2.
2. McQuestion M. Evidence-based skin care management in radiation therapy. Semin Oncol Nurs. 2006;22:163–73. doi:10.1016/j.soncn.2006.04.004.
3. McQuestion M. Evidence-based skin care management in radiation therapy: clinical update. Semin Oncol Nurs. 2011;27:e1–17. doi:10.1016/j.soncn.2011.02.009.
4. Hymes SR, Strom EA, Fife C. Radiation dermatitis: clinical presentation, pathophysiology, and treatment 2006. J Am Acad Dermatol. 2006;54:28–46. doi:10.1016/j.jaad.2005.08.054.
5. Schnur JB, Graff Zivin J, Mattson Jr DM, Green S, Jandorf LH, Wernicke AG, et al. Acute skin toxicity-related, out-of-pocket expenses in patients with breast cancer treated with external beam radiotherapy: a descriptive, exploratory study. Support Care Cancer. 2012;20:3105–13. doi:10.1007/s00520-012-1435-6.
6. Di Franco R, Sammarco E, Calvanese MG, De Natale F, Falivene S, Di Lecce A, et al. Preventing the acute skin side effects in patients treated with radiotherapy for breast cancer: the use of corneometry in order to evaluate the protective effect of moisturizing creams. Radiat Oncol. 2013;8:57. doi:10.1186/1748-717X-8-57.
7. Wells M, Macmillan M, Raab G, MacBride S, Bell N, MacKinnon K, et al. Does aqueous or sucralfate cream affect the severity of erythematous radiation skin reactions? A randomised controlled trial. Radiother Oncol. 2004;73:153–62. doi:10.1016/j.radonc.2004.07.032.
8. Meghrajani CF, Co HC, Ang-Tiu CM, Roa FC. Topical corticosteroid therapy for the prevention of acute radiation dermatitis: a systematic review of randomized controlled trials. Expert Rev Clin Pharmacol. 2013;6:641–9. doi:10.1586/17512433.2013.841079.
9. Hindley A, Zain Z, Wood L, Whitehead A, Sanneh A, Barber D, et al. Mometasone furoate cream reduces acute radiation dermatitis in patients receiving breast

radiation therapy: results of a randomized trial. Int J Radiat Oncol Biol Phys. 2014;90:748–55. doi:10.1016/j.ijrobp.2014.06.033.
10. Heggie S, Bryant GP, Tripcony L, Keller J, Rose P, Glendenning M, et al. A Phase III study on the efficacy of topical aloe vera gel on irradiated breast tissue. Cancer Nurs. 2002;25:442–51.
11. Graham P, Browne L, Capp A, Fox C, Graham J, Hollis J, et al. Randomized, paired comparison of no-sting barrier film versus sorbolene cream (10% glycerine) skin care during postmastectomy irradiation. Int J Radiat Oncol Biol Phys. 2004;58:241–6.
12. Loden M. Role of topical emollients and moisturizers in the treatment of dry skin barrier disorders. Am J Clin Dermatol. 2003;4:771–88.
13. Kraft JN, Lynde CW. Moisturizers: what they are and a practical approach to product selection. Skin Therapy Lett. 2005;10:1–8.
14. Lotion Soft Skin Conditioner Skin Cream Safety Data Sheet. Steris. 2015. http://webapi.steris.com/api/alesconnection/getdocumentbynumber?id=1029&fileName=LOTIONSOFTSKINCONDITIONER.pdf. Accessed 20 July 2015.
15. Remedy Basics Moisturizing Lotion. Medline. 2015. https://www.medline.com/product/Remedy-Basics-Moisturizing-Body-Lotion/Lotions/Z05-PF44875?question=&index=P7&indexCount=7. Accessed 20 July 2015.
16. Remedy Phytoplex Nourishing Skin Cream. Medline Industries, Inc. 2015. https://www.medline.com/jump/product/x/Z05-PF06510. Accessed 23 July 2015.
17. Spotlight on Marigold. The Complete Herbal. 2015. http://www.complete-herbal.com/details/marigold.html. Accessed 27 May 2015.
18. Pommier P, Gomez F, Sunyach MP, D'Hombres A, Carrie C, Montbarbon X. Phase III randomized trial of Calendula officinalis compared with trolamine for the prevention of acute dermatitis during irradiation for breast cancer. J Clin Oncol. 2004;22:1447–53. doi:10.1200/JCO.2004.07.063.
19. Kassab S, Cummings M, Berkovitz S, van Haselen R, Fisher P. Homeopathic medicines for adverse effects of cancer treatments. Cochrane Database Syst Rev. 2009:CD004845. doi: 10.1002/14651858.CD004845.pub2.
20. Schneider F, Danski MT, Vayego SA. Usage of Calendula officinalis in the prevention and treatment of radiodermatitis: a randomized double-blind controlled clinical trial. Rev Esc Enferm USP. 2015;49:221–8. doi:10.1590/S0080-623420150000200006.
21. Fisher J, Scott C, Stevens R, Marconi B, Champion L, Freedman GM, et al. Randomized phase III study comparing Best Supportive Care to Biafine as a prophylactic agent for radiation-induced skin toxicity for women undergoing breast irradiation: Radiation Therapy Oncology Group (RTOG) 97–13. Int J Radiat Oncol Biol Phys. 2000;48:1307–10.
22. Fenig E, Brenner B, Katz A, Sulkes J, Lapidot M, Schachter J, et al. Topical Biafine and Lipiderm for the prevention of radiation dermatitis: a randomized prospective trial. Oncol Rep. 2001;8:305–9.
23. Laffin N, Smyth W, Heyer E, Fasugba O, Abernethy G, Gardner A. Effectiveness and acceptability of a moisturizing cream and a barrier cream during radiation therapy for breast cancer in the tropics: a randomized controlled trial. Cancer Nurs. 2015;38:205–14. doi:10.1097/NCC.0000000000000161.
24. Coderch L, Lopez O, de la Maza A, Parra JL. Ceramides and skin function. Am J Clin Dermatol. 2003;4:107–29.
25. Information for Physicians: Atopic Dermatitis Treatments. PuraCap® Pharmaceutical, LLC. . 2015. http://epiceram-us.com/physician-information-2/. Accessed 223 July 2015.
26. Pinnix C, Perkins GH, Strom EA, Tereffe W, Woodward W, Oh JL, et al. Topical hyaluronic acid vs. standard of care for the prevention of radiation dermatitis after adjuvant radiotherapy for breast cancer: single-blind randomized phase III clinical trial. Int J Radiat Oncol Biol Phys. 2012;83:1089–94. doi:10.1016/j.ijrobp.2011.09.021.
27. Liguori V, Guillemin C, Pesce GF, Mirimanoff RO, Bernier J. Double-blind, randomized clinical study comparing hyaluronic acid cream to placebo in patients treated with radiotherapy. Radiother Oncol. 1997;42:155–61.
28. Rollmann DC, Novotny PJ, Petersen IA, Garces YI, Bauer HJ, Yan ES, et al. Double-blind, placebo-controlled pilot study of processed ultra emu oil versus placebo in the prevention of radiation dermatitis. Int J Radiat Oncol Biol Phys. 2015;92:650–8. doi:10.1016/j.ijrobp.2015.02.028.
29. Jeengar MK, Kumar PS, Thummuri D, Shrivastava S, Guntuku L, Sistla R, et al. Review on emu products for use as complementary and alternative medicine. Nutrition. 2015;31:21–7. doi:10.1016/j.nut.2014.04.004.
30. Burnett CL, Bergfeld WF, Belsito DV, Klaassen CD, Marks Jr JG, Shank RC, et al. Final report on the safety assessment of Cocos nucifera (coconut) oil and related ingredients. Int J Toxicol. 2011;30:5S–16. doi:10.1177/1091581811400636.
31. DebMandal M, Mandal S. Coconut (Cocos nucifera L.: Arecaceae): in health promotion and disease prevention. Asian Pac J Trop Med. 2011;4:241–7. doi:10.1016/S1995-7645(11)60078-3.
32. Lexicomp: Coconut Oil (Natural Products Database). Wolters Kluwer. 2015. http://www.crlonline.com/lco/action/doc/retrieve/docid/fc_rnp2/4044543. Accessed 22 June 2015.
33. Lexicomp: Olive Oil (Natural Products Database). Wolters Kluwer. 2015. http://www.crlonline.com/lco/action/doc/retrieve/docid/fc_rnp2/3750282. Accessed 22 June 2015.
34. Danby SG, AlEnezi T, Sultan A, Lavender T, Chittock J, Brown K, et al. Effect of olive and sunflower seed oil on the adult skin barrier: implications for neonatal skin care. Pediatr Dermatol. 2013;30:42–50. doi:10.1111/j.1525-1470.2012.01865.x.
35. Nayak BS, Raju SS, Chalapathi Rao AV. Wound healing activity of Persea Americana (avocado) fruit: a preclinical study on rats. J Wound Care. 2008;17:123–6. doi:10.12968/jowc.2008.17.3.28670.

36. Carson CF, Hammer KA, Riley TV. Melaleuca alternifolia (Tea Tree) oil: a review of antimicrobial and other medicinal properties. Clin Microbiol Rev. 2006;19:50–62. doi:10.1128/CMR.19.1.50-62.2006.
37. Pazyar N, Yaghoobi R, Bagherani N, Kazerouni A. A review of applications of tea tree oil in dermatology. Int J Dermatol. 2013;52:784–90. doi:10.1111/j.1365-4632.2012.05654.x.
38. Hammer KA, Carson CF, Riley TV, Nielsen JB. A review of the toxicity of Melaleuca alternifolia (tea tree) oil. Food Chem Toxicol. 2006;44:616–25. doi:10.1016/j.fct.2005.09.001.
39. RadiaGel Hydrogel. Medline Industries, Inc. 2015. http://www.medline.com/product/RadiaGel-Hydrogel/Z05-PF00180#. Accessed 23 July 2015.
40. RadiaPlex®Rx Gel. MPM Medical, Inc. 2014. http://www.mpmmedicalinc.com/productdetails.aspx?pin=c.OC.3.p.7. Accessed 23 July 2015.
41. My Girls™ Skin Care is Available at Oncology Boutiques, Post-Surgery Specialty Retailers, & Pharmacies. Business Wire. 2015. http://www.businesswire.com/news/home/20110914005265/en/Girls%E2%84%A2-Skin-Care-Oncology-Boutiques--Post-Surgery-Specialty#.VbfdCk2h35p. Accessed 23 July 2015.
42. Oakley A. Soaps and Cleansers. DermaNet NZ. 2014. http://www.dermnetnz.org/treatments/cleansers.html. Accessed 5 June 2015.
43. Karki S, Cheng AC. Impact of non-rinse skin cleansing with chlorhexidine gluconate on prevention of healthcare-associated infections and colonization with multi-resistant organisms: a systematic review. J Hosp Infect. 2012;82:71–84. doi:10.1016/j.jhin.2012.07.005.
44. Lexicomp: Chlorhexidine Gluconate. Wolters Kluwer. 2015. http://www.crlonline.com/lco/action/doc/retrieve/docid/sfcomb_f/386209. Accessed 5 June 2015.
45. Main RC. Should chlorhexidine gluconate be used in wound cleansing? J Wound Care. 2008;17:112–4. doi:10.12968/jowc.2008.17.3.28668.
46. Drosou A, Falabella A, Kirsner RS. Antiseptics on wounds: an area of controversy. Wounds: A Compendium Clin Res Pract. 2003;15:149–66.
47. HIBICLENS®. Mölnlycke Health Care. 2015. http://www.hibiclens.com/. Accessed 23 July 2015.
48. Skintegrity Hydrogel. Medline Industries, Inc. 2015. https://www.medline.com/product/Skintegrity-Hydrogel/Gel/Z05-PF00182. Accessed 23 July 2015.
49. Hyo Y, Yamada S, Ishimatsu M, Fukutsuji K, Harada T. Antimicrobial effects of Burow's solution on Staphylococcus aureus and Pseudomonas aeruginosa. Med Mol Morphol. 2012;45:66–71. doi:10.1007/s00795-011-0540-9.
50. Lexicomp: Aluminum Acetate (AHFS Essentials (Adult and Pediatric)). Wolters Kluwer. 2015. http://www.crlonline.com/lco/action/doc/retrieve/docid/essential_ashp/988219. Accessed 27 May 2015.
51. Shelton RM. Aloe vera. Its chemical and therapeutic properties. Int J Dermatol. 1991;30:679–83.
52. Vogler BK, Ernst E. Aloe vera: a systematic review of its clinical effectiveness. Br J Gen Pract. 1999;49:823–8.
53. Olsen DL, Raub Jr W, Bradley C, Johnson M, Macias JL, Love V, et al. The effect of aloe vera gel/mild soap versus mild soap alone in preventing skin reactions in patients undergoing radiation therapy. Oncol Nurs Forum. 2001;28:543–7.
54. clotrimazole. Lexicomp. 2015. http://www.crlonline.com/lco/action/search?q=clotrimazole&t=name. Accessed 23 July 2015.
55. miconazole. Lexicomp. 2015. http://www.crlonline.com/lco/action/search?q=miconazole&t=name. Accessed 23 July 2015.
56. bacitracin. Lexicomp. 2015. http://www.crlonline.com/lco/action/search?q=bacitracin&t=name. Accessed 23 July 2015.
57. Mandal MD, Mandal S. Honey: its medicinal property and antibacterial activity. Asian Pac J Trop Biomed. 2011;1:154–60. doi:10.1016/S2221-1691(11)60016-6.
58. Jull AB, Cullum N, Dumville JC, Westby MJ, Deshpande S, Walker N. Honey as a topical treatment for wounds. Cochrane Database Syst Rev. 2015;3, CD005083. doi:10.1002/14651858.CD005083.pub4.
59. George NM, Cutting KF. Antibacterial honey (medihoney): in-vitro activity against clinical isolates of MRSA, VRE, and other multiresistant gram-negative organisms including Pseudomonas aeruginosa. Wounds. 2007;19:231–6.
60. Molan PC. Honey as a topical antibacterial agent for treatment of infected wounds World Wide Wounds. 2001. http://www.worldwidewounds.com/2001/november/Molan/honey-as-topical-agent.html. Accessed 27 May 2015.
61. Kwakman PH, te Velde AA, de Boer L, Speijer D, Vandenbroucke-Grauls CM, Zaat SA. How honey kills bacteria. Federation of the American Societies for. Exp Biol. 2010;24:2576–82. doi:10.1096/fj.09-150789.
62. Armstrong DG, Meyr DPM. UpToDate: Basic principles of wound management Wolters Kluwer. 2015. http://www.uptodate.com/contents/basic-principles-of-wound-management. Accessed 27 May 2015.
63. Zbuchea A. Up-to-date use of honey for burns treatment. Ann Burns Fire Disasters. 2014;27:22–30.
64. Medihoney® Products. Derma Sciences. 2015. http://www.dermasciences.com/medihoney-products. Accessed 28 Apr 2015.
65. Lexicomp: Silver Sulfadiazine. Wolters Kluwer. 2015. http://www.crlonline.com/lco/action/doc/retrieve/docid/sfcomb_f/386934. Accessed 5 June 2015.
66. Muangman P, Pundee C, Opasanon S, Muangman S. A prospective, randomized trial of silver containing hydrofiber dressing versus 1% silver sulfadiazine for the treatment of partial

thickness burns. Int Wound J. 2010;7:271–6. doi:10.1111/j.1742-481X.2010.00690.x.
67. Silverstein P, Heimbach D, Meites H, Latenser B, Mozingo D, Mullins F, et al. An open, parallel, randomized, comparative, multicenter study to evaluate the cost-effectiveness, performance, tolerance, and safety of a silver-containing soft silicone foam dressing (intervention) vs silver sulfadiazine cream. J Burn Care Res. 2011;32:617–26. doi:10.1097/BCR.0b013e318236fe31.
68. Black JS, Drake DB. A prospective randomized trial comparing silver sulfadiazine cream with a water-soluble polyantimicrobial gel in partial-thickness burn wounds. Plast Surg Nurs. 2015;35:46–9. doi:10.1097/PSN.0000000000000081.
69. Silver Sulfadiazine. Lexicomp. 2015. http://www.crlonline.com/lco/action/doc/retrieve/docid/patch_f/7668. Accessed 23 July 2015.
70. Storm-Versloot MN, Vos CG, Ubbink DT, Vermeulen H. Topical silver for preventing wound infection. Cochrane Database Syst Rev. 2010:CD006478. doi: 10.1002/14651858.CD006478.pub2.
71. Schuren J, Becker A, Sibbald RG. A liquid film-forming acrylate for peri-wound protection: a systematic review and meta-analysis (3M Cavilon no-sting barrier film). Int Wound J. 2005;2:230–8. doi:10.1111/j.1742-4801.2005.00131.x.
72. Herst PM, Bennett NC, Sutherland AE, Peszynski RI, Paterson DB, Jasperse ML. Prophylactic use of Mepitel Film prevents radiation-induced moist desquamation in an intra-patient randomised controlled clinical trial of 78 breast cancer patients. Radiother Oncol. 2014;110:137–43. doi:10.1016/j.radonc.2014.01.005.
73. Twardella D, Popanda O, Helmbold I, Ebbeler R, Benner A, von Fournier D, et al. Personal characteristics, therapy modalities and individual DNA repair capacity as predictive factors of acute skin toxicity in an unselected cohort of breast cancer patients receiving radiotherapy. Radiother Oncol. 2003;69:145–53.
74. Elgharably H, Ganesh K, Dickerson J, Khanna S, Abas M, Ghatak PD, et al. A modified collagen gel dressing promotes angiogenesis in a preclinical swine model of chronic ischemic wounds. Wound Repair Regen. 2014;22:720–9. doi:10.1111/wrr.12229.
75. Morgan N. Wound Care Advisor; What you need to know about collagen wound dressings. HealthCom Media. 2015. http://woundcareadvisor.com/what-you-need-to-know-about-collagen-wound-dressings/. Accessed 27 May 2015.
76. Mak SS, Molassiotis A, Wan WM, Lee IY, Chan ES. The effects of hydrocolloid dressing and gentian violet on radiation-induced moist desquamation wound healing. Cancer Nurs. 2000;23:220–9.
77. Macmillan MS, Wells M, MacBride S, Raab GM, Munro A, MacDougall H. Randomized comparison of dry dressings versus hydrogel in management of radiation-induced moist desquamation. Int J Radiat Oncol Biol Phys. 2007;68:864–72. doi:10.1016/j.ijrobp.2006.12.049.
78. Gollins S, Gaffney C, Slade S, Swindell R. RCT on gentian violet versus a hydrogel dressing for radiotherapy-induced moist skin desquamation. J Wound Care. 2008;17:268–75. doi:10.12968/jowc.2008.17.6.29589.
79. Bordered Granuflex. Surgical Materials Testing Lab. 2002. http://www.dressings.org/Dressings/granufl-brd.html. Accessed 27 May 2015.
80. Morgan N. Wound Care Advisor; What you need to know about hydrocolloid dressings. HealthCom Media. 2015. http://woundcareadvisor.com/apple-bites_vol2_no3/. Accessed 27 May 2015.
81. Morgan N. Wound Care Advisor; What you need to know about hydrogel dressings. HealthCom Media. 2015. http://woundcareadvisor.com/apple-bites-vol2-no6/. Accessed 27 May 2015.
82. Coats TJ, Edwards C, Newton R, Staun E. The effect of gel burns dressings on skin temperature. Emerg Med J. 2002;19:224–5.
83. Morgan N. Wound Care Advisor; Calcium alginate. HealthCom Media. 2015. http://woundcareadvisor.com/apple-bites-vol1-no2/. Accessed 27 May 2015.
84. Thomas S. Alginate dressings in surgery and wound management—part 1. J Wound Care. 2000;9:56–60. doi:10.12968/jowc.2000.9.2.26338.
85. Thin foam dressing for low exuding acute and chronic wounds. Mölnlycke Health Care. 2015. http://www.molnlycke.com/advanced-wound-care-products/foam-dressings/mepilex-lite/#confirm. Accessed 23 July 2015.
86. Fong J, Wood F. Nanocrystalline silver dressings in wound management: a review. Int J Nanomedicine. 2006;1:441–9.
87. Leaper D, Ayello EA, Carville K, Fletcher J, Keast D, Lindholm C, et al. International Consensus; Appropriate use of silver dressings in wounds. An expert working group consensus. Wounds International. 2012. http://www.woundsinternational.com/media/issues/567/files/content_10381.pdf. Accessed 4 June 2015.
88. Hurlow J. AQUACEL(R) Ag dressing with Hydrofiber(R) technology. Adv Wound Care (New Rochelle). 2012;1:104–7. doi:10.1089/wound.2011.0286.
89. Vuong T, Franco E, Lehnert S, Lambert C, Portelance L, Nasr E, et al. Silver leaf nylon dressing to prevent radiation dermatitis in patients undergoing chemotherapy and external beam radiotherapy to the perineum. Int J Radiat Oncol Biol Phys. 2004;59:809–14. doi:10.1016/j.ijrobp.2003.11.031.
90. Glat PM, Zhang SH, Burkey BA, Davis WJ. Clinical evaluation of a silver-impregnated foam dressing in paediatric partial-thickness burns. J Wound Care. 2015;24(Suppl 4a):S4–10. doi:10.12968/jowc.2015.24.Sup4a.S4.
91. Wasiak J, Cleland H, Campbell F, Spinks A. Dressings for superficial and partial thickness burns. Cochrane Database Syst Rev. 2013;3, CD002106. doi:10.1002/14651858.CD002106.pub4.

Part II

Site-Specific Recommendations

5 Head and Neck Cancer

Sue S. Yom, Florence Yuen, and Joyce Tang

Head and neck cancers (HNC) are frequently cited as the sixth most common type of cancer worldwide [1] but may number among the top cancers in endemic geographic areas. It is challenging to estimate the true incidence of the total category of head and neck cancers because of the diversity of head and neck anatomic subsites and the substantial variation in incidence by geographic region. For example, oral cavity cancers, larynx cancers, and thyroid cancers are all classified as among the top 15 cancers worldwide, but oral cavity and nasopharyngeal cancers are among the very top cancer diagnoses among males in endemic areas of South and Southeast Asia [2].

In any case, in the United States, cancers of the oral cavity, larynx, pharynx, salivary glands, and nose and nasal passages account for about 3 % of all cancer diagnoses yearly [3]. There is some indication that the incidence of human papillovirus-associated oropharyngeal cancer will continue to rise over the next several years [4]. Based on current trends, the National Cancer Institute estimates that in 2014, an estimated $3.6 billion will be spent on care for these cancers in the United States [5].

In addition, thyroid and skin cancers, for which multimodality treatment may be required for aggressive or advanced presentations and which usually fall into the range of cancers managed by the HNC radiation specialist, are exceedingly common. As a comparison, there were 45,780 oral cavity and pharyngeal cancers and 13,560 larynx cancers in 2015, versus 62,450 thyroid cancers and more than 3.5 million cases of nonmelanomatous skin cancer diagnosed in the United States in that same year [3, 6].

Radiation is a critical part of the multimodality treatment of advanced stage HNC, often following surgery, and can be employed in a monotherapeutic fashion for early stage presentations or advanced stage pharyngeal cancers. For very early stage head and neck, thyroid, and skin cancers, surgery alone may be perfectly adequate treatment, but postoperative radiation or chemoradiation will be used if negative prognostic features are discovered at the time of operation [7]. When upfront radiation is used for advanced stage cases, it is frequently delivered with concurrent systemic therapy, which can increase the mucosal and hematologic toxicity burden and level of supportive care required [8].

Radiation is often used as palliation for head and neck tumors that are incurable, recurrent, or metastatic. Radiation is an effective tool to reduce symptoms of bleeding, dysphagia, and especially

S.S. Yom, MD, PhD (✉) • F. Yuen, RN, MSN, AOCNP
J. Tang, RN, MN
Department of Radiation Oncology,
University of California, San Francisco,
1600 Divisadero Street, Suite H1031, Box 1708,
San Francisco, CA 94143, USA
e-mail: yoms@radonc.ucsf.edu

B. Fowble et al. (eds.), *Skin Care in Radiation Oncology*, DOI 10.1007/978-3-319-31460-0_5

pain, and in 80 % of cases can result in an improvement of symptoms or reduction of opioid analgesics [9].

5.1 Types and Frequency of Skin Reactions

Skin reactions are considered among the dose-limiting toxicities of HNC radiation, and these effects have a major impact on the level of acute pain and the duration of recovery experienced by the patient during the treatment course. Prospectively collected data obtained in Radiation Therapy Oncology Group cooperative group studies included clinician-graded assessments of skin toxicity (Table 5.1) [10–19]. However, in these studies, the true impact was likely underestimated due to the relative insensitivity and non-specificity of the grading scales that are commonly used and the generally lower prioritization in these therapeutically directed protocols of acute management of skin toxicity as compared to mucositis and dysphagia. Furthermore, while the RTOG defines the period of less than 90 days as the acute period, the designation of acute effects versus prolonged acute effects versus late effects was not classified in these studies and the grading scales differed depending on the attribution of the toxicity to radiation therapy or chemotherapy. In some of the studies, the authors reported only minimal data pertaining to skin toxicity and others reported only grade 3 or higher toxicity.

The probable underestimation of toxicity and heterogeneity of reporting in what could be considered to rank among the highest quality head and neck cancer data available indicates the ongoing, substantial challenges to the reliability of clinician-based skin toxicity assessment. Complete recording requires a highly sensitive instrument, dedicated training of the clinical team in standardized procedures for this special type of assessment, perhaps including high-quality photography, and designation of additional time and care for this activity. It is understandable that this level of effort may not be the highest immediate priority for very ill patients. Nonetheless, if we are to gain a better understanding of skin toxicity in the HNC radiotherapy population, these elements will be required to move forward. The developing specialty of dermatologic oncology may make contributions in this area in the future.

One can make a few generalizations from the available data. First, in the RTOG 9512 study, which reported the most detailed data on grade 1–2 skin toxicity, the hyperfractionated arm seemed to produce slight increases in acute grade 3 toxicity and late grade 2 toxicity. While the radiation fields in this study were small and the level of grade 3 toxicity was limited, these results are consistent with radiobiologic models predicting increased acute effects from hyperfractionation [20]. Second, one cannot clearly conclude from the overall data that concurrent platinum-based chemotherapy increases rates of clinician-graded skin toxicity. In RTOG 9111 and RTOG 9501, the arms in which patients received concurrent cisplatin-based chemotherapy did not produce notably higher rates of reported observable skin toxicity. A moderate acceleration of radiation therapy within the context of a concurrent chemoradiation program, whether enacted using a concomitant boost as in RTOG 0129 or as a simultaneous integrated boost with IMRT as in RTOG 0022, 0522, or 0225, also did not produce notable reported changes in grade 3 toxicity. Third, the addition of certain types of targeted therapy agents to a concurrent chemoradiotherapy platform did seem to increase skin toxicity. Most importantly, in a trial incorporating cetuximab, RTOG 0522, grade 3 toxicity within the RT field was comparable or higher and there were additional out-of-field toxicities attributable to the added drug. A nasopharyngeal chemoradiation trial incorporating bevacizumab, RTOG 0615, showed increases in high-grade skin toxicities as compared to a very similar earlier trial, RTOG 0225, that did not include bevacizumab. It should be noted that for cetuximab, the development of a clinically significant skin rash has been correlated to improved clinical response and survival benefit [21], and there are two case reports of this nature related to bevacizumab as well [22, 23].

Table 5.1 Acute and late skin toxicity as assessed in RTOG radiation therapy-based clinical trials in head and neck cancer

#	Description	Scale	Acute					Late				
			1	2	3	4	5	1	2	3	4	5
9512 [1]	Hyperfractionation vs. Conventional Fractionation in T2 Laryngeal Cancer	RTOG/EORTC criteria	QD: 45/119 (38 %), BID: 44/120 (37 %)	QD: 56/119 (47 %), BID: 55/120 (46 %)	QD: 6/119 (5 %), BID 13/120 (11 %)	0	0	QD: 41/118 (35 %), BID: 41/119 (34 %)	QD: 5/118 (4 %), BID: 14/119 (12 %)	QD: 0/118 (0 %), BID: 1/119 (1 %)	0	0
9111 [2, 3]	Induction Chemotherapy and Radiation vs. Concurrent Chemoradiation vs. Radiation for Advanced Stage Laryngeal Cancer	Induction phase only: NCI CTC v 1.0, All else: RTOG/EORTC criteria	NR	NR	Induction: 16/156 (10 %), CRT: 10/171 (6 %), RT: 15/171 (9 %)	Induction: 0/156 (0 %), CRT: 2/171 (1 %), RT: 0/171 (0 %)	0	Induction: 51/154 (33 %), CRT: 58/157 (37 %), RT: 59/158 (37 %)	Induction: 16/154 (10 %), CRT: 16/157 (10 %), RT: 20/158 (13 %)	Induction: 5/154 (3 %), CRT: 1/157 (1 %), RT: 2/158 (1 %)	Induction: 1/154 (1 %), CRT: 0/157 (0 %), RT: 1/158 (1 %)	0
9501 [4, 5]	Surgical Resection Followed by Radiation vs. Concurrent Chemoradiation	Chemotherapy: NCI CTC v 2.0, RT: RTOG criteria	NR	NR	RT: 20/209 (10 %), combined: 14/204 (7 %)	RT: 1/209 (<1 %), CRT: 0	0	NR	NR	RT: 2/208 (1 %), CRT: 2/201 (1 %)	RT: 0/208 (0 %), CRT: 3/201 (1 %)	0
0129 [6]	Concurrent Chemotherapy and Standard Radiation vs. Accelerated Concomitant Boost Radiation	Acute: NCI CTC v 2.0, Late: RTOG criteria	NR	NR	Standard: 31/361 (9 %), CCB: 35/360 (10 %)		NR	NR	NR	Standard: 5/351 (1 %), CCB: 2/343 (<1 %)		NR
0022 [7]	IMRT for Oropharyngeal Cancer	Acute: NCI CTC v 2.0, Late: RTOG/ EORTC criteria	NR	21 %	10 %	0	0	NR	5 %	0	0	0
0522 [8]	Concurrent Accelerated Radiation and Cisplatin (P) vs. Concurrent Accelerated Radiation with Cisplatin and Cetuximab (P-X)	NCI CTCAE v 3	NR	NR	Outside RT portal: P: 1 %, P-X: 20 % Inside RT portal: P: 15 %, P-X: 25 %		0	NR	NR	Outside RT portal: P: 2 %, P-X: 4 % Inside RT portal: P: <1 %, P-X: <1%P-X:		0

(continued)

Table 5.1 (continued)

#	Description	Scale	Acute					Late				
			1	2	3	4	5	1	2	3	4	5
0225 [9]	IMRT with Concurrent and Adjuvant Chemotherapy for Nasopharyngeal Cancer	Systemic and acute: NCI CTC v 2.0, Late: RTOG criteria	16/68 (24 %)	30/68 (44 %)	9/68 (13 %)	0	0	16/64 (25 %)	3/64 (5 %)	0	0	0
0615 [10]	Radiation with Concurrent and Adjuvant Chemotherapy and Bevacizumab for Nasopharyngeal Cancer	NCI CTCAE v 3	12/44 (27 %)	18/44 (41 %)	9/44 (20 %)	0	0	16/41 (39 %)	5/41 (12 %)	0	0	0

RTOG radiation therapy oncology group, *vs.* versus, *EORTC* European Organization for Research and Treatment of Cancer, *QD* daily, *BID* twice daily, *v* version, *NR* not reported, *CRT* concurrent chemoradiation, *RT* radiation therapy, *IMRT* intensity modulated radiation therapy

5.2 Management of Skin Reaction

Radiation-induced skin reaction in the head and neck region can usually be visibly detected within the first few weeks of treatment as a mild erythema, to be followed by a period of hyperpigmentation ("tanning") and dry desquamation or peeling. In the fifth to seventh week of treatment, this reaction can progress rapidly to moist desquamation. In some cases, if the reaction is not controlled aggressively by means of supportive care or adjustment of the radiation plan, the result can be a large-scale deep desquamation and even necrosis of the underlying soft tissues. When a skin reaction begins, it will typically accumulate in severity, so the areas that begin to manifest reaction earliest in the treatment course will be those that are most severely affected in the last third of the treatment course. The peak reaction will occur at the time of the maximum dose delivery to that area of tissue and will continue for another few weeks. The time to resolution is variable but can be prolonged, over the course of several weeks in the case of the most severe reactions.

Historically, skin reactions were quite severe as a routine in HNC, but with the advent of more sophisticated planning techniques and improvements in preventive and supportive care, the level of suffering during HNC radiation can now be managed more effectively. While most practitioners will start a preventive program to try to delay the onset of severe skin reactions, no high-quality data has established the efficacy of these interventions. There is very likely some degree of individual variation in patients' responses to radiation therapy; in the future, genomic approaches may yield measures of sensitivity to predict patients' skin reactions [24]. In the clinical setting, it is key to recognize an unusual degree of sensitivity in a particular individual early in the treatment course, and if the reaction is highly out of proportion to past experience with similar patients, to consider an adjustment accordingly.

Once a skin reaction has begun, the immediate goal should be to delay its progression to a higher level. An important component of management is the proper identification of the reaction's severity. In practice, most radiation oncologists are generally familiar with the RTOG grading scale, which labels the level of skin reaction as: grade 1, erythema or dry desquamation; grade 2, tender or bright erythema or patchy moist desquamation; grade 3, confluent moist desquamation outside of skin folds; grade 4, ulceration or hemorrhagic necrosis; grade 5, death related to treatment effects. Table 5.2 presents the evolution of skin reactions as recorded in some case series as well as selected examples of special cases of skin toxicity.

Clinical practice guidelines on the management of skin toxicity remain quite limited. For example, the MASCC Skin Toxicity Study Group conducted an extensive literature review on the management of acute and late radiation-related skin reactions. It is important to note that the majority of these recommendations were based on studies from the breast cancer literature. The recommendations included washing with water with or without a mild soap, allowing the use of antiperspirants, and topical prophylactic corticosteroids such as mometasone to reduce discomfort and itching. The group found some evidence supporting the use of silver sulfadiazine cream and insufficient evidence to support the use of trolamine, topical sulcrate, hyaluronic acid, ascorbic acid, silver leaf dressing, light-emitting diode lasers, Theta cream, dexpanthenol, calendula, proteolytic enzymes, sucralfate, oral zinc, and pentoxifylline. For telangiectasia, the panel recommended pulse dye laser for improvement of visual appearance and the use of pentoxifylline and vitamin E for fibrosis [25]. These are more limited recommendations than can be found in the nursing and wound care literature.

5.3 Impact of Technical Choices on the Skin

The widespread adoption of intensity modulated radiation therapy (IMRT) for HNC irradiation has resulted in characteristic patterns of effects on the skin surface. Conventional three-dimensional (3D) treatments with large collimated fields resulted in a more uniform level of dose delivery to large swathes of skin; these effects could not be easily manipulated in the planning process. With IMRT, areas of skin may be deliberately spared during the planning process (by drawing the external skin as a structure to avoid), but superficial external areas which are not spared, or which are deliberately targeted, are at a very high risk of reaction. The doses to the skin, particularly around the lateral aspects of the lower neck, in a "collar" region, can be much higher with IMRT because of the multiple beam angles typically used in step and shoot or rotational plan designs, which tangentially glance off the surface of the skin (Table 5.3) [26]. Furthermore, unanticipated "beam path" effects, such as alopecia to the occipital scalp, have been documented occurring at the exit points of the IMRT beams [27].

Some special technical notes apply to IMRT. When scars are targeted for high dosage, such as in cases of extracapsular extension, there will be an accordant skin reaction in that area and anticipatory management should be part of the plan (Table 5.3). Or, in some cases, IMRT plans may be matched to abutting conventional fields, such as the commonly used technique of the anteroposterior conventional field used to treat the low neck. In these cases, special care must be taken not to allow the skin to be "hot" at the junction. Of course, this same caveat also should be strongly applied to any abutting conventional photon fields and particularly to the rarely used situation of abutting electron fields. In these situations, thermoluminescent dosimeter measurements are highly encouraged to confirm the dose delivered in the junctional areas, as most treatment planning systems cannot model the skin dose as accurately as they model the deep tissue doses.

5.4 Patient-Related Factors Affecting Acute Skin Toxicity

5.4.1 Age

In a study of breast cancer patients, younger age was found to be a predisposing factor to greater skin toxicity [28]. A confounding factor may be that older patients are less likely to receive concurrent chemotherapy or more aggressive forms of radiation therapy.

5.4.2 Nutrition

A poor nutritional status will prevent repair of tissue damage. This is a common and serious risk for head and neck cancer patients, as undernourished patients are at high risk for skin damage and prolonged wound healing [29].

5.4.3 Ethnicity

The "redhead" phenotype, which is associated with polymorphisms in the melanocortin-1 receptor gene, has been found to produce unexpectedly severe acute reactions to radiation therapy [30]. Furthermore, dark-skinned persons will frequently show earlier and more severe desquamation and late onset of hypopigmentation in severely damaged areas [31].

5.4.4 Rheumatologic Disorders

Patients who have diagnoses of lupus, rheumatoid arthritis, dermatomyositis, or other collagen-vascular disorders may tolerate the treatment course relatively well but suffer from greater late toxicity. The radiation therapy can result in prolonged healing and greater degree of fibrosis [32].

5.4.5 Medical Conditions

Poor circulation affects the ability of the cutaneous tissue to heal. These factors include diabetes, hypertension, vascular compromise, renal insufficiency, and smoking [33–35].

5.4.6 Obesity

Obese patients will be at higher risk for medical comorbidities that limit healing potential but also have the physical disadvantage of increased skin folds, which may trap moisture and infection. Furthermore, an excess of tissue is a predisposing factor for increased risk of trauma and friction [36].

5.4.7 Prior UV Damage or Reirradiation

Patients who have extensive history of UV skin damage are prone to greater skin reactions during therapeutic radiotherapy [28]. Patients who are reirradiated are also at risk for skin reactions because of the reduction in skin integrity that has already occurred from previous treatment and the preexisting damage to the basal layers of the skin.

5.4.8 Antioxidants

It is very frequent that patients will ask to use a topical or oral antioxidant during their radiation treatment course in an attempt to reduce side effects. The interaction of these substances with radiation therapy is not well characterized although there is a theoretical basis and animal models suggest that these substances could block the oxygen-dependent mechanism by which therapeutic radiation operates [37].

In our clinic, high-dose topical and oral antioxidants are discouraged as they may exert systemic interactions with chemotherapy or radiation that are unknown. For topical applications, it may be reasonable to allow use in non-treated areas where there is no need to achieve therapeutic radiation dosage. Examples could include patients who are receiving radiation only to the upper part of the neck or one side of the neck, who may wish to apply topical antioxidants to the untreated areas of the neck, or who are being treated electively to deeper regions within the neck without substantial cancer risk to the superficial skin. These fine distinctions may be difficult to understand and accurately implement but can be carried out if there is a very clear understanding of the radiotherapy technique and goals and sufficient individualized counseling time is spent with the patient. Given the uncertainty about the concomitant use of these substances during radiation, patients should be counseled to the best of the physician's ability about the risk level of their choice of action.

5.5 Treatment-Related Factors Affecting Acute Skin Toxicity

5.5.1 Location and Volume of Irradiated Tissue

A larger volume of irradiated skin will increase the risk of toxicity and increase the effects felt by the patient. Most importantly, a wider extent of the radiation high-dose region will usually expand to encompass areas that are sensitive to radiation effects, such as skin folds or deeper subcutaneous tissues. The postauricular area and the "collar" encircling the low neck are typical areas where the combined effects of a curved surface, skin folds, and tangential radiation beam angles will frequently result in wet desquamation. The use of very low-energy photon beams or electron beams will localize the volume receiving the highest radiation dose to the surface of skin and thus also are associated with increased reaction [38].

5.5.2 Dose and Fraction Size

A higher total dose of radiation therapy and the use of fraction sizes larger than 200 cGy/fraction are both associated with a higher risk of skin reaction [33, 38].

5.5.3 Surgery and/or Reconstruction

Surgical procedures result in a loss of skin integrity; the incision site is more likely to be at risk for radiation reaction compounded by risks of infection and slow healing [34]. Post-surgical reconstruction may take a wide variety of forms including skin grafts, which should be considered extremely fragile especially if placed directly over bone, or myocutaneous and osseomyocutaneous flaps, which are inset into an area of a major tissue deficit. Additional time may be required after surgery to allow for adequate healing of any breakdown in skin integrity prior to starting radiation therapy; however, the oncologic dangers of excessive delay of initiation of postoperative therapy should take priority over the real potential complications of skin or flap necrosis and patients must be counseled about these relative considerations [34, 39]. Often the center of the flaps will show less reaction to radiotherapy [40], but the edges of the reconstruction, while at the most risk for necrosis, are precisely the areas at highest risk for recurrence (Table 5.3). Many practitioners use bolus materials or IMRT-based dose deposition over areas of surgical scar where tumor infiltration is suspected; both the use of bolus and physical targeting are highly associated with increased skin reaction in the intended area (Table 5.3).

5.5.4 Interactions with Systemic Therapy

Cisplatin is the most common radiosensitizer that is given concurrently with radiation therapy, but its effects on the skin, even when delivered concurrently with radiation therapy, appear to be minimal. However, cisplatin and carboplatin are sometimes delivered in conjunction with 5-fluorouracil (5-FU), which has been associated with cutaneous effects on the palms and soles ("hand-foot syndrome"), trunk and extremities, and fingernails. 5-FU has also been associated with photosensitivity and radiation recall phenomena [41].

It is important to be aware that the portfolio of systemic therapies that are being employed in combination with radiation therapy is expanding. The taxane class in particular has entered clinical trials in the induction chemotherapy setting as well as in the concurrent chemoradiation setting. Taxanes are considered excellent radiosensitizers and a potential alternative or additional agent to be used in platinum-refractory cancers. However, taxanes are associated with an incidence of dermatologic side effects as high as 81 % and are known to produce many of the effects associated with 5-FU with occasional clinical symptoms of subungual abscess, confluent and erosive hand-foot eruptions, and rarely, scleroderma or lupus-like reactions [41].

Cetuximab and other inhibitors of the epidermal growth factor receptor are widely recognized for their predominant side effect of skin reaction. Cetuximab is now approved for concurrent administration during HNC radiation therapy. The original study that resulted in this approval reported that grade 3–5 radiation dermatitis was 18 % in the radiation-only arm and 23 % in the radiation-cetuximab combined modality arm [42]. Subsequent clinical experience with cetuximab and a growing awareness of the severe effects of epidermal growth factor receptor (EGFR) inhibitors on the skin have led to continued evaluation of cetuximab's dermatologic effects, with some arguing that these are underappreciated. For instance, a survey conducted by the EORTC revealed that 49 % of HNC patients treated with cetuximab and concurrent radiation therapy experienced grade 3 or 4 dermatitis within the radiation portals, as judged by the NCI CTC version 2.0 grading scale [43]. While the usual effects of cetuximab are mild to moderate, including skin rash, skin dryness, xerosis, pruritus, hair abnormality, and nail changes, the classic finding of papulopustular rash, which affects 60–80 % of patients, can be severe in 5–20 % [44] (Table 5.3).

There is some indication that there may be an underlying biologic predisposition to very high-grade toxicity related to cetuximab. A high rate of hypersensitivity reactions in patients from the Southeast led to a laboratory-based investigation demonstrating a higher prevalence of IgE antibodies specific for an oligosaccharide present on the Fab portion of the cetuximab heavy chain [45].

As a result of the special dermatologic needs of patients receiving cetuximab (or EGFR inhibitor), the MASCC Skin Toxicity Study Group has developed an EGFR inhibitor-specific grading scale for dermatologic adverse events [46] as well as clinical practice guidelines for the management of these patients [47]. There is also a consensus guideline on the management of skin reactions in the presence of EGFR inhibition that was developed by a group of experienced clinical trial leaders in Europe and the United States [48]. The basic recommendations by MASCC to prevent worsening of papulopustular rash were to combine 1 % hydrocortisone with moisturizer, sunscreen, and oral doxycycline 100 mg twice a day, for the first 6 weeks of EGFR inhibition treatment. Schools of thought vary on whether to start doxycycline only at the onset of grade 2 rash or whether prophylactic doxycycline is the most practical course of action.

Finally, the rapidly evolving area of immunotherapy in HNC treatment is likely to require additional dermatologic evaluation. Only initial reports exist thus far for cytotoxic T-lymphocyte antigen-4 (CTLA-4) or anti-PD1 antibodies, but it is known that there are distinct immune-related effects that commonly do occur in the skin, most commonly as a maculopapular rash that may or may not be pruritic [49]. As these agents are increasingly combined, either sequentially or concurrently, with radiation therapy, their dermatologic effects will require further characterization.

5.6 Late Reactions

Acute skin reactions may signal a risk for higher late toxicity. Major late effects to the superficial skin include dryness and aging of the skin, alopecia, changes in pigmentation, telangiectasia, and superficial fibrosis. A severe superficial skin reaction is a signal of the risk of late fibrosis to the underlying soft tissues in that area.

5.7 Preventive Interventions

Early prevention of skin reactions, when the skin is intact and dry, is based on the dual principles of maintenance of skin integrity and protection of the skin from trauma or environmental stress or exposure as well as moisturization. Cleanliness is encouraged; washing the skin with lukewarm water or saline soaks is encouraged. A mild, nonalkaline, unscented soap may be used. Moisturization with an unscented, lanolin-free, water-based moisturizing lotion is important to maintain the natural barriers of the skin surface and prevent dry cracking. Emollients in a lotion form are probably easier for patients to apply and more readily absorbed than more heavily oil-based cream or ointment preparations. Gels are usually drying and stinging. Aloe vera gel, while it has anti-inflammatory and antibacterial properties, is not a moisturizer [50] and well-designed studies have failed to establish benefit from its use [51]. For male patients, an electric razor is encouraged to avoid cuts to the skin, and perfumes and aftershave should be avoided as they are irritating to microabrasions. Likewise, although many patients enjoy swimming, exposure to chlorine can be irritating and drying to the skin; if the patient really wishes to swim, the skin should be rinsed and moisturized immediately after [52].

Most of the literature concerning skin care during radiotherapy has focused on breast cancer patients. However, in trials including head and neck cancer patients, a number of preventive topical applications, such as trolamine [53, 54], hyaluronic acid [55], allantoin [56], and pentoxifylline [57], may be beneficial but have either produced conflicting results in clinical trials or been inadequately tested [58]. Sucralfate does not appear to be helpful [59, 60]. In a phase III study of breast cancer patients receiving postoperative radiotherapy, calendula was found to be superior to trolamine in reducing incidence of RTOG grade 2 dermatitis, but the ointment formulation in this particular study was considered difficult to apply by some patients [61] and a subsequent randomized blinded study of calendula cream showed no improvement over an aqueous cream [62]. A recent Brazilian study in head and neck cancer patients, however, showed that 4 % calendula oil prevented or delayed the onset of grade 2 radiodermatitis more effectively than oil containing essential fatty acids [63].

High-potency corticosteroids such as mometasone [64] have been shown to be effective in soothing irritative symptoms and reducing the severity of moist desquamation in the breast cancer population, but in the head and neck cancer population outside of the group receiving EGFR inhibition, we prefer to use very low-potency formulations (1 % simple hydrocortisone, in formulations without urea or salicylic acid which increase the steroid absorption) only as required to address itching, to avoid thinning and atrophy of the skin as well as other long-term effects such as telangiectasia, striae, and hypopigmentation [65]. Corticosteroid-induced skin atrophy begins in as little as a few days and is evident at 2 weeks. Its effects are most potent on the skin of the face (due to the thin stratum corneum in this area, which allows for tenfold higher absorption than on the arm, with the arm manifesting clinical effects threefold higher than the back or abdomen) and in areas of creases, such as can be found in the neck [66]. In particular, steroids should not be applied near the eyelids where side effects can include glaucoma and cataracts [67]. Even in cases of cetuximab-induced rash, the use of topical low-potency steroids should be restricted to less than 6 weeks. We prefer to restrict use to minimal application and only as absolutely necessary to prevent patients who would otherwise scratch themselves. Furthermore, a small study of head and neck cancer patients was stopped early due to clinically obvious worsening skin reaction and worsened outcomes determined by the RTOG and Radiation-Induced Skin Reaction Scale (RISRAS) scales on the side of the neck where patients were applying 1 % hydrocortisone twice daily [68].

Because dermatitis reactions commonly occur around the neck, patients should wear loose, open-neck clothing that does not rub against this area and cause friction and irritation against the skin surface. Cotton is absorbent and non-clinging, whereas polyester fabrics are hydrophobic and cling due to local electrostatic potentials on the surface of the skin, which also inhibit hair regrowth [69]. In any case, any kind of coarse or rough woven clothing should be strictly avoided in proximity to the face, neck, and chest. To reduce friction in areas of skin that rub or fold on themselves, we recommend films or spray barriers (Mepitel film, Cavilon No-Sting spray), as opposed to bulky or adherent dressings that cannot easily be removed from the skin prior to daily treatment. If necessary to guard against rubbing by clothes or other sources of external friction, an easily removable lightweight dressing can be applied to the low neck to provide protection from bacteria and repeated friction and trauma. A recent study of a thin silicone foam dressing (Mepilex Lite) in nasopharyngeal cancer patients who had developed erythema showed more rapid wound healing and improvement of sleep as compared to standard procedures of salt-water washing [70].

It is very challenging to prevent physical trauma to the skin in patients who wear tracheostomy appliances or collars. If the appliances are clearly not situated in an area of high risk for recurrence of cancer, it may be worth considering additional sparing of these areas during the radiation planning process to provide relief to the skin in those areas that will experience a bolus effect and repeated trauma from the appliance against the skin. A reduction of the radiation dose to less than 50–55 Gy to the skin surface will prevent very severe reactions; confirmatory thermoluminescent dosimetry can be considered to gauge the true effect. Furthermore, these areas of the skin should be kept as clean as possible; the typically recommended hydrogen peroxide solution can be very irritating and drying, so we recommend gentle soap or wound cleansers. Gauze soaked in sterile normal saline and left on the area for a few minutes may be a useful technique to loosen and remove mucus or crusting if there are excessive secretions.

In the peri-wound region, a barrier ointment (Ilex, Calmoseptine) is recommended. While zinc oxide can work well for this function around both tracheostomy and gastrostomy tube sites, it will potentially worsen any fungal infection present. If there is redness and itchiness (similar to "athlete's foot") indicative of fungal infection, clotrimazole should be applied to the area for several days followed by the barrier ointment.

A thin absorptive dressing can be placed around the wound site to prevent excessive moisture from or around the wound from softening and weakening the skin. Preventive lightweight or foam nonadherent dressings (Telfa, Mepilex Lite, Lyofoam) can be used to cushion and protect the skin underneath; absorbing properties of the dressing can be tailored to the level of secretions and wetness. Patients, following standard recommendations, will often use dry gauze ("4×4" squares) to try to cushion the areas around the tracheostomy appliance, which is appropriate when the skin is dry and intact, but in the setting of radiation-induced skin desquamation, gauze can adhere to moisture and act in a traumatic skin-stripping manner, much like a wet-to-dry dressing, when removed each day. Similar principles of trauma and friction avoidance and cushioning where possible should be applied to care of a gastrostomy or nasogastric tube insertion site, although these appliances are not typically being radiated.

Gastric acid leakage from the gastrostomy site may result from balloon malfunction or tube migration and these correctable issues should be handled promptly. Acid leakage causes chronic moisture and acid excoriation and maceration of the surrounding skin. For severe cases that cannot be mechanically corrected, consider ranitidine or omeprazole to reduce the acid. Magnesium-aluminum hydroxide (Mylanta) can be placed on irritated areas. If the reaction is chronic in nature, shielding of the peri-wound region can be achieved with an impermeable hydrocolloid powder or dressing (DuoDERM).

5.7.1 Management of Dry Desquamation

After 30 Gy of radiation has been delivered, sebaceous glands can be permanently destroyed and the skin suffers from reduced lubrication. Treatment of dry desquamation, which may often result in flaking or peeling, requires very frequent use of moisturizing emollient. Care should be taken that these lotions, or possibly creams, are applied after treatments or well ahead of radiation treatments so that there is not a bolus effect on the skin from the moisturizer itself. For this reason, water-based light lotions and creams tend to be strongly favored as they are tolerated well and absorbed into the skin surface more readily and rapidly than heavier oil-based creams or ointments. To avoid this bolus effect, any tape, adhesives, or bandages should be removed from the skin prior to radiation delivery.

If dry slough can be seen on the surface of a wound, it should be debrided by manual (tweezers, scalpel, curette), enzymatic (collagenase SANTYL, Accuzyme papain-urea), or autolytic (using the body's own enzymes) (medical grade honey such as MediHoney, prescription sugar paste, amorphous hydrogel) means or with a wound cleansing agent (Skintegrity) designed for this purpose. Mechanical means (friction/rubbing, pulsating water jet, or wet-to-dry dressing) are less preferred as they induce more trauma. Necrotic tissue in particular should be removed as it is a source of bacterial proliferation. The wound should be thoroughly cleansed after debridement. Antimicrobial wound cleansers should be avoided as they are frequently cytotoxic and antimitotic and will inhibit fibroblast and keratinocyte activity needed for cellular regeneration. For cleansing an open wound, normal saline or a noncytotoxic wound cleanser is preferred over tap water, as the quality, contaminant level, and levels of chlorine and fluorine additives in tap water are variable.

5.7.2 Management of Moist Desquamation

The application of drying antiseptics (povidone-iodine spray, proflavine lotion) and mechanical means for drying out the skin (hair dryers on a cool setting) remain popular for common skin reactions despite recent recommendations to the contrary, with one older survey in the United Kingdom revealing usage of these outdated techniques in about 60 % of radiotherapy departments [71]. Another study found gentian violet application to be a continuing common practice that resulted in drying and discomfort [72]. Gentian violet is potentially carcinogenic and not recommended for routine use. As compared to a nonadherent polyamide dressing, gentian violet was nonsignificantly associated with higher wound pain scores in a study of nasopharyngeal cancer patients [73]. In our clinic, we engage in daily debridement of dry peeling tissue and cleansing of any moist or crusted exudate from the surface of the wound with noncytotoxic wound cleansers (sterile normal saline, Skintegrity) but we do not try to "dry a wet wound" (Table 5.3).

Once a reaction has progressed, we believe that topical dressings are absolutely needed to provide greater protection from friction and external trauma and to keep the area clean. These dressings should always be removed at the time of delivery of radiation treatment to avoid a bolus effect. Two important additional principles should be observed more stringently at this point: prevention of infection and promotion of a moist wound-healing environment. In the wound-healing literature, it has been well established since the 1960s that an open wound that is kept moist will heal 50 % faster than one that is dried out or scabbed over [74]. The moisture enhances fibroblast proliferation and keratinocyte differentiation necessary for healing. However, excessive moisture is very detrimental, resulting in maceration injury and excessive levels of enzymes such as matrix metalloproteinases (MMPs) within the fluid. Furthermore, an excess of fluid causes mechanical softening and increased friction against clothing [75]. Newer absorptive dressings, such as alginate or hydrofiber dressings, donate optimal moisture to the wounded area but resorb excessive moisture.

5.7.3 Common Types of Wound Dressings

Wet-to-dry dressings consist of gauze dampened in saline that is allowed to dry against the wound and then removed, stripping off the surface of the wound. For many reasons, while it remains very popular, especially in the surgical community [76], this is not an optimal strategy. It results in repeated painful trauma to the area, leaves foreign bodies within the wound, and at least for some time the wound bed will be dried out preventing the optimal healing environment. This approach increases the risk of infection into the wound and repeatedly disrupts granulation and epithelization. We discourage this approach to wound care and favor other means of debridement.

Hydrocolloids (DuoDERM) consist of hydrophilic colloid particles bound to polyurethane foam. They form an impermeable, adherent, yellow, malodorous gel in contact with the surface of the wound. Due to the color and odor that results, these areas can look as if they are infected but are actually highly protective against infection because of their complete barrier properties. Hydrocolloids are highly adherent and conforming and thus can be used for autolytic debridement but are difficult to remove gently and thus are inappropriate if ongoing radiation requires daily removal. These are appropriate for use to chronically ulcerated, relatively dry wounds [77].

Hydrated polymer dressings, or hydrogels, consist of 80–99 % water on a cross-linked polymer. They are minimally absorptive and thus are only recommended for dry or minimally exudative wounds. Due to their high water content, they cool and rehydrate the wound. Hydrogel formulations include amorphous gels (Intrasite, Regenecare, RadiaCare), nonadherent sheets (CoolMagic, NuGel, RadiaCare), and impregnated gauze (Skintegrity). Amorphous formulations are commonly used to promote autolytic debridement of sloughing or necrotic wounds but not exudative ones. As hydrogels are nonadherent, they can be changed daily but a secondary dressing may be needed on top [77]. We have used hydrogel sheets occasionally as a simple maneuver to cool the skin or to provide a protective and hydrating barrier for very early dry desquamation. We also use a silver-containing amorphous hydrogel formulation for very early skin cracking that is dry or has minimal moistness but increasing redness, heat, swelling, or pain indicative of infection (SilvaSorb).

Alginates (Kaltostat, Sorbsan) comprise a composite of brown seaweed cellulose fibers and dissolve on contact with the wound to form a soft hydrophilic gel. The calcium of the seaweed is exchanged with the sodium in the fluid of the wound to transform the dressing into a gel. Alginates may absorb 10–15 times their weight and are only appropriate for moderately or heavily exudative wounds but not for drier wounds where they will dry out the wound further and damage the tissues due to adherence. For the appropriate type of wound, these have excellent properties of facile non-traumatic removal as a gel-forming dressing. Alginates high in mannuronic acid will wash off easily but alginates high in guluronic acid can be removed from the wound bed retaining their one-piece structure. In addition, alginates have hemostatic properties if there is mild bleeding from the wound [77]. We have employed silver-containing alginates (Algicell Ag, Tegaderm Alginate Ag) with remarkable success in deep, highly exudative wound surfaces.

Very similar to alginates, the new technology of hydrofiber dressings (Aquacel, Versiva) utilizes sodium carbomethylcellulose to combine with wound exudate, thus forming a soft conforming gel sheet. Hydrofiber dressings are increasingly being used in place of alginates. Similar to alginates, hydrofiber dressings are highly absorbent, nonadherent, and most appropriate for exudative wounds [77]. At present, one of the main strategies in our clinic for wet, desquamating neck wounds is to use silver-containing alginate or hydrofiber dressings (Aquacel Ag, Tegaderm Alginate Ag).

A variety of silver-impregnated dressings exploit the antimicrobial properties of ionic silver. Unlike antibiotics, because of its multiple facets of antibacterial action, silver does not tend to produce resistance and thus is an excellent choice for long-standing wounds at high risk of infection or colonization. Alginate and hydrofiber silver-containing dressings bring the added benefit of an absorptive and moisture balancing capacity restoring the optimal wound-healing environment. The application of silver sulfadiazine cream (Silvadene, Flamazine) does not achieve this second purpose. Silver sulfadiazine is considered a standard treatment for thermal burns, but randomized studies have demonstrated that in comparison to silver sulfadiazine, silver-impregnated dressings are associated with less pain on application, lower total treatment costs, and in some studies, improved re-epithelization and wound healing [78–80]. A small phase 2 study of silver leaf dressing versus silver sulfadiazine applied to opposite sides of the neck in head and neck cancer radiation patients failed to show a reduction in the global RTOG toxicity grade, but observers noted improvement within the same grade. Furthermore, patients reported improved pain control on the side treated with silver leaf dressing, and wound healing was thought to be accelerated [81]. Silver dressings obviously cannot be used on patients who have sensitivity to silver and the silver may leave a visible black stain in the wound area as it oxidizes, which should not be of concern as this is temporary.

In our clinic, for an area of minimal skin breakdown that is at some risk for infection, we will use a silver-containing hydrogel formulation (SilvaSorb), which was shown in a randomized study to reduce pain in comparison to silver sulfadiazine cream [82]. For a small area, it can be overwhelming for the patient to secure a large size silver-impregnated dressing to the neck and these sheet-based dressings can impair mobility, are expensive, and are complicated to manage daily. For the more serious scenario of large-scale wet desquamation, we have a fairly standard policy of using silver-impregnated alginate or hydrofiber dressings with excellent results. Except for special situations, such as dry eschar, we do not tend to use iodine-containing wound dressings, as the iodine potentiates hypothyroidism, a common problem in head and neck cancer patients, interacts with medications such as lithium and warfarin, and may be associated with more pain and less efficacy than silver-containing hydrofiber dressing [83].

5.7.4 Post-treatment and Chronic Management

Re-epithelization should occur within 10–14 days after the last dose of radiation is given. A number of conditions can result in failure to improve for more than 2 weeks. Poor nutrition, concomitant medications, infection, or compromised vascularity resulting from hypertension, diabetes, or smoking can impair healing. If a patient's skin shows no improvement after 10 days, serious consideration should be given to which factors may be preventing healing, especially infection, and corrective action or an altered treatment plan should be attempted. It is often helpful to consult with the hospital wound care specialty service in this type of situation.

Culture of any wound should be considered for worsening pain, edema, or warmth over a centimeter from the wound edges, or for failure to show improvement over a course of active therapy lasting more than 2 weeks. In these cases, a tissue culture should be obtained by the most noninvasive means possible such as a scraping, aspiration, or swab. Prior to swabbing, the wound bed should be cleansed with saline, the culture should be obtained from an area free of necrotic tissue, and pressure should be applied to the area to obtain fresh wound fluid.

Eschar is a brown or black, leathery-appearing dead tissue over the surface. It should usually be removed, unless removal would result in exposure of bone and risk of osteomyelitis. In this special case, if the eschar does not feel boggy and is dry and appears intact without drainage, it can be left in place, soaked with povidone-iodine (Betadine) twice daily, and covered with dry gauze in hopes that epithelization may occur underneath. If the eschar becomes boggy or drains, removal should be reconsidered. Consultation with a specialized wound care team and plastic surgery team should be strongly considered.

5.8 Photographs and Recommendations

Below are general skin care recommendations (Table 5.2), as well as week by week treatment instructions and photographs that demonstrate typical skin reactions over time (Table 5.3). Photographs of special reactions and instructions on how to treat these more uncommon cases are also provided (Table 5.4). Figure 5.1 is a general suggested treatment algorithm for skin care for head and neck cancer patients.

Table 5.2 General principles of skin care for head and neck patients

Patient should:
• Cleanse daily with a non-perfumed mild soap and water
• Moisturize the skin
• Protect the radiated site from sun exposure by using a soft, wide-brimmed, sun blocking hat or scarf
• Apply sunscreen with SPF >25 to exposed treatment area if in the sun. Ensure this is washed off prior to daily radiation treatment
• Monitor weight during treatment and have access to nutritional consults, to promote wound and skin healing
• Remove all dressings or films, prior to treatment
Patient should not:
• Rub, put pressure on, or scratch radiated area
• Expose the treatment area to direct sunlight when undergoing radiation treatments
• Take hot water showers, hot baths, use wash cloths
• Use a razor in the radiation site for shaving
• Apply astringents, facial toners, after shave lotions or colognes to the radiation site
• Apply any lotion, cream, or ointment in the 3 hours prior to radiation treatment
• Wash off lotion, cream, or ointments if applied three or more hours before radiation treatment
• Use drying agents to the skin unless instructed to do so
• Use any tape or adhesives on the radiated skin

Table 5.3 Examples of acute skin reactions and recommended interventions for head and neck patients undergoing external beam radiation

Week	Skin reaction	Reaction type	Treatment and intervention
1 and 2	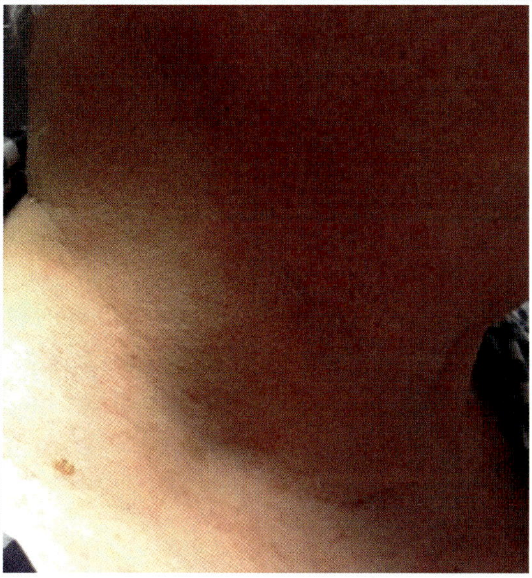 A 69-year-old male with base of tongue squamous cell cancer, receiving weekly cisplatin and concurrent radiation to 70 Gy	No reaction	• Cleanse daily with a mild non-perfumed soap and water • Apply a light moisturizing lotion two times per day • Avoid application within 3 h prior to receiving radiation • Protect the radiation site from sun exposure • Avoid any rubbing or friction to the skin surface
3	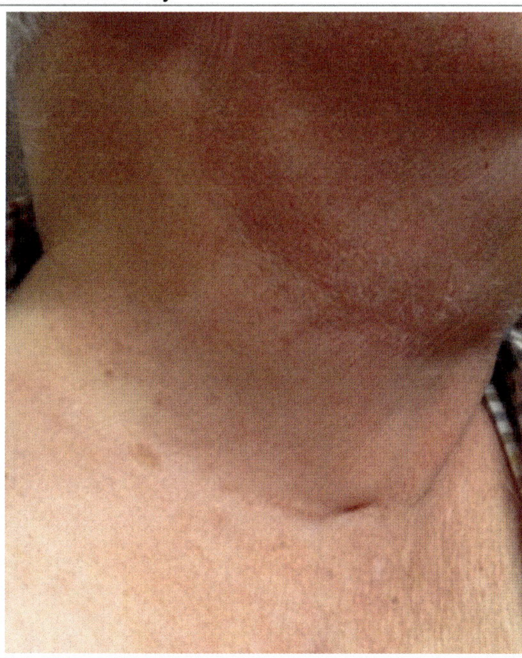	Mild hyperpigmentation with mild erythema	• Cleanse daily with mild non-perfumed soap and water • Consider initiating Skintegrity wound cleanser (or similar product) • Switch to a thicker moisturizing cream such as calendula. Apply a thin layer two times per day • Avoid application within 3 h prior to receiving radiation • Apply Mepilex Lite to areas experiencing rubbing or friction. Remove this dressing prior to radiation treatment

(continued)

Table 5.3 (continued)

Week	Skin reaction	Reaction type	Treatment and intervention
4	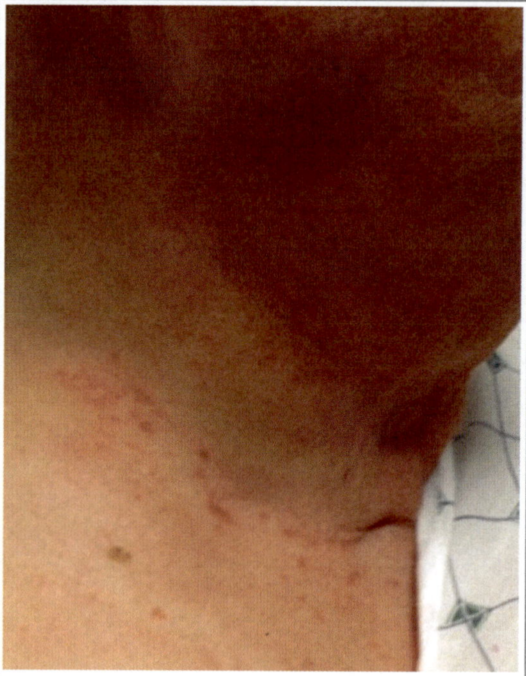	Moderate erythema and dry desquamation	• Begin Skintegrity spray if not already using. Spray it liberally on the radiation site. Allow it to remain on the skin for 1–2 min and then rinse it off • Apply a thin coat of calendula cream to the area on to two times a day or discontinue and switch to the ointments below • Add Aquaphor or A+D Ointment. Liberally apply Aquaphor or A+D to the radiation site once a day before bed. It does not need to be washed off in the morning • Apply Mepilex Lite to any areas experiencing rubbing or friction. Remove this dressing prior to radiation treatment • Apply cooling compresses (cool towel or thick towel with ice pack on top) to the areas that are inflamed twice a day. Do NOT inflict cold thermal trauma to the skin • Consider a hydrogel sheet dressing (Nugel, Xtrasorb HCS, or Medihoney HCS) to intact briskly erythematous areas. This dressing can be placed following radiation and left in place until the next treatment or removed when the patient showers. Use care when removing the dressing as to not traumatize or tear the skin. Not recommended on skin that is fragile or likely to lift off. Remove this dressing prior to radiation treatment

(continued)

Table 5.3 (continued)

Week	Skin reaction	Reaction type	Treatment and intervention
5	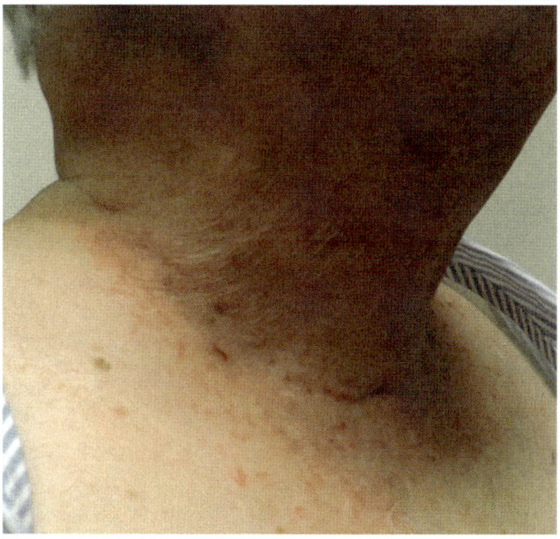	Progressive erythema and hyperpigmentation with areas of dry desquamation	• Continue daily cleansing with Skintegrity spray • Manually debride peeling skin once a day if needed (patients should not do this) • Discontinue calendula • Moisturize with A+D or Aquaphor ointment twice a day • Apply Mepilex Lite to protect the skin and allow healing to the site • Remove all dressings prior to radiation treatment • May continue cooling compresses and/or hydrogel treatments to briskly erythematous areas for comfort
6	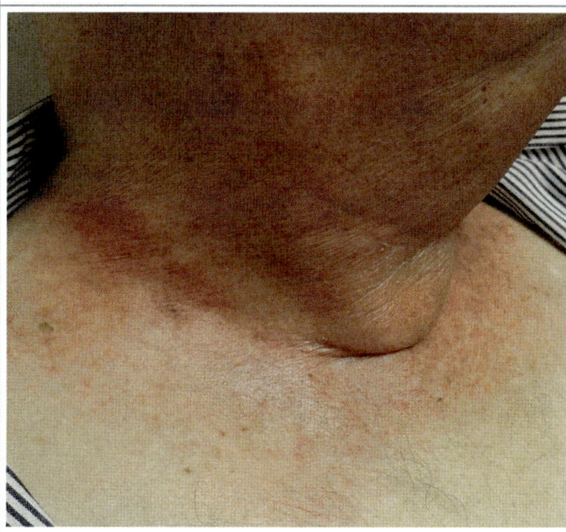	Dry fissures/ dry desquamation of skin and early focal moist desquamation with minimal exudate	• Continue to cleanse and moisturize as above • Apply a small amount of bacitracin mixed with Aquaphor (1:2 ratio) to the dry cracking/desquamated area 2× a day • Apply Silvasorb hydrogel to this area • Cover with a secondary dressing such as Mepilex lite • Gently wash off Silvasorb if used prior to treatment • May continue cooling compresses to dry, erythematous areas

(continued)

Table 5.3 (continued)

Week	Skin reaction	Reaction type	Treatment and intervention
7	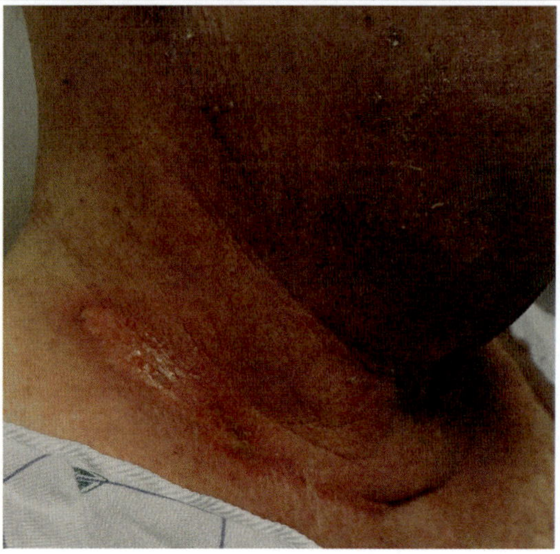	Moist desquamation along the neck fold	• Continue daily cleansing with Skintegrity spray • Manually debride peeling skin once a day if needed (patients should not do this) • Apply Aquacel Ag/Algicel Ag/Mepitel Ag (or similar dressing). Cut to fit over the edges of moist desquamation. Cover this with a secondary dressing such as Mepilex lite • Do not use tape or adhesives on the radiated skin • May place a flexible netting (Flexinet) or scarf over the dressing to keep it in place • Continue A + D or Aquaphor or A + D ointment to undressed skin • Change dressing every 24–48 h while undergoing treatment • Wet the primary dressing down thoroughly if it does not come off easily to avoid traumatizing new skin with dressing removal

(continued)

Table 5.3 (continued)

Week	Skin reaction	Reaction type	Treatment and intervention
8	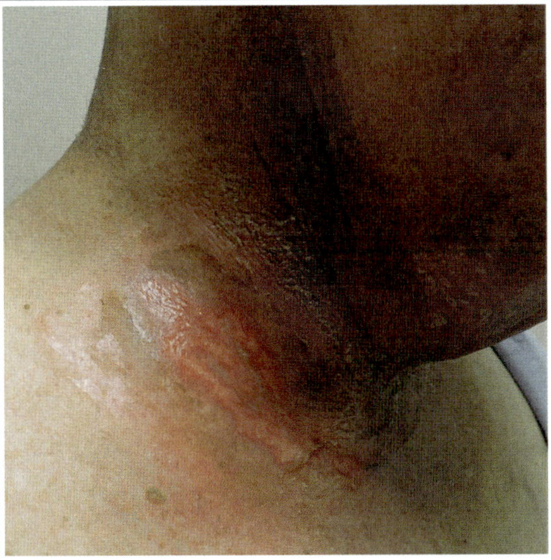	Confluent dry and resolving moist desquamation (with the formation of new skin islands)	• Continue daily cleansing with Skintegrity spray • Continue dressings as above to moist desquamation • Discontinue Aquacel Ag/alginate dressings as wound begins to dry • May transition to Mepilex Ag, Mepilex transfer Ag, Silvasorb gel, or Medihoney gel with a nonstick cover dressing • Continue to moisturize the remaining undressed skin with A + D or Aquaphor ointment twice daily
10 weeks post-radiation completion	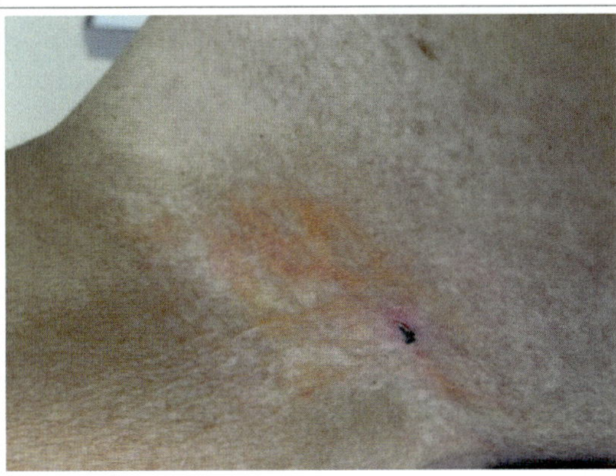	Induration with residual hyperpig-mentation and resolving erythema of the radiation site	• Continue to moisturize the area one to two times a day • Continue to apply sunscreen and protect the area when exposed to direct sunlight as this can prolong the hyperpigmentation • Consider pentoxifylline and vitamin E for fibrosis prevention

Table 5.4 Special cases and reactions

Week 7	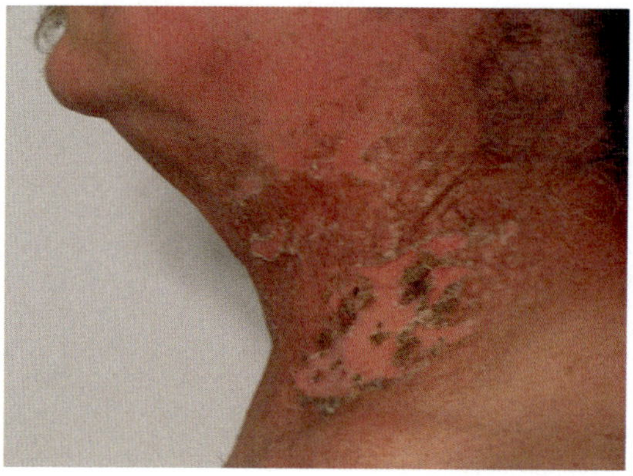	"Collar" reaction in low neck with dry desquamation	• Spray Skintegrity or similar on the area and allow it to remain on the skin for 1–2 min then rinse. Manually or enzymatically or autolytically debride any remaining loose, dry skin • Apply calendula twice daily • Protect the "collar area" radiation site with Mepilex lite or a soft cotton scarf. Remove daily prior to radiation • Avoid the application of drying agents to the site
Week 5	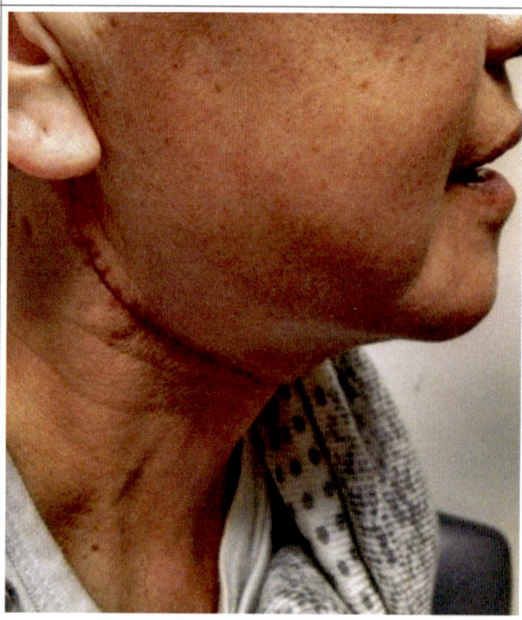 A 64-year-old Asian woman with high-grade adenocarcinoma of right parapharyngeal space, with positive margins after resection, treated postoperatively to 6600 cGy with weekly cisplatin. Reaction shown at mid-course	Enhanced erythema around surgical incision	• Cleanse the site daily with mild soap and water • Moisturize the site twice daily with a mild lotion (such as Lotion Soft or Remedy) • Monitor the incision site over the course of radiation • Be alert for any signs of infection such as redness, heat, fluctuance, swelling or dehiscence • Scar reduction products not recommended while on treatment

(continued)

Table 5.4 (continued)

Week 3	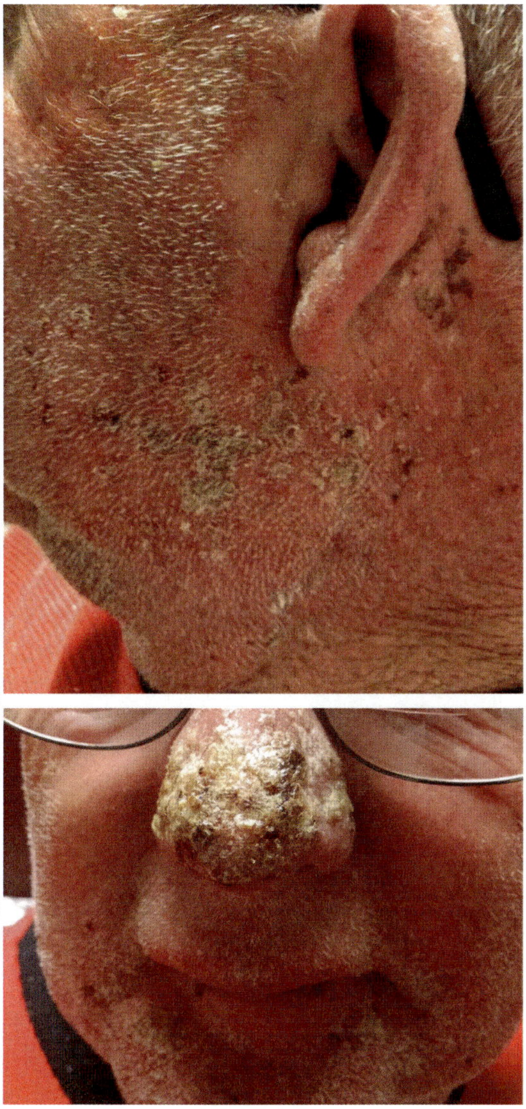 A 65-year-old man with stage III squamous cell carcinoma of the lower lip with extracapsular extension, receiving 66 Gy in 33 fractions with concurrent cetuximab, in fourth week of radiation treatment	Cetuximab-associated rash seen during concurrent radiation	• Apply or spray Skintegrity (or similar) to the hyperkeratotic plaques. Use care to not get the spray into the eyes. Allow Skintegrity to remain on the skin for 1–2 min then rinse • Gently debride any remaining loose, dry debris • Apply 1 % clindamycin lotion twice daily for 35 days • Apply 1 % hydrocortisone lotion or cream for pruritis, two times a day • Doxycycline 100 mg by mouth twice a day for 21 days or oral antibiotics per institutional guidelines for coverage of Staphylococcus Aureus • Moisturize with Aquaphor ointment liberally applied over entirety of face and neck twice a day

(continued)

Table 5.4 (continued)

	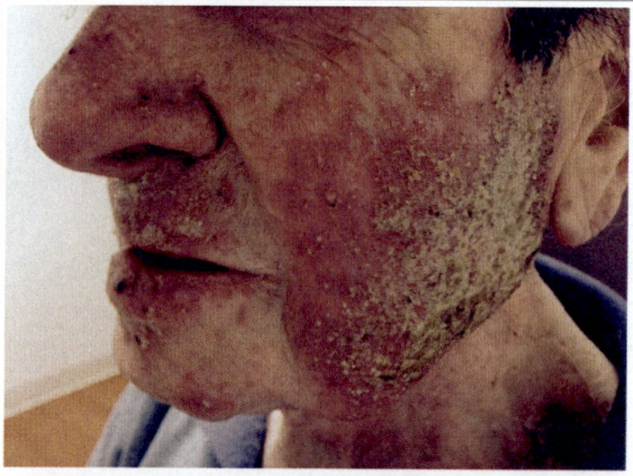 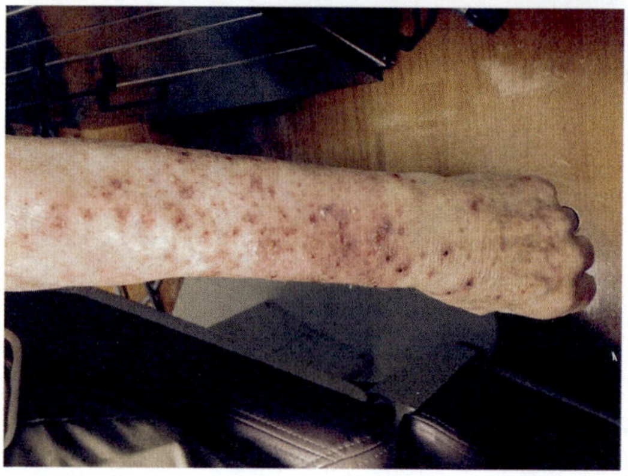 A 72-year-old man with aplastic anemia and history of squamous cell carcinoma of the base of tongue, treated with definitive radiotherapy and cetuximab and then, following metastasis, salvage cetuximab. Reactions from cetuximab intensify with the cumulative number of cycles given. Reactions are not confined to the head and neck region only. The chest, back, and extremities should be inspected		

(continued)

Table 5.4 (continued)

Week 3	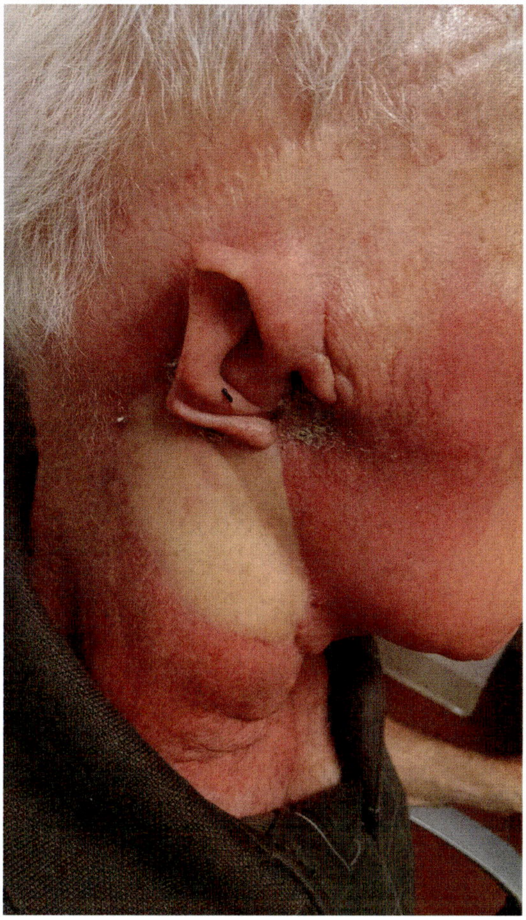 An 80-year-old man with squamous cell carcinoma of the skin, recurrent and metastatic to the parotid gland, treated with surgery and neck dissection with positive margin followed by re-excision, then postoperative radiation to 66 Gy	Differential reaction of flap versus normal skin	• Cleanse daily with mild soap and water or Skintegrity • Moisturize twice daily with A+ D or Aquaphor ointment • Flap edges should be monitored carefully over the course of radiation for potential breakdown, infection, or necrosis • Protect the area from friction with Mepilex Lite or soft scarf

(continued)

Table 5.4 (continued)

Bolus or targeting reaction around surgical incision	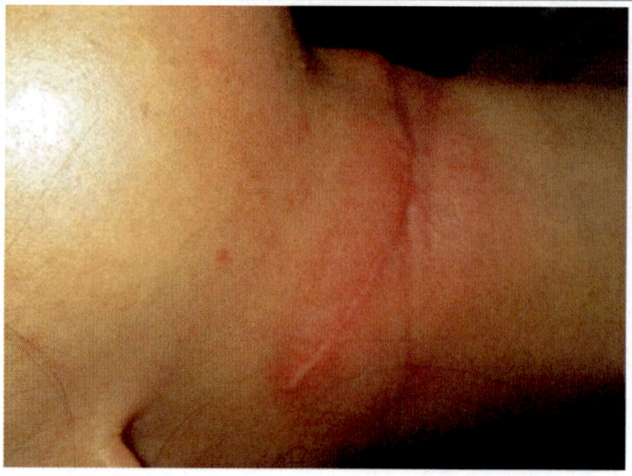 A 30-year-old female with multiply recurrent stage IVB hyalinizing clear cell carcinoma of right parapharyngeal space, resected with close margins, undergoing postoperative radiation therapy to 64 Gy	Moderate erythema over incision bolus site	• Measure delivered surface dose with thermoluminescent dosimetry • Cleanse daily with mild soap and water or Skintegrity • Moisturize twice daily with A + D or Aquaphor ointment • Incisions should be monitored carefully over the course of radiation for potential breakdown, infection • Protect the area from friction with Mepilex lite or soft scarf • Review plan or remeasure surface dose if the reaction is excessive

(continued)

Table 5.4 (continued)

Debride-ment and cleansing of wound	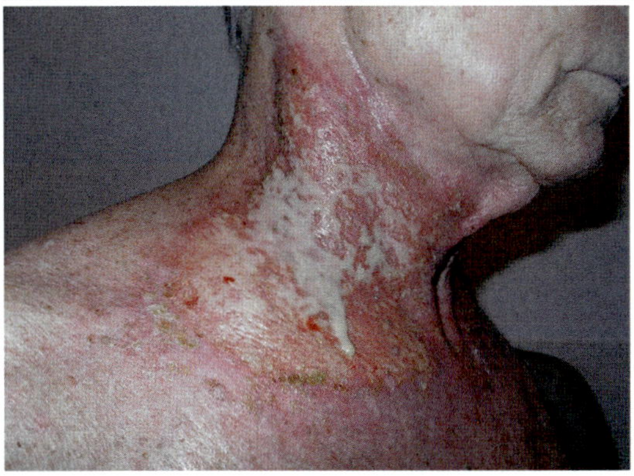	Moist desquamation with purulent exudate	• Spray Skintegrity (or similar) on the area and allow it to remain on the skin for 1–2 min then rinse • Manually or enzymatically or autolytically debride any remaining nonviable tissue or dry skin • Begin oral antibiotics to cover for Staphylococcus Aureus • Apply a dressing that will absorb exudate and reduce bioburden. Assess site every 24 h
	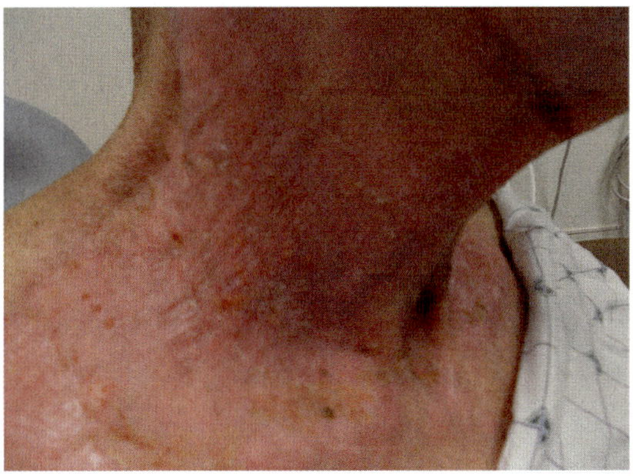	Resolution of moist desquamation	*Dressing options* 1. Apply Aquacel Ag (or similar dressing) • The dressing may be cut to size as needed. Aquacel Ag should extend about one-half to one inch over the area of desquamation • The dressing can be left in place for 24–48 h (or longer per manufacturer's recommendation) • If the dressing is dry and sticking to the wound bed, moisten with sterile water or saline before removing it so as to not disturb the wound bed • Cover the Aquacel Ag dressing with Mepilex Lite or similar nonstick dressing • Secure this with additional dressing such as flexible netting (Flexinet), or roller gauze (Kerlix) • Do not use tape on radiated skin 2. Apply Mepilex Ag alone over moist desquamated area. Secure with flexible netting (Flexinet) or roller gauze (Kerlix)

Week	Apply to Radiated Area			Notes
1-3	Cleanse daily with mild soap and water → 1x/day		Light moisturizer → Apply 2x/day	Apply thin lotion such as Lotion Soft or Remedy that is quickly absorbed, leaves no residue and is not comedogenic.
3+	Switch to calendula or continue with light moisturizer → Apply 2x/day			A thicker cream can be used to help maintain moisture. Continue until skin erythema resolves usually 2 weeks post radiation.
4 - 5+ Without moist desquamation	Skintegrity → Spray 1x/day	A+D Ointment OR Aquaphor → Apply 2x/day	Bacitracin & Aquaphor OR Silvasorb → Apply 2x/day	Begin applying this combination as erythema progresses and moisture loss becomes apparent Spray Skintegrity and wash off after 1 - 2 minutes. Apply A+D until 1 week post radiation.
4-6 (With Moist Desquamation)	Skintegrity (or similar wound cleanser) Skintegrity OR Preservative free normal saline	A+D Ointment OR Aquaphor → Apply 2x/day	Dressing Aquacel Ag (or similar) with Mepilex Lite cover dressing OR Mepilex Ag	Cleanser Options 1. Skintegrity and wash off after 1 - 2 minutes. 2. Preservative free normal saline rinse if the above not tolerated. Dressings Options 1. Apply Aquacel Ag/Algicell Ag/Mepitel Ag or transfer Ag (or similar) and cover with Mepilex lite. 2. Apply Mepilex Ag alone over desquamated area. No cover dressing required.
1-3 Weeks Post Radiation	A+D Ointment OR Aquaphor → Apply 2x day		Skintegrity (or similar wound cleanser) or return to mild soap and water → Daily	Apply A+D or Aquaphor for 2 to 3 weeks post radiation. Continue Skintegrity until dry desquamation is resolved then may discontinue.

Fig. 5.1 Suggested treatment algorithm for skin care

References

1. Parkin DM, Stjernsward J, Muir CS. Estimates of the worldwide frequency of twelve major cancers. Bull World Health Organ. 1984;62:163–82.
2. Joshi P, Dutta S, Chaturvedi P, Nair S. Head and neck cancers in developing countries. Rambam Maimonides Med J. 2014;5, e0009. doi:10.5041/RMMJ.10143.
3. Cancer Facts and Figures 2015. American Cancer Society. 2015. http://www.cancer.org/acs/groups/content/@editorial/documents/document/acspc-044552.pdf. Accessed 29 Apr 2015.
4. Chaturvedi AK, Engels EA, Pfeiffer RM, Hernandez BY, Xiao W, Kim E, et al. Human papillomavirus and rising oropharyngeal cancer incidence in the United States. J Clin Oncol. 2011;29:4294–301. doi:10.1200/JCO.2011.36.4596.
5. Mariotto AB, Yabroff KR, Shao Y, Feuer EJ, Brown ML. Projections of the cost of cancer care in the United States: 2010–2020. J Natl Cancer Inst. 2011;103:117–28. doi:10.1093/jnci/djq495.
6. Rogers HW, Weinstock MA, Harris AR, Hinckley MR, Feldman SR, Fleischer AB, et al. Incidence estimate of nonmelanoma skin cancer in the United States, 2006. Arch Dermatol. 2010;146:283–7. doi:10.1001/archdermatol.2010.19.
7. Yom SS. Radiation treatment of head and neck cancer. Surg Oncol Clin N Am. 2015;24:423–36. doi:10.1016/j.soc.2015.03.015.
8. Trotti A, Pajak TF, Gwede CK, Paulus R, Cooper J, Forastiere A, et al. TAME: development of a new method for summarising adverse events of cancer treatment by the Radiation Therapy Oncology Group. Lancet Oncol. 2007;8:613–24. doi:10.1016/S1470-2045(07)70144-4.
9. Stevens CM, Huang SH, Fung S, Bayley AJ, Cho JB, Cummings BJ, et al. Retrospective study of palliative radiotherapy in newly diagnosed head and neck carcinoma. Int J Radiat Oncol Biol Phys. 2011;81:958–63. doi:10.1016/j.ijrobp.2010.06.055.
10. Trotti 3rd A, Zhang Q, Bentzen SM, Emami B, Hammond ME, Jones CU, et al. Randomized trial of hyperfractionation versus conventional fractionation in T2 squamous cell carcinoma of the vocal cord (RTOG 9512). Int J Radiat Oncol Biol Phys. 2014;89:958–63. doi:10.1016/j.ijrobp.2014.04.041.
11. Forastiere AA, Goepfert H, Maor M, Pajak TF, Weber R, Morrison W, et al. Concurrent chemotherapy and radiotherapy for organ preservation in advanced laryngeal cancer. N Engl J Med. 2003;349:2091–8. doi:10.1056/NEJMoa031317.
12. Forastiere AA, Zhang Q, Weber RS, Maor MH, Goepfert H, Pajak TF, et al. Long-term results of RTOG 91–11: a comparison of three nonsurgical treatment strategies to preserve the larynx in patients with locally advanced larynx cancer. J Clin Oncol. 2013;31:845–52. doi:10.1200/JCO.2012.43.6097.
13. Cooper JS, Pajak TF, Forastiere AA, Jacobs J, Campbell BH, Saxman SB, et al. Postoperative concurrent radiotherapy and chemotherapy for high-risk squamous-cell carcinoma of the head and neck. N Engl J Med. 2004;350:1937–44. doi:10.1056/NEJMoa032646.
14. Cooper JS, Zhang Q, Pajak TF, Forastiere AA, Jacobs J, Saxman SB, et al. Long-term follow-up of the RTOG 9501/intergroup phase III trial: postoperative concurrent radiation therapy and chemotherapy in high-risk squamous cell carcinoma of the head and neck. Int J Radiat Oncol Biol Phys. 2012;84:1198–205. doi:10.1016/j.ijrobp.2012.05.008.
15. Fakhry C, Zhang Q, Nguyen-Tan PF, Rosenthal D, El-Naggar A, Garden AS, et al. Human papillomavirus and overall survival after progression of oropharyngeal squamous cell carcinoma. J Clin Oncol. 2014;32:3365–73. doi:10.1200/JCO.2014.55.1937.
16. Eisbruch A, Harris J, Garden AS, Chao CK, Straube W, Harari PM, et al. Multi-institutional trial of accelerated hypofractionated intensity-modulated radiation therapy for early-stage oropharyngeal cancer (RTOG 00–22). Int J Radiat Oncol Biol Phys. 2010;76:1333–8. doi:10.1016/j.ijrobp.2009.04.011.
17. Ang KK, Zhang Q, Rosenthal DI, Nguyen-Tan PF, Sherman EJ, Weber RS, et al. Randomized phase III trial of concurrent accelerated radiation plus cisplatin with or without cetuximab for stage III to IV head and neck carcinoma: RTOG 0522. J Clin Oncol. 2014;32:2940–50. doi:10.1200/JCO.2013.53.5633.
18. Lee N, Harris J, Garden AS, Straube W, Glisson B, Xia P, et al. Intensity-modulated radiation therapy with or without chemotherapy for nasopharyngeal carcinoma: radiation therapy oncology group phase II trial 0225. J Clin Oncol. 2009;27:3684–90. doi:10.1200/JCO.2008.19.9109.
19. Lee NY, Zhang Q, Pfister DG, Kim J, Garden AS, Mechalakos J, et al. Addition of bevacizumab to standard chemoradiation for locoregionally advanced nasopharyngeal carcinoma (RTOG 0615): a phase 2 multi-institutional trial. Lancet Oncol. 2012;13:172–80. doi:10.1016/S1470-2045(11)70303-5.
20. Kaanders JH, Ang KK. Early reactions as dose-limiting factors in radiotherapy. Semin Radiat Oncol. 1994;4:55–67. doi:10.1053/SRAO00400055.
21. Bonner JA, Harari PM, Giralt J, Cohen RB, Jones CU, Sur RK, et al. Radiotherapy plus cetuximab for locoregionally advanced head and neck cancer: 5-year survival data from a phase 3 randomised trial, and relation between cetuximab-induced rash and survival. Lancet Oncol. 2010;11:21–8. doi:10.1016/S1470-2045(09)70311-0.
22. Gotlib V, Khaled S, Lapko I, Mar N, Saif MW. Skin rash secondary to bevacizumab in a patient with advanced colorectal cancer and relation to response. Anticancer Drugs. 2006;17:1227–9. doi:10.1097/01.cad.0000231481.07654.fc.
23. Saif MW, Longo WL, Israel G. Correlation between rash and a positive drug response associated with

Bevacizumab in a patient with advanced colorectal cancer. Clin Colorectal Cancer. 2008;7:144–8. doi:10.3816/CCC.2008.n.020.
24. West CM, Barnett GC. Genetics and genomics of radiotherapy toxicity: towards prediction. Genome Med. 2011;3:52. doi:10.1186/gm268.
25. Wong RK, Bensadoun RJ, Boers-Doets CB, Bryce J, Chan A, Epstein JB, et al. Clinical practice guidelines for the prevention and treatment of acute and late radiation reactions from the MASCC Skin Toxicity Study Group. Support Care Cancer. 2013;21:2933–48. doi:10.1007/s00520-013-1896-2.
26. Lee N, Chuang C, Quivey JM, Phillips TL, Akazawa P, Verhey LJ, et al. Skin toxicity due to intensity-modulated radiotherapy for head-and-neck carcinoma. Int J Radiat Oncol Biol Phys. 2002;53:630–7.
27. Rosenthal DI, Chambers MS, Fuller CD, Rebueno NC, Garcia J, Kies MS, et al. Beam path toxicities to non-target structures during intensity-modulated radiation therapy for head and neck cancer. Int J Radiat Oncol Biol Phys. 2008;72:747–55. doi:10.1016/j.ijrobp.2008.01.012.
28. Porock D, Kristjanson L, Nikoletti S, Cameron F, Pedler P. Predicting the severity of radiation skin reactions in women with breast cancer. Oncol Nurs Forum. 1998;25:1019–29.
29. Nayel H, el-Ghoneimy E, el-Haddad S. Impact of nutritional supplementation on treatment delay and morbidity in patients with head and neck tumors treated with irradiation. Nutrition. 1992;8:13–8.
30. Fogarty GB, Muddle R, Sprung CN, Chen W, Duffy D, Sturm RA, et al. Unexpectedly severe acute radiotherapy side effects are associated with single nucleotide polymorphisms of the melanocortin-1 receptor. Int J Radiat Oncol Biol Phys. 2010;77:1486–92. doi:10.1016/j.ijrobp.2009.07.1690.
31. Ryan JL, Bole C, Hickok JT, Figueroa-Moseley C, Colman L, Khanna RC, et al. Post-treatment skin reactions reported by cancer patients differ by race, not by treatment or expectations. Br J Cancer. 2007;97:14–21. doi:10.1038/sj.bjc.6603842.
32. Lin A, Abu-Isa E, Griffith KA, Ben-Josef E. Toxicity of radiotherapy in patients with collagen vascular disease. Cancer. 2008;113:648–53. doi:10.1002/cncr.23591.
33. Porock D. Factors influencing the severity of radiation skin and oral mucosal reactions: development of a conceptual framework. Eur J Cancer Care. 2002;11:33–43.
34. McQuestion M. Evidence-based skin care management in radiation therapy: clinical update. Semin Oncol Nurs. 2011;27:e1–17. doi:10.1016/j.soncn.2011.02.009.
35. McNees P. Skin and wound assessment and care in oncology. Semin Oncol Nurs. 2006;22:130–43. doi:10.1016/j.soncn.2006.04.003.
36. Herst PM. Protecting the radiation-damaged skin from friction: a mini review. J Med Radiat Sci. 2014;61:119–25. doi:10.1002/jmrs.46.
37. Lawenda BD, Kelly KM, Ladas EJ, Sagar SM, Vickers A, Blumberg JB. Should supplemental antioxidant administration be avoided during chemotherapy and radiation therapy? J Natl Cancer Inst. 2008;100:773–83. doi:10.1093/jnci/djn148.
38. Sitton E. Early and late radiation-induced skin alterations. Part II: nursing care of irradiated skin. Oncol Nurs Forum. 1992;19:907–12.
39. Porock D, Nikoletti S, Cameron F. The relationship between factors that impair wound healing and the severity of acute radiation skin and mucosal toxicities in head and neck cancer. Cancer Nurs. 2004;27:71–8.
40. Belum VR, Hill A, Matros E, Lacouture ME, Barker CA. Differential radiation dermatitis in native skin and an autologous transplanted myocutaneous flap. JAMA Dermatol. 2014;150:1365–7. doi:10.1001/jamadermatol.2014.888.
41. Payne AS, James WD, Weiss RB. Dermatologic toxicity of chemotherapeutic agents. Semin Oncol. 2006;33:86–97. doi:10.1053/j.seminoncol.2005.11.004.
42. Bonner JA, Harari PM, Giralt J, Azarnia N, Shin DM, Cohen RB, et al. Radiotherapy plus cetuximab for squamous-cell carcinoma of the head and neck. N Engl J Med. 2006;354:567–78. doi:10.1056/NEJMoa053422.
43. Giro C, Berger B, Bolke E, Ciernik IF, Duprez F, Locati L, et al. High rate of severe radiation dermatitis during radiation therapy with concurrent cetuximab in head and neck cancer: results of a survey in EORTC institutes. Radiother Oncol. 2009;90:166–71. doi:10.1016/j.radonc.2008.09.007.
44. Cante D, La Porta MR, Franco P, Sciacero P, Girelli GF, Marra A, et al. Management of 'in-field' skin toxicity in head and neck cancer patients treated with combined cetuximab and radiotherapy. Oncology. 2013;85:257–61. doi:10.1159/000355579.
45. Chung CH, Mirakhur B, Chan E, Le QT, Berlin J, Morse M, et al. Cetuximab-induced anaphylaxis and IgE specific for galactose-alpha-1,3-galactose. N Engl J Med. 2008;358:1109–17. doi:10.1056/NEJMoa074943.
46. Lacouture ME, Maitland ML, Segaert S, Setser A, Baran R, Fox LP, et al. A proposed EGFR inhibitor dermatologic adverse event-specific grading scale from the MASCC skin toxicity study group. Support Care Cancer. 2010;18:509–22. doi:10.1007/s00520-009-0744-x.
47. Lacouture ME, Anadkat MJ, Bensadoun RJ, Bryce J, Chan A, Epstein JB, et al. Clinical practice guidelines for the prevention and treatment of EGFR inhibitor-associated dermatologic toxicities. Support Care Cancer. 2011;19:1079–95. doi:10.1007/s00520-011-1197-6.
48. Bernier J, Bonner J, Vermorken JB, Bensadoun RJ, Dummer R, Giralt J, et al. Consensus guidelines for the management of radiation dermatitis and coexisting acne-like rash in patients receiving radiotherapy plus EGFR inhibitors for the treatment of squamous

cell carcinoma of the head and neck. Ann Oncol. 2008;19:142–9. doi:10.1093/annonc/mdm400.
49. Lacouture ME, Wolchok JD, Yosipovitch G, Kahler KC, Busam KJ, Hauschild A. Ipilimumab in patients with cancer and the management of dermatologic adverse events. J Am Acad Dermatol. 2014;71:161–9. doi:10.1016/j.jaad.2014.02.035.
50. Vogler BK, Ernst E. Aloe vera: a systematic review of its clinical effectiveness. Br J Gen Pract. 1999; 49:823–8.
51. Richardson J, Smith JE, McIntyre M, Thomas R, Pilkington K. Aloe vera for preventing radiation-induced skin reactions: a systematic literature review. Clin Oncol. 2005;17:478–84.
52. Boot-Vickers M, Eaton K. Skin care for patients receiving radiotherapy. Prof Nurse. 1999;14:706–8.
53. Abbas H, Bensadoun RJ. Trolamine emulsion for the prevention of radiation dermatitis in patients with squamous cell carcinoma of the head and neck. Support Care Cancer. 2012;20:185–90. doi:10.1007/s00520-011-1110-3.
54. Elliott EA, Wright JR, Swann RS, Nguyen-Tan F, Takita C, Bucci MK, et al. Phase III Trial of an emulsion containing trolamine for the prevention of radiation dermatitis in patients with advanced squamous cell carcinoma of the head and neck: results of Radiation Therapy Oncology Group Trial 99–13. J Clin Oncol. 2006;24:2092–7. doi:10.1200/JCO.2005.04.9148.
55. Liguori V, Guillemin C, Pesce GF, Mirimanoff RO, Bernier J. Double-blind, randomized clinical study comparing hyaluronic acid cream to placebo in patients treated with radiotherapy. Radiother Oncol. 1997;42:155–61.
56. Chan RJ, Mann J, Tripcony L, Keller J, Cheuk R, Blades R, et al. Natural oil-based emulsion containing allantoin versus aqueous cream for managing radiation-induced skin reactions in patients with cancer: a phase 3, double-blind, randomized, controlled trial. Int J Radiat Oncol Biol Phys. 2014;90:756–64. doi:10.1016/j.ijrobp.2014.06.034.
57. Aygenc E, Celikkanat S, Kaymakci M, Aksaray F, Ozdem C. Prophylactic effect of pentoxifylline on radiotherapy complications: a clinical study. Otolaryngol Head Neck Surg. 2004;130:351–6. doi:10.1016/j.otohns.2003.08.015.
58. Salvo N, Barnes E, van Draanen J, Stacey E, Mitera G, Breen D, et al. Prophylaxis and management of acute radiation-induced skin reactions: a systematic review of the literature. Curr Oncol. 2010;17:94–112.
59. Lievens Y, Haustermans K, Van den Weyngaert D, Van den Bogaert W, Scalliet P, Hutsebaut L, et al. Does sucralfate reduce the acute side-effects in head and neck cancer treated with radiotherapy? A double-blind randomized trial. Radiother Oncol. 1998; 47:149–53.
60. Wells M, Macmillan M, Raab G, MacBride S, Bell N, MacKinnon K, et al. Does aqueous or sucralfate cream affect the severity of erythematous radiation skin reactions? A randomised controlled trial. Radiother Oncol. 2004;73:153–62. doi:10.1016/j.radonc.2004.07.032.
61. Pommier P, Gomez F, Sunyach MP, D'Hombres A, Carrie C, Montbarbon X. Phase III randomized trial of Calendula officinalis compared with trolamine for the prevention of acute dermatitis during irradiation for breast cancer. J Clin Oncol. 2004;22:1447–53. doi:10.1200/JCO.2004.07.063.
62. Sharp L, Finnila K, Johansson H, Abrahamsson M, Hatschek T, Bergenmar M. No differences between Calendula cream and aqueous cream in the prevention of acute radiation skin reactions—results from a randomised blinded trial. Eur J Oncol Nurs. 2013;17: 429–35. doi:10.1016/j.ejon.2012.11.003.
63. Schneider F, Danski MT, Vayego SA. Usage of Calendula officinalis in the prevention and treatment of radiodermatitis: a randomized double-blind controlled clinical trial. Rev Esc Enferm USP. 2015;49:221–8. doi:10.1590/S0080-623420150000200006.
64. Miller RC, Schwartz DJ, Sloan JA, Griffin PC, Deming RL, Anders JC, et al. Mometasone furoate effect on acute skin toxicity in breast cancer patients receiving radiotherapy: a phase III double-blind, randomized trial from the North Central Cancer Treatment Group N06C4. Int J Radiat Oncol Biol Phys. 2011;79:1460–6. doi:10.1016/j.ijrobp.2010.01.031.
65. Fisher DA. Adverse-effects of topical corticosteroid use. Western J Med. 1995;162:123–6.
66. Ference JD, Last AR. Choosing topical corticosteroids. Am Fam Physician. 2009;79:135–40.
67. Renfro L, Snow JS. Ocular effects of topical and systemic steroids. Dermatol Clin. 1992;10:505–12.
68. Sperduti A, Cashell A, Rocca C, Hirji A, Billingsley S, Waldron J, et al. A feasibility study of an internal control methodology using hydrocortisone cream for the management of skin reactions in patients receiving radical radiation therapy for cancers of the head and neck. J Radiother Pract. 2006;5:211–8. doi:10.1017/S1460396906000306.
69. Shafik A. Polyester but not cotton or wool textiles inhibit hair growth. Dermatology. 1993;187:239–42.
70. Zhong WH, Tang QF, Hu LY, Feng HX. Mepilex Lite dressings for managing acute radiation dermatitis in nasopharyngeal carcinoma patients: a systematic controlled clinical trial. Med Oncol. 2013;30:761. doi:10.1007/s12032-013-0761-y.
71. Thomas S. Current practices in the management of fungating lesions and radiation damaged skin. Bridgend, South Wales: Surgical Materials Testing Laboratory; 1992.
72. Mak SS, Molassiotis A, Wan WM, Lee IY, Chan ES. The effects of hydrocolloid dressing and gentian violet on radiation-induced moist desquamation wound healing. Cancer Nurs. 2000;23:220–9.
73. Mak SS, Zee CY, Molassiotis A, Chan SJ, Leung SF, Mo KF, et al. A comparison of wound treatments in nasopharyngeal cancer patients receiving radiation therapy. Cancer Nurs. 2005;28:436–45.

74. Winter GD. Formation of the scab and the rate of epithelization of superficial wounds in the skin of the young domestic pig. Nature. 1962;193:293–4.
75. Gerhardt LC, Strassle V, Lenz A, Spencer ND, Derler S. Influence of epidermal hydration on the friction of human skin against textiles. J R Soc Interface. 2008;5:1317–28. doi:10.1098/rsif.2008.0034.
76. Cowan LJ, Stechmiller J. Prevalence of wet-to-dry dressings in wound care. Adv Skin Wound Care. 2009;22:567–73. doi:10.1097/01.ASW.0000363469.25740.74.
77. Jones V, Grey JE, Harding KG. Wound dressings. BMJ. 2006;332:777–80. doi:10.1136/bmj.332.7544.777.
78. Caruso DM, Foster KN, Blome-Eberwein SA, Twomey JA, Herndon DN, Luterman A, et al. Randomized clinical study of Hydrofiber dressing with silver or silver sulfadiazine in the management of partial-thickness burns. J Burn Care Res. 2006;27:298–309. doi:10.1097/01.BCR.0000216741.21433.66.
79. Muangman P, Pundee C, Opasanon S, Muangman S. A prospective, randomized trial of silver containing hydrofiber dressing versus 1% silver sulfadiazine for the treatment of partial thickness burns. Int Wound J. 2010; 7:271–6. doi:10.1111/j.1742-481X.2010.00690.x.
80. Silverstein P, Heimbach D, Meites H, Latenser B, Mozingo D, Mullins F, et al. An open, parallel, randomized, comparative, multicenter study to evaluate the cost-effectiveness, performance, tolerance, and safety of a silver-containing soft silicone foam dressing (intervention) vs silver sulfadiazine cream. J Burn Care Res. 2011;32:617–26. doi:10.1097/BCR.0b013e318236fe31.
81. Vavassis P, Gelinas M, Chabot Tr J, Nguyen-Tan PF. Phase 2 study of silver leaf dressing for treatment of radiation-induced dermatitis in patients receiving radiotherapy to the head and neck. J Otolaryngol Head Neck Surg. 2008;37:124–9.
82. Glat PM, Kubat WD, Hsu JF, Copty T, Burkey BA, Davis W, et al. Randomized clinical study of SilvaSorb gel in comparison to Silvadene silver sulfadiazine cream in the management of partial-thickness burns. J Burn Care Res. 2009;30:262–7. doi:10.1097/BCR.0b013e318198a2e8.
83. Jurczak F, Dugre T, Johnstone A, Offori T, Vujovic Z, Hollander D, et al. Randomised clinical trial of Hydrofiber dressing with silver versus povidone-iodine gauze in the management of open surgical and traumatic wounds. Int Wound J. 2007;4:66–76. doi:10.1111/j.1742-481X.2006.00276.x.

Thoracic Cancers

6

Sue S. Yom and Florence Yuen

Lung cancer is the number one cancer killer in the United States for both men and women and ranks in the top such cancers around the world as well [1, 2]. In the United States, an estimated 221,200 new lung cancers will be diagnosed in 2015, and an estimated 158,040 deaths will result from lung cancer [3]. However, there is substantial variation in prognosis depending on the stage at diagnosis. For example, for stage I non-small cell lung cancers (NSCLC), the overall survival rate at 5 years is 53 %, compared to 31 % for stage II cancers, 9 % for stage III cancers, and 2 % for stage IV cancers [4]. Thus, the treatments delivered for lung cancer vary widely depending on anatomic location, surgical resectability, medical fitness of the patient, and, above all, stage.

A number of other types of tumors in the thorax may require radiation therapy as part of the treatment plan. For example, other tumors and cancers arising in the chest, for which radiation may be employed, include carcinoid, thymoma or thymic carcinoma, salivary gland tumor or carcinoma, lymphoma, germ cell tumor, sarcomas, neurogenic tumors, and mesothelioma.

S.S. Yom, MD, PhD (✉)
F. Yuen, RN, MSN, AOCNP
Department of Radiation Oncology,
University of California, San Francisco,
1600 Divisadero Street, Suite H1031, Box 1708,
San Francisco, CA 94143, USA
e-mail: yoms@radonc.ucsf.edu

6.1 Thoracic Radiation Treatment

For early-stage NSCLC, surgery is most frequently the frontline treatment, but in cases of limited medical fitness or other factors precluding surgery, these cancers may be treated with stereotactic radiation therapy. Three randomized trials directly comparing stereotactic radiation therapy (SRT) to surgery in early-stage operable patients have failed to accrue, but a fourth such trial has recently launched in the United States using a novel pre-randomization design [5], and others are in early development. Patients who have early-stage NSCLC with limited lymph node involvement may be treated with either surgery with perioperative chemotherapy or conventionally fractionated radiation therapy potentially combined with concurrent chemotherapy.

Stage III NSCLC are typically treated with a multimodality treatment plan involving various combinations of chemotherapy, surgery, and radiation therapy. A variety of different sequences may be used depending on the clinical situation. Radiation may be used in these cases as preoperative treatment in combination with concurrent chemotherapy or as a postoperative treatment preceding or following chemotherapy. For patients who cannot undergo surgery, concurrent chemoradiation is considered the standard of care for patients who are medically fit for it and may be followed by a couple of cycles of additional chemotherapy. For patients who cannot tolerate concurrent chemoradiation,

B. Fowble et al. (eds.), *Skin Care in Radiation Oncology*, DOI 10.1007/978-3-319-31460-0_6

which actually may comprise the majority of stage III patients [6], a sequential regimen of chemotherapy and radiation is the next best option [7], with radiation or chemotherapy monotherapy reserved mostly for palliative purposes.

Small cell lung cancers (SCLC) are usually treated with concurrent chemoradiation, if the patient is medically fit for it [8]. These radiation fields can sometimes be very large and are sometimes located high in the upper thorax. Historically, the radiation dosages for this disease have been moderate, but recent investigations are emphasizing doses as high as 70 Gy for this histology [9]. Patients who are not able to undergo concurrent chemoradiation or who have extensive stage disease at presentation often receive palliative chemotherapy and often achieve very dramatic if temporary responses. These patients are considered eligible for consolidative radiation therapy to the chest following their chemotherapy [10, 11].

Over 40 % of lung cancer patients present with stage IV disease [12]. In these cases, in the presence of distant metastasis, chemotherapy or targeted therapy will be the mainstay for treatment, but radiation may be used as a local palliative treatment. Radiation has an established role in the treatment of bronchial obstruction, bleeding, or pain [13].

6.2 Types and Frequency of Skin Reactions

The skin reaction has more to do with technical aspects of the radiation therapy plan than the specific intrathoracic cancer diagnosis. Therefore, while a large variety of cancers in the thorax may be treated with radiation, the principles of skin care can be applied based on a thorough understanding of the treatment area in question and the technical aspects of the radiation delivery.

Patients treated with radiation to the thorax for definitive or curative intent often receive high dosages (60–70 Gy) fractionated over several weeks to deep-seated areas within the thorax, and they frequently will receive concurrent chemotherapy. These patients are simultaneously at risk for multiple, very serious symptoms that take clinical priority, and these potentially life threatening, dosimetrically related risks are usually emphasized in the radiation planning process over consideration of skin reactions. The premier risks to be minimized include pneumonitis, esophagitis, and occasionally pericarditis [14]. Thus, in the typical high-dose radiotherapy treatment planning process, the chest wall or skin is only rarely considered as a formal avoidance structure to consider explicitly.

Nonetheless, an experienced clinician will proactively anticipate some level of skin reaction. Patients receiving radiation to relatively deep-seated areas within the thorax can still be expected to experience dryness, erythema, pruritus, tanning, and freckling, often on the mid-back. While these symptoms often remain at relatively tolerable levels, patients may have some moderate discomfort due to increasing dryness, and some may scratch at the area with their fingernails in an attempt to relieve the itchiness, which risks creating deep furrows in the skin or encouraging a superficial skin infection. On rare occasions, the area may become hot and uncomfortable with associated inflammation and pain. Over the long term, moderately hyperpigmented tanning or even mild telangiectasia may be permanent in the highest dose radiation area on the skin, especially if a number of beams enter and exit in one area. It should of course be understood that in clinical practice, there can be a fair degree of idiosyncrasy in the relative sensitivity of one patient versus another. If any patient manifests with an unusual degree of skin reaction early in the treatment course, it should be examined and documented regularly, and the radiotherapy plan should be reviewed with the possibility of altering the technical factors to forestall a severe reaction from developing.

Postoperative radiation therapy is generally given to a lower dose than curative-intent radiation therapy (45–54 Gy). The reasons for limiting the dosages given to postoperative patients are that the combined effects of large-scale surgery and postoperative chemotherapy and radiation therapy can result in excessive morbidity if the doses exceed a moderate level [15]. These patients are not usually expected to develop high-grade skin reactions, but many may experience a focal dryness and moderate tanning localized around the targeted areas. The thoracotomy scar may darken to a greater degree than the surrounding skin.

Stereotactic radiation therapy (SRT) is based on the delivery of a small number of very high-dose fractions (extreme hypofractionation). Typically the patient will receive 1–5 fractions at a dosage per fraction that might be 10–34 Gy. These high doses per fraction produce a higher rate of acute and late effects, as would be expected. One study reported a rate of acute grade 2 or higher skin toxicity reaching 14 % following thoracic SRT [16]. Several reported series have documented new risks for long-term chest wall injury or pain, not previously seen in patients receiving fractionated thoracic radiotherapy, especially in obese or diabetic patients or when the intercostal nerves lie in close proximity to the high-dose treatment field [17, 18].

Whole-brain radiation therapy (WBRT) is given for any type of lung cancer that has spread to the brain. For small cell cancers, prophylactic cranial irradiation (PCI, essentially WBRT but usually given to slightly lower doses) is part of the standard of care for any limited stage patient who achieves a complete response to chemoradiation or extensive stage patient who shows response to chemotherapy [19, 20]. Temporary alopecia should be expected after PCI with some regrowth of hair in 2–3 months [21]. After WBRT, hair regrowth will be less, and many patients will experience regrowth of hair in a specific pattern called "reverse Mohawk," meaning that the vertex area of the scalp may receive the highest doses and remain bald [22].

6.3 Impact of Technical Choices on the Skin

For treatments using megavoltage photons treating lung parenchymal or mediastinal regions, the skin reactions due to irradiation tend to be moderate in nature, because of the inherently skin-sparing physical characteristics of megavoltage energy beams and the central nature of these areas within the chest cavity. However, the skin-sparing effects can be negated if the overall field size is very large, which creates a high buildup of electrons at the surface, or if an excessive number of devices such as blocking trays or multileaf collimation are introduced into the beam pathway such as may be used in an attempt to make the radiation doses very conformal to the tumor shape, or, finally, if the entry of one highly penetrating beam coincides with the exit point of another [23]. Therefore, it is important that the prescribing physician has familiarity with the characteristics of the radiation to be employed and inspect the arrangement of the beams that comprise the total plan for the patient.

Even in relatively simple plans, the choices of beam arrangement can have impact on the skin. For example, the use of exclusively anteroposteriorly angled beams may increase the risk of a local dermatitis because of the coincidence of entry and exit of simultaneously delivered beams in the same area. When planning a high-dose treatment, it can be worth considering an arrangement of beam angles that do not all enter through the same exact region of skin. With more complex and conformal treatments, whether given using a 3D conformal or intensity-modulated technique, consideration should be given to the superficial effect of so-called *glancing* beams. With an increasing number of beams that are intended to produce a more conformal dose distribution around the target, there is a higher likelihood of employing beams that are obliquely angled to the surface of the skin. Oblique beams increase the surface dose and, when multiplied, can create a local area of intense skin reaction [24], especially because the beams are sometimes extensively blocked and collimated for greater conformality. This is seen more and more frequently with the advent of high-dose radiation delivered with intensity-modulated techniques.

In particular, these effects can be more pronounced depending on the distance of the skin from the targeted high-dose region. For instance, if areas in the thoracic inlet or supraclavicular region are included in the treatment field, especially in a thinner patient, more severe reactions may be seen because of the proximity of the skin to these relatively superficially located regions. This phenomenon of increased reactions around and above the collar bone has long been recognized and studied in breast cancer radiation treatment [25], although there is less of a focus on the issue in thoracic oncology because of the greater rarity of a clinical situation justifying high-dose supraclavicular radiotherapy. In any case, special care should be taken when radiation of any type is to be delivered to the supraclavicular or mid-upper neck regions, as dermatitis in these areas tends to be more severe and also more disabling and painful to the patient than reactions on the skin of the thorax proper. These neck treatments can result in painful erythema and dry and wet desquamation, in a manner similar to that seen when treatments are given for breast or head and neck cancers (see related chapters on these issues).

Conversely, in patients who are obese (the standard definition would include patients with a body mass index >30 kg/m^2), more severe reactions may be observed in any part of the body due to the quantifiably larger amount of body surface area [26], the physical presence of skin folds, and the excessive number of monitor units (actual machine output) that must be delivered through the surface to achieve the full amount of the dose prescribed to the deeply located targeted regions. Patients who are obese often have comorbid medical conditions that impede healing from acute tissue injury, and thus they may suffer from a longer duration of skin-related or other severe effects.

Certain special clinical situations may incur an increased risk of radiation-related skin or chest wall reaction. For example, the use of superficially directed electron therapy, which is occasionally used to treat scars (sarcoma, mesothelioma), will deliberately increase superficially located dermatitis in a dose-dependent manner [27, 28].

In stereotactically directed treatments, the proximal chest wall may need to be defined as a dosimetrically defined avoidance structure due to the risks of long-term toxicity to the chest wall musculature, ribs, and intercostal nerves. Creating a formal chest wall avoidance structure in this manner is usually considered a standard practice only for tumors that are to be treated to high doses in close proximity to the chest wall [29–31]. However, there may be a role for increased attention to superficial skin toxicity as a more general practice. In regard specifically to acute skin reaction, SRT-related acute toxicity was reported by one group as most accentuated by the same technical factors widely recognized as risks in traditionally fractionated external beam therapy; identified factors associated with Common Terminology Criteria for Adverse Event (CTCAE)-defined grade 2 or higher acute skin toxicity included using only three beams (due to the convergence of their exit and entry points in one area), distance from the tumor to the posterior chest wall skin of less than 5 cm (due to superficial location of the high-dose region near the skin surface and the added bolus effect of a stabilizing immobilization cradle in which the patient lies down), and a maximum skin dose of 50 % or higher of the prescribed dose [16].

Furthermore, dosimetric precautions to the external skin surface or chest wall, while they mostly apply to the superficial tissues in close proximity to the target of a stereotactic or high-dose treatment, should be kept in mind as potentially useful to evaluate all subcutaneous tissues where beams enter or exit. For example, in one clinical trial of SRT given for liver metastases, the investigators reported a grade 3 severe reaction with overlying skin breakdown in the subcutaneous tissue of an area remote from the posteriorly located target [32]. As a result, some SRT lung cancer trials, such as RTOG 0618, have mandated contouring of a 5 mm ring at the entire external surface of the body to check for high-dose regions that may be unintentionally delivered to focal spots remote from the areas of highest interest [33].

There is a substantial body of evidence that individual patient-related factors also play a role in chest wall toxicities and should be considered in anticipating a severe reaction. Patients with conditions predisposing to poor healing, such as diabetes, obesity, vascular compromise, or osteoporosis, are at highest risk for nerve damage, rib fracture, long-term inflammation, fibrosis, or pain [17, 18, 34]. In these patients, consideration may be given to treatment courses lasting 4–5 fractions as opposed to 3 fractions or less, to try to reduce toxicity [35]. This patient population represents an area of ongoing clinical investigations to develop medical or technical strategies to reduce the potential for high-grade effects.

Not just unique to lung cancer but also in other areas of focal radiotherapy, the study of hypofractionated treatments is a very rapidly growing area of medicine; as these practices becomes more widespread for all stages of lung cancer treatments, the immediate effect of their dissemination will likely be some increase in both acute and late toxicity incidence. Strategies to prevent and manage these toxicities are likely to be an area of greater interest as these approaches become widespread. Hypofractionated approaches are not isolated to lung cancer but are being used in all areas of medicine including palliation [36].

Proton therapy is beginning to be used for patients with intrathoracic conditions such as lymphoma, sarcoma, and lung cancer. Proton therapy poses a special risk of skin toxicity due to a typical arrangement utilizing fewer beams and the relatively higher percentage of dose deposited at the entry point of each beam. Especially if the number of entry beams is limited and/or if the treatment is hypofractionated, the expected reaction can be notably higher than what is seen with megavoltage photon-based treatments. One small case report anecdotally noted a higher incidence of grade 2–3 skin reactions being observed with the use of thoracic proton therapy and proposed the use of a transparent film which seemed to decrease effects to the surface via an unclear mechanism [37]. Other forms of particle therapy, such as neutron or carbon ion therapy, are less well known but have also been associated with higher rates of skin toxicity.

6.4 Other Factors Affecting Acute Skin Toxicity

6.4.1 Concurrent Chemotherapy

Concurrent use of systemic chemotherapy in combination with radiation therapy is very common in treating lung cancers. Concurrent chemotherapy does increase the incidence of other acute toxicities, such as esophagitis, although whether there is an effect on acute dermatitis is unknown [38]. Taxanes, which are frequently used in concurrent chemoradiation regimens, result in hair loss [39].

In the advanced stage population, where traditionally fractionated 3D conformal and intensity-modulated radiation therapy treatments are often combined with concurrent chemotherapy, there has been a relatively low incidence of severe dermatitis because of the usual deep-seated nature of these tumors, so this has not usually been an area of focused concern. However, with newer developments such as hypofractionation or proton therapy, the effects of concurrent systemic therapy will require closer evaluation.

In metastatic patients who start with radiation but later receive chemotherapy at some point in their course, recall phenomena may be seen with certain chemotherapy agents if they are given prior to radiation. Gemcitabine is the best-known systemic agent in producing these recall phenomena, but erlotinib and pemetrexed, both very commonly used in metastatic lung cancer, have also been reported in this context [40, 41].

6.4.2 Concurrent Targeted Therapy

Targeted therapies have not been used concurrently with radiation except in a few circumstances. The most substantial concurrent uses of targeted therapies (cetuximab, erlotinib) have occurred as add-ons to the basic chemoradiation platform for stage III disease. For example, in the large randomized trial RTOG 0617, there were four arms arranged in a two-by-two design including 74 Gy versus 60 Gy, with or without cetuximab [42]. Across the four arms, there was no clearly noticeable pattern of increased general dermatologic effects or specific effects such as dermatitis, dryness, and pruritus. The rate of dermatitis across the four arms ranged from 18 to 26 % for grade 1, 6 to 12 % for grade 2, and 1 to 3 % for grade 3, which was the highest grade attained. However, the two cetuximab-containing arms did have higher rates of dry skin, approximately 25–27 % and 11–12 % for grades 1 and 2, compared to the non-cetuximab-containing arms, which had rates of 7–9 % and 2–3 %, respectively, as well as pruritus, which was counted at rates of 10–12 % and 0–1 % for grades 1 and 2 in the non-cetuximab-containing arms, versus 17–26 % and 6–8 % in the cetuximab-containing arms. It is unclear how rigorously these effects were graded, and it is likely that there may have been some underreporting of these somewhat more subtle and less clinically significant effects. The largest level of difference between the non-cetuximab and cetuximab arms was seen in the rates of desquamating rash, perhaps because of its more clinically evident nature. The cetuximab arms had rates of 14–15 %, 12–13 %, and 4 % for grades 1, 2, and 3, respectively, versus rates of 4–7 %, 2–3 %, and 0–1 % in the non-cetuximab-containing arms.

Targeted therapies (such as erlotinib) have been very rarely used with SRT. The one prospective trial that has been published did not report dermatologic or chest wall toxicity [43].

6.4.3 Reirradiation

For patients being reirradiated to the chest for palliative purposes, skin reaction has not been reported as a dose-limiting toxicity [44]. However, patients who have been previously radiated to the thorax and are treated again with curative intent can be at higher risk for radiation skin toxicity, especially if the second treatment is given with stereotactic technique. One study of this specific clinical scenario reported an incidence of grade 2 or higher chest wall pain in 18 % and skin toxicity in 5 % [45]. For these patients, the original plan should be reviewed, and consideration should be given to avoid excessive skin and chest wall dosages to areas treated previously. Particular attention should be paid if the reirradiation will include the supraclavicular region or neck. For these cases, thermoluminescent dosimetry is advised to gauge the delivered dose to the areas at highest risk.

6.5 Management of Skin Reaction

Most thoracic radiation patients will not require very extensive management. Ongoing self-care activities should be encouraged to minimize the reaction and not allow it to progress. Most of the time, the program will require relatively simple interventions such as moisturization to relieve dryness as well as consideration of light cotton clothing or dressings (Mepilex Lite) to reduce friction and sun exposure to the area. Itching is an issue that should be very actively managed; if the patient scratches the area, there is increased irritation and exacerbation of the reaction, with risk for dry desquamation as well as infection. These patients should be given soothing emollients, 1 % topical hydrocortisone lotion, and if the reaction is truly very severe, antipruritic medication can be prescribed or intermediate potency steroid creams may be required. All patients should be generally counseled to avoid sun exposure to the chest area, and, if swimming is desired, moisturization is advised after completion of activity (a partner may be needed to help apply the moisturizer over the back, where tanning is typically the most pronounced).

For patients who experience severe brisk erythema, cooling hydrogels should be used to increase comfort. The rare patients who demonstrate a very intense level of this reaction are at high risk for wet desquamation and should be monitored closely. For severe wet desquamation, control of potential skin infection may be required. In our clinic, we will consider the use of silver-containing amorphous hydrogel (Silvasorb) or, in very severe cases, silver-impregnated hydrofiber or alginate dressings.

6.6 Photographs and Recommendations

Below are general skin care recommendations (Table 6.1), week-by-week treatment instructions, and photographs that demonstrate typical skin reactions over time for patients undergoing external beam radiation to the thorax (Table 6.2). Photographs of special reactions and instructions on how to treat these more uncommon cases are also provided (Table 6.3). Figure 6.1 is a general suggested treatment algorithm for skin care for patients undergoing external beam radiation to the thorax.

Table 6.1 General principles of skin care for patients with skin reactions involving the thorax

Patient should:
• Cleanse daily with mild soap and water
• Use lotions and creams recommended by your provider
• Continue to wear soft under garments that provide support and control moisture
Patient should not:
• Rub, put pressure on, or scratch radiated area
• Take hot water showers, hot baths, use wash cloths, or use loofahs
• Apply any lotion, cream, or ointment within the 3 hours prior to radiation treatment
• Wash off lotion, cream, or ointments if applied three or more hours before radiation treatment
• Apply drying agents to the skin unless instructed to do so
• Use any tape or adhesives on the radiated skin

Table 6.2 Examples of typical acute skin reactions and recommended interventions for patients undergoing external beam radiation to the thorax

Week	Skin reaction	Reaction type	Intervention
1–2	Caucasian male lung cancer patient receiving IMRT to a dose of 45 Gy in 25 fractions with a reaction on the thorax 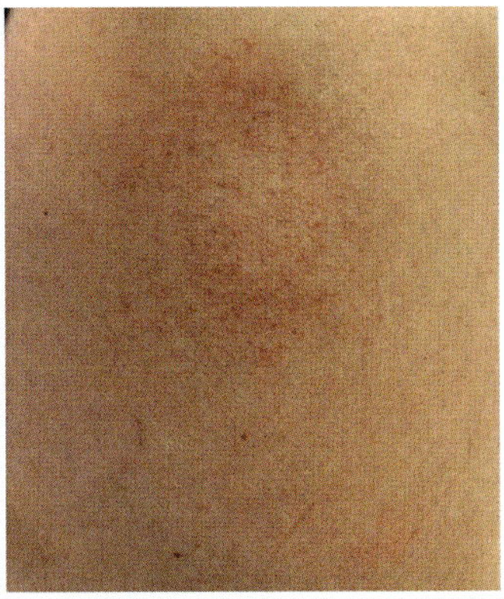	Development of mild hyperpigmentation	• Cleanse daily with mild soap and water • Apply Lotion Soft twice a day
3	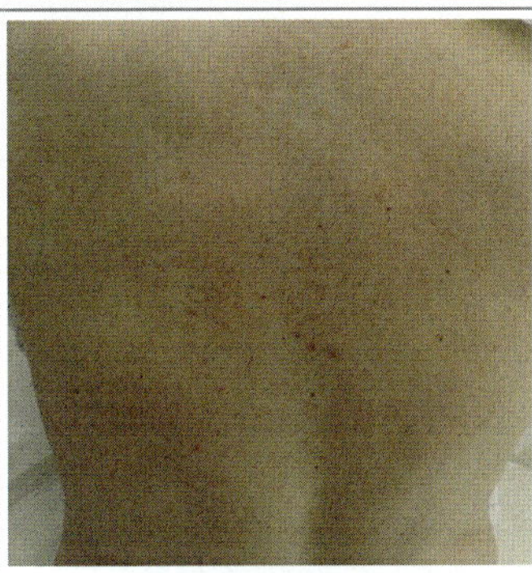	Hyperpigmentation and onset of mild erythema	• Cleanse daily with mild soap and water • Apply Lotion Soft twice a day
4	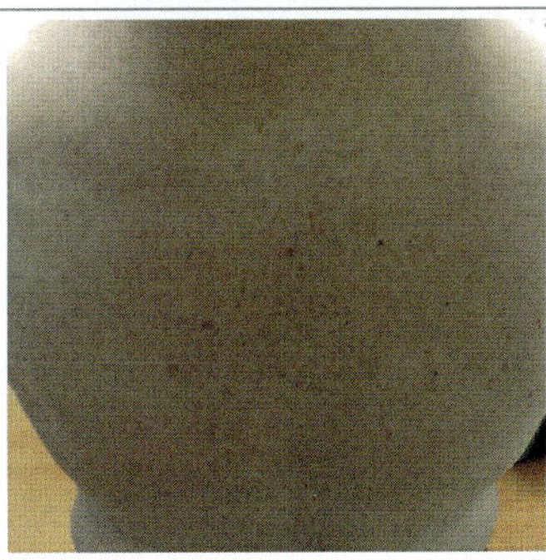	Mild erythema	• Cleanse daily with mild soap and water • Apply calendula twice a day

(continued)

Table 6.2 (continued)

Week	Skin reaction	Reaction type	Intervention
5	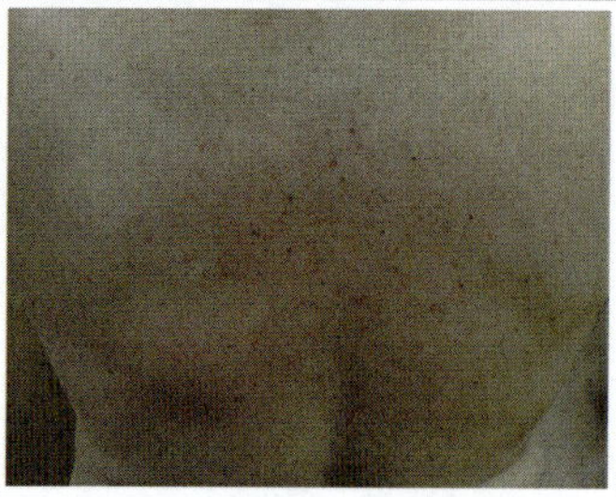	Mild to moderate erythema	• Cleanse daily with mild soap and water • Apply calendula twice a day • Apply A&D Ointment or Aquaphor before bedtime
1	78-year-old male with newly diagnosed metastatic prostate cancer with a thoracic spine vertebral metastasis s/p resection and stabilization, followed by postoperative radiotherapy with 3000 cGy in 10 daily fractions 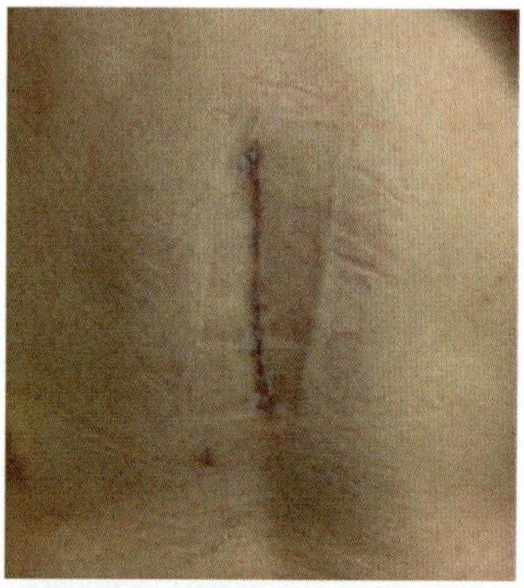	No reaction	• Cleanse daily with mild soap and water • Apply Lotion Soft twice a day
2	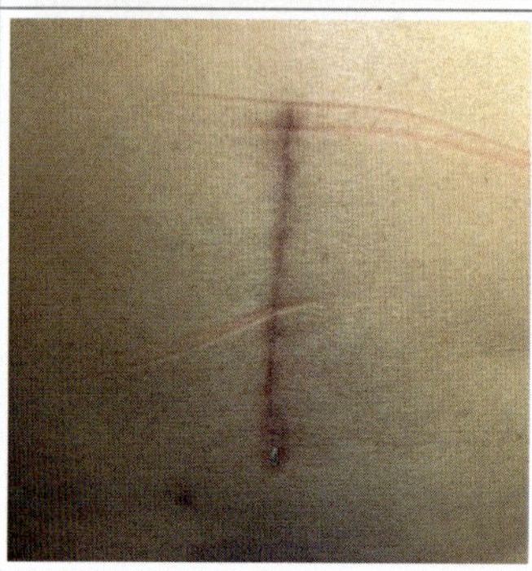	No reaction	• Continue to cleanse daily with mild soap and water • Apply Lotion Soft twice a day for 1 week post XRT, then as needed

Table 6.3 Special cases and reactions

Description	Reaction type	Treatment and intervention
Primary adenocarcinoma lung cancer stage IIIB treated with carboplatin, paclitaxel, and cetuximab 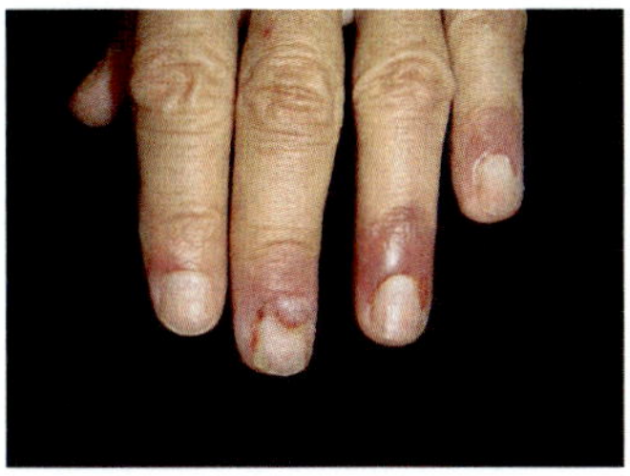	Cetuximab-induced paronychia	• This side effect may occur in 10–15 % of patients, especially those treated for longer than 2 months • It is painful and results in functional impairment • Prevention should include frequent inspection, gentle cleansing, moisturization, and avoidance of trauma • Treatment requires topical antiseptics and oral antibiotics
62-year-old male with adenocarcinoma of the superior sulcus, treated 3.5 years earlier with 15 Gy of 3D conformal external beam radiotherapy and 15 Gy of neutron therapy 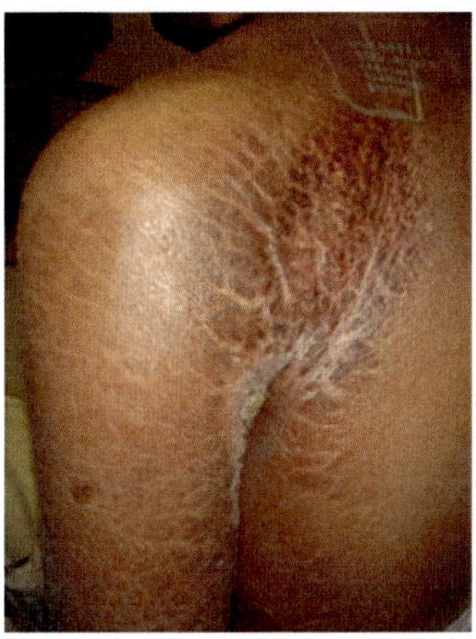	Hyperpigmentation, fibrosis, atrophy, and plexopathy	• Cleanse with mild soap and water • Moisturize daily following bath
Stage IIIA adenocarcinoma at 45 Gy/25 fx preoperative radiation treatment, with carboplatin/paclitaxel 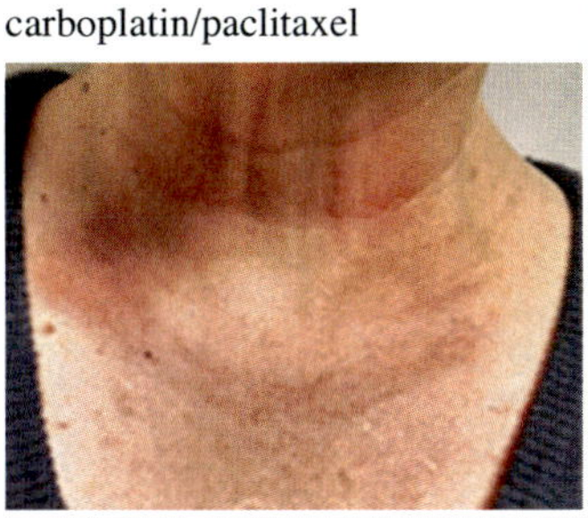	Example of reaction at the thoracic inlet/low neck	

(continued)

Table 6.3 (continued)

Description	Reaction type	Treatment and intervention
Asian patient with stage IIIB adenocarcinoma being treated to high dose for curative intent, with involved nodes in the supraclavicular region, receiving definitive concurrent chemoradiation (60 Gy) 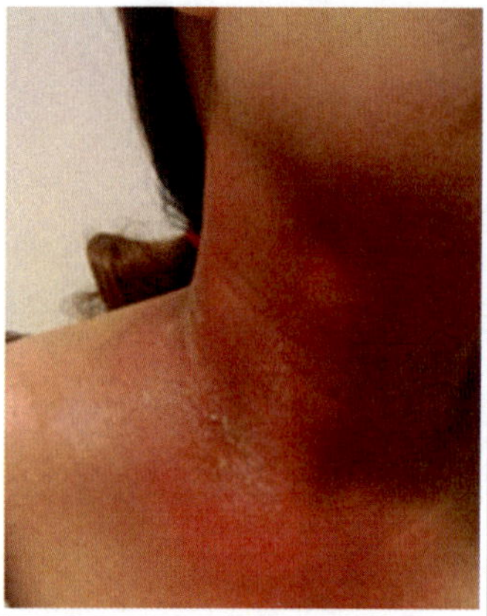	Example of mid-neck reaction, moderate/marked erythema	• Cleanse with soap and water or Skintegrity and moisturize twice daily with calendula or Aquaphor • Mepilex Lite for comfort as needed
Stage IIB cavitary squamous cell carcinoma at 50 Gy 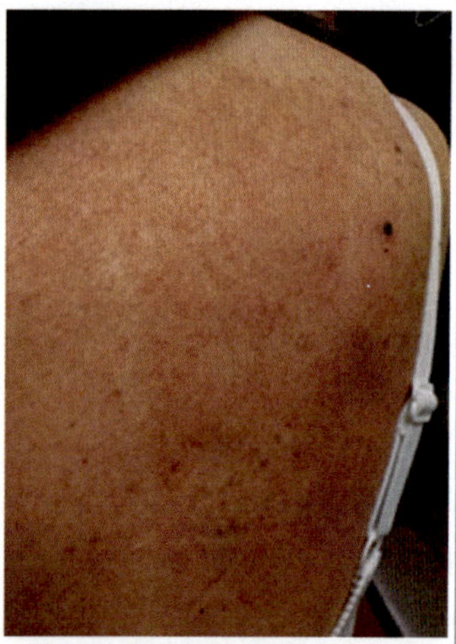 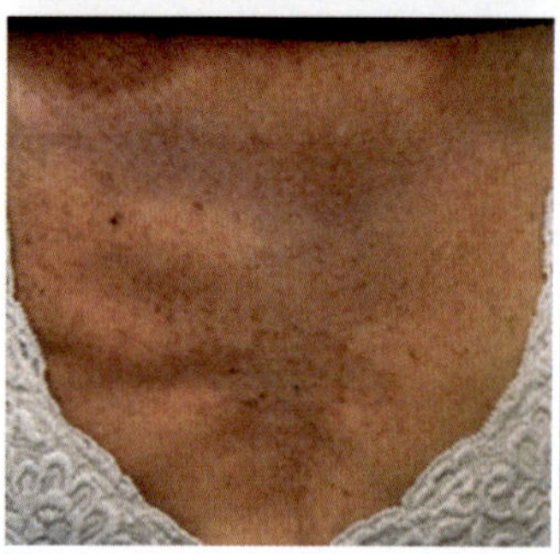	While most patients will develop reactions of erythema, dryness, freckling, and tanning on the back, occasionally patients will develop skin reactions anteriorly as well	• Cleanse with soap and water or Skintegrity and moisturize twice daily with calendula or Aquaphor

Week	Apply to Radiated Area		Notes
1-3	Lotion Soft ↓ Apply 2x/day		Thin lotion that is quickly absorbed, leaves no residue and does not clog pores.
3+	Switch to calendula ↓ Apply 2x/day		Thicker cream to help maintain moisture. Continue until skin erythema resolves, typically 2 weeks post radiation.
4+	Skintegrity Wound Cleansing Spray,		Begin applying this combination as erythema progression and moisture loss become apparent. Apply A&D until one week post radiation. Apply calendula until normal skin color returns. Mepilex Lite can be used for comfort.
	Calendula ↓ Apply 1x/day	A&D Ointment OR Aquaphor ↓ Apply 1x/day before bed	

Fig. 6.1 Suggested treatment algorithm for skin care

References

1. Cancer Facts and Figures 2015. American Cancer Society. 2015. http://www.cancer.org/research/cancer-factsstatistics/cancerfactsfigures2015/index. Accessed 16 Apr 2015
2. Stewart BW, Wild CP (eds). World Cancer Report 2014 (PDF). International Agency for Research on Cancer, United Nations, 2014.
3. Siegel RL, Miller KD, Jemal A. Cancer statistics, 2015. CA Cancer J Clin. 2015;65:5–29. doi:10.3322/caac.21254.
4. Gloeckler Ries LA, Reichman ME, Lewis DR, Hankey BF, Edwards BK. Cancer survival and incidence from the Surveillance, Epidemiology, and End Results (SEER) program. Oncologist. 2003;8:541–52.
5. Chang JY, Senan S, Paul MA, Mehran RJ, Louie AV, Balter P, et al. Stereotactic ablative radiotherapy versus lobectomy for operable stage I non-small-cell lung cancer: a pooled analysis of two randomised trials. Lancet Oncol. 2015;16:630–7. doi:10.1016/S1470-2045(15)70168-3.
6. De Ruysscher D, Botterweck A, Dirx M, Pijls-Johannesma M, Wanders R, Hochstenbag M, et al. Eligibility for concurrent chemotherapy and radiotherapy of locally advanced lung cancer patients: a prospective, population-based study. Ann Oncol. 2009;20:98–102. doi:10.1093/annonc/mdn559.
7. Dillman RO, Herndon J, Seagren SL, Eaton Jr WL, Green MR. Improved survival in stage III non-small-cell lung cancer: seven-year follow-up of cancer and leukemia group B (CALGB) 8433 trial. J Natl Cancer Inst. 1996;88:1210–5.
8. Turrisi 3rd AT, Kim K, Blum R, Sause WT, Livingston RB, Komaki R, et al. Twice-daily compared with once-daily thoracic radiotherapy in limited small-cell lung cancer treated concurrently with cisplatin and etoposide. N Engl J Med. 1999;340:265–71. doi:10.1056/NEJM199901283400403.
9. Salama JK, Hodgson L, Pang H, Urbanic JJ, Blackstock AW, Schild SE, et al. A pooled analysis of limited-stage small-cell lung cancer patients treated with induction chemotherapy followed by concurrent platinum-based chemotherapy and 70 Gy daily radiotherapy: CALGB 30904. J Thorac Oncol. 2013;8:1043–9. doi:10.1097/JTO.0b013e318293d8a4.
10. Slotman BJ, van Tinteren H, Praag JO, Knegjens JL, El Sharouni SY, Hatton M, et al. Use of thoracic radiotherapy for extensive stage small-cell lung cancer: a phase 3 randomised controlled trial. Lancet. 2015;385:36–42. doi:10.1016/S0140-6736(14)61085-0.
11. Jeremic B, Shibamoto Y, Nikolic N, Milicic B, Milisavljevic S, Dagovic A, et al. Role of radiation therapy in the combined-modality treatment of patients with extensive disease small-cell lung cancer: a randomized study. J Clin Oncol. 1999;17:2092–9.
12. Halpern MT, Ward EM, Pavluck AL, Schrag NM, Bian J, Chen AY. Association of insurance status and ethnicity with cancer stage at diagnosis for 12 cancer sites: a retrospective analysis. Lancet Oncol. 2008;9:222–31. doi:10.1016/S1470-2045(08)70032-9.
13. Toy E, Macbeth F, Coles B, Melville A, Eastwood A. Palliative thoracic radiotherapy for non-small-cell

lung cancer: a systematic review. Am J Clin Oncol. 2003;26:112–20.
14. Fogh S, Yom SS. Symptom management during the radiation oncology treatment course: a practical guide for the oncology clinician. Semin Oncol. 2014;41:764–75. doi:10.1053/j.seminoncol.2014.09.020.
15. Machtay M, Lee JH, Shrager JB, Kaiser LR, Glatstein E. Risk of death from intercurrent disease is not excessively increased by modern postoperative radiotherapy for high-risk resected non-small-cell lung carcinoma. J Clin Oncol. 2001;19:3912–7.
16. Hoppe BS, Laser B, Kowalski AV, Fontenla SC, Pena-Greenberg E, Yorke ED, et al. Acute skin toxicity following stereotactic body radiation therapy for stage I non-small-cell lung cancer: who's at risk? Int J Radiat Oncol Biol Phys. 2008;72:1283–6. doi:10.1016/j.ijrobp.2008.08.036.
17. Welsh J, Thomas J, Shah D, Allen PK, Wei X, Mitchell K, et al. Obesity increases the risk of chest wall pain from thoracic stereotactic body radiation therapy. Int J Radiat Oncol Biol Phys. 2011;81:91–6. doi:10.1016/j.ijrobp.2010.04.022.
18. Woody NM, Videtic GM, Stephans KL, Djemil T, Kim Y, Xia P. Predicting chest wall pain from lung stereotactic body radiotherapy for different fractionation schemes. Int J Radiat Oncol Biol Phys. 2012;83:427–34. doi:10.1016/j.ijrobp.2011.06.1971.
19. Auperin A, Arriagada R, Pignon JP, Le Pechoux C, Gregor A, Stephens RJ, et al. Prophylactic cranial irradiation for patients with small-cell lung cancer in complete remission. Prophylactic Cranial Irradiation Overview Collaborative Group. N Engl J Med. 1999;341:476–84. doi:10.1056/NEJM199908123410703.
20. Slotman B, Faivre-Finn C, Kramer G, Rankin E, Snee M, Hatton M, et al. Prophylactic cranial irradiation in extensive small-cell lung cancer. N Engl J Med. 2007;357:664–72. doi:10.1056/NEJMoa071780.
21. Slotman BJ, Mauer ME, Bottomley A, Faivre-Finn C, Kramer GW, Rankin EM, et al. Prophylactic cranial irradiation in extensive disease small-cell lung cancer: short-term health-related quality of life and patient reported symptoms: results of an international Phase III randomized controlled trial by the EORTC Radiation Oncology and Lung Cancer Groups. J Clin Oncol. 2009;27:78–84. doi:10.1200/JCO.2008.17.0746.
22. Lawenda BD, Gagne HM, Gierga DP, Niemierko A, Wong WM, Tarbell NJ, et al. Permanent alopecia after cranial irradiation: dose-response relationship. Int J Radiat Oncol Biol Phys. 2004;60:879–87. doi:10.1016/j.ijrobp.2004.04.031.
23. Butson MJ, Mathur JN, Metcalfe PE. Skin dose from radiotherapy X-ray beams: the influence of energy. Australas Radiol. 1997;41:148–50.
24. Chow JC, Grigorov GN. Surface dosimetry for oblique tangential photon beams: a Monte Carlo simulation study. Med Phys. 2008;35:70–6.
25. Tho LM, McIntyre A, Rosst A, Gallagher C, Yap C, Ritchie DM, et al. Acute supraclavicular skin toxicity in patients undergoing radiotherapy for breast cancer: an evaluation of the 'T'-grip method of patient positioning. Clin Oncol (R Coll Radiol). 2006;18:133–8.
26. Verbraecken J, Van de Heyning P, De Backer W, Van Gaal L. Body surface area in normal-weight, overweight, and obese adults. A comparison study. Metabolism. 2006;55:515–24. doi:10.1016/j.metabol.2005.11.004.
27. Doyle LA, Showalter TN, Werner-Wasik M, Weksler B, Xiao Y, Yu Y, et al. High-dose-rate surface brachytherapy to boost elongated, curvilinear incisional scars after extrapleural pneumonectomy for malignant pleural mesothelioma treated with adjuvant intensity-modulated radiation therapy. Brachytherapy. 2010;9:86–90. doi:10.1016/j.brachy.2009.08.009.
28. Tapley ND, Fletcher GH. Skin reactions and tissue heterogeneity in electron beam therapy. I. Clinical experience. Radiology. 1965;84:812–6. doi:10.1148/84.5.812.
29. Stephans KL, Djemil T, Tendulkar RD, Robinson CG, Reddy CA, Videtic GM. Prediction of chest wall toxicity from lung stereotactic body radiotherapy (SBRT). Int J Radiat Oncol Biol Phys. 2012;82:974–80. doi:10.1016/j.ijrobp.2010.12.002.
30. Mutter RW, Liu F, Abreu A, Yorke E, Jackson A, Rosenzweig KE. Dose-volume parameters predict for the development of chest wall pain after stereotactic body radiation for lung cancer. Int J Radiat Oncol Biol Phys. 2012;82:1783–90. doi:10.1016/j.ijrobp.2011.03.053.
31. Andolino DL, Forquer JA, Henderson MA, Barriger RB, Shapiro RH, Brabham JG, et al. Chest wall toxicity after stereotactic body radiotherapy for malignant lesions of the lung and liver. Int J Radiat Oncol Biol Phys. 2011;80:692–7. doi:10.1016/j.ijrobp.2010.03.020.
32. Kavanagh BD, Schefter TE, Cardenes HR, Stieber VW, Raben D, Timmerman RD, et al. Interim analysis of a prospective phase I/II trial of SBRT for liver metastases. Acta Oncol. 2006;45:848–55. doi:10.1080/02841860600904870.
33. RTOG 0618 Protocol Information. RTOG. 2015. https://www.rtog.org/ClinicalTrials/ProtocolTable/StudyDetails.aspx?study=0618. Accessed 11 Sept 2015.
34. Thibault I, Chiang A, Erler D, Yeung L, Poon I, Kim A, et al. Predictors of chest wall toxicity after lung stereotactic ablative radiotherapy. Clin Oncol (R Coll Radiol). 2015;28(1):28–35. doi:10.1016/j.clon.2015.06.009.
35. Lo SS, Fakiris AJ, Wang JZ, Mayr NA. In regard to Hoppe et al. (Int J Radiat Oncol Biol Phys 2008;72:1283–1286). Int J Radiat Oncol Biol Phys. 2009;74:977. doi:10.1016/j.ijrobp.2009.02.046; author reply 8.
36. Mitera G, Chan G, Mah K, Law R, Deangelis C, Dent R, et al. A rare adverse skin reaction after 8 Gy of radiation therapy to the thoracic spine: case report and review of the literature. Curr Oncol. 2010;17:70–3.
37. Whaley JT, Kirk M, Cengel K, McDonough J, Bekelman J, Christodouleas JP. Protective effect of transparent film dressing on proton therapy induced skin reactions. Radiat Oncol. 2013;8:19. doi:10.1186/1748-717X-8-19.
38. Werner-Wasik M, Pequignot E, Leeper D, Hauck W, Curran W. Predictors of severe esophagitis include use of concurrent chemotherapy, but not the length of irra-

diated esophagus: a multivariate analysis of patients with lung cancer treated with nonoperative therapy. Int J Radiat Oncol Biol Phys. 2000;48:689–96.
39. Yeager CE, Olsen EA. Treatment of chemotherapy-induced alopecia. Dermatol Ther. 2011;24:432–42. doi:10.1111/j.1529-8019.2011.01430.x.
40. Dauendorffer JN, Dupuy A. Radiation recall dermatitis induced by erlotinib. J Am Acad Dermatol. 2009;61:1086. doi:10.1016/j.jaad.2009.04.033.
41. Khanfir K, Anchisi S. Pemetrexed-associated radiation recall dermatitis. Acta Oncol. 2008;47:1607–8. doi:10.1080/02841860802120036.
42. Bradley JD, Paulus R, Komaki R, Masters G, Blumenschein G, Schild S, et al. Standard-dose versus high-dose conformal radiotherapy with concurrent and consolidation carboplatin plus paclitaxel with or without cetuximab for patients with stage IIIA or IIIB non-small-cell lung cancer (RTOG 0617): a randomised, two-by-two factorial phase 3 study. Lancet Oncol. 2015;16:187–99. doi:10.1016/S1470-2045(14)71207-0.
43. Iyengar P, Kavanagh BD, Wardak Z, Smith I, Ahn C, Gerber DE, et al. Phase II trial of stereotactic body radiation therapy combined with erlotinib for patients with limited but progressive metastatic non-small-cell lung cancer. J Clin Oncol. 2014;32:3824–30. doi:10.1200/JCO.2014.56.7412.
44. Ebara T, Tanio N, Etoh T, Shichi I, Honda A, Nakajima N. Palliative re-irradiation for in-field recurrence after definitive radiotherapy in patients with primary lung cancer. Anticancer Res. 2007;27:531–4.
45. Reyngold M, Wu AJ, McLane A, Zhang Z, Hsu M, Stein NF, et al. Toxicity and outcomes of thoracic re-irradiation using stereotactic body radiation therapy (SBRT). Radiat Oncol. 2013;8:99. doi:10.1186/1748-717X-8-99.

7 Breast Cancer

Barbara Fowble, Catherine Park, and Florence Yuen

Breast cancer is the most common cancer in women. It is estimated that 231,840 women in the United States will be diagnosed with breast cancer in 2015 [1]. Radiation is an integral component of the treatment of early-stage breast cancer and in the majority of women is administered after breast-conserving surgery. However, recent studies have reported increased trends for mastectomy with or without reconstruction [2, 3]. Postmastectomy radiation is received by almost 80 % of women with established indications for treatment and 47 % of those with weaker indications [4]. Radiation may also be used to palliate sites of metastatic disease such as the lung, bone, or brain. Inoperable locally advanced tumors may benefit from radiation with a resultant decrease in bleeding, ulceration, drainage, and odor and in some cases may be rendered operable.

7.1 Types and Frequency of Skin Reactions

The majority of the literature on the prevention and treatment of acute radiation dermatitis has focused on breast cancer patients. Radiation dermatitis is common in these women and ranges from mild erythema which occurs in 90–95 % to brisk erythema with or without moist desquamation and dry desquamation [5]. The skin reaction increases throughout treatment as the dose is cumulative. The peak reaction occurs 1–2 weeks post treatment [6–8]. Therefore, studies which evaluate skin toxicity at 6 weeks post treatment will underestimate the maximum acute reaction. The effectiveness of an intervention will vary with the treatment interval at which it is tested. Some interventions may be effective earlier in the treatment but not later as the reaction peaks.

Modifications of the Radiation Therapy Oncology Group (RTOG) [9] and Common Terminology Criteria for Adverse Event (CTCAE) [10] skin toxicity scoring systems have been proposed to better reflect the changes observed in breast cancer patients [11–13]. Moist desquamation is the most clinically significant skin reaction in women with breast cancer. However, in the RTOG and CTCAE scoring systems, moist desquamation in the inframammary fold is classified as a grade 2 toxicity. Wright et al. [13] added three subcategories to grade 2 toxicity of the CTCAE scale. The authors recommended the use of the following scores: grade 1 (faint or dull erythema and/or follicular reaction and/or itching), grade 2 (bright erythema and/or tender to touch), grade 3 (dry desquamation with or without erythema), grade 4 (small or moderate moist desquamation), grade 5 (confluent moist), and grade 6 (ulceration, hemorrhage, or necrosis).

B. Fowble, MD, FACR, FASTRO (✉) • C. Park, MD
F. Yuen, RN, MSN, AOCNP
Department of Radiation Oncology, University of California, San Francisco, 1600 Divisadero, H1031, San Francisco, CA 94115, USA
e-mail: BFowble@radonc.ucsf.edu

B. Fowble et al. (eds.), *Skin Care in Radiation Oncology*, DOI 10.1007/978-3-319-31460-0_7

Table 7.1 [5, 6, 12–24] presents series reporting acute skin toxicity in breast cancer patients receiving radiation. The incidence of grade 2–3 toxicity ranges from 23 to 80 % with the incidence of moist desquamation ranging from 15 to 48 %. This variation reflects the type of surgery (breast-conserving surgery vs. mastectomy) and the extent of moist desquamation (any moist desquamation vs. extensive). Bolus is often used on the skin surface to increase dose in the postmastectomy setting. In the absence of bolus, TLD (thermoluminescent dosimeter) measurements for surface dose are similar for the intact breast (inframammary fold) and mastectomy patients (inferior lateral) and average 3400–3900 cGy for conventional fractionation [14] with 6 or 6/18 MV photon tangential beams. With the use of bolus, Graham et al. [21] recorded TLD surface dose measurements of 203–215 cGy per fraction.

Breast edema has been reported to be present in 5–20 % of women before the initiation of radiation [5, 15, 25]. It has been correlated with the extent of the surgical resection and axillary surgery (axillary dissection vs. sentinel node biopsy) and post-surgery edema and infection [15]. Freedman et al. [25] reported that with IMRT it peaks 3–6 months after treatment and generally resolves within 3 years. At 3–6

Table 7.1 Acute skin toxicity; breast cancer

Study	Number of patients	Fractionation	Technique	Toxicity GR 2–3 (%)	Toxicity GR 3 (%)	Moist desquamation (%)	Scoring system
Breast-conserving surgery							
RTOG 9713 [14]	172	Conventional	2D	37			RTOG
Freedman [12]	804	Conventional	Wedge-based IMRT	75 52			CTCAE
Pignol [5]	331	Conventional	Wedge-based IMRT			48 31	CTCAE
Back [15]	223	Conventional	Not stated			31	RTOG
Rutter [16]	69	Conventional	3D			33	[none]
Freedman [17]	75	Hypofractionated	IMRT	23			CTCAE
De Langhe [18]	377	Hypofractionated	IMRT	58		15	CTCAE
McDonald [19]	240	Conventional	Wedge-based vs. IMRT	52 39			RTOG
Harsolia [20]	172	Conventional	Wedge-based vs. IMRT	85 41	6 1		CTCAE
Postmastectomy							
Graham, PH [21]	318	Not stated	Not stated		41		CTCAE
Pignol [6]	257	Conventional	3D		33	28	CTCAE
Wright [13]	110	Conventional	3D	80	8		CTCAE
Ma [22]	85	Conventional	IMRT	42		41	CTCAE
Spierer [23]	118	Conventional	Electrons		52		RTOG
Cuaron [24]	26	Conventional	Protons			29	CTCAE

CTCAE common terminology criteria for adverse events, *2D* two dimensional, *3D* three dimensional conformal, *IMRT* intensity-modulated radiation therapy

months, 26 % of women were noted to have breast edema. At 3 years 3.7 % had persistent breast edema. Vicini et al. [26] reported a 54 % incidence of breast edema in African-American women compared to 43 % in Caucasian women. A systematic review of breast edema following breast-conserving surgery and radiation reported significant variation in the incidence of breast edema (0–90 %) depending on the method of assessment (patient, physician, imaging) [27]. Factors which contributed to the incidence of breast edema include larger breast size or separation, higher boost dose and larger boost volume, conventional wedge-based tangents, and a shorter interval between intraoperative radiation and external beam radiation [27]. Harsolia et al. [20] reported chronic breast edema in 25 % of large breasted women treated with wedge-based radiation compared to 1 % for those treated with IMRT. The influence of systemic therapy on breast edema has varied. Some studies have reported an increased incidence of breast edema with chemotherapy [25, 28], while others have not [29]. Tamoxifen has been associated with an increased incidence of breast edema [29, 30]. However, the incidence of breast edema has not been influenced by whether tamoxifen was given concurrently or sequentially with radiation [31].

7.2 Factors Affecting Acute Skin Toxicity

7.2.1 Intact Breast

Patient-related factors that have been associated with increased acute skin reactions include higher body mass index (BMI), larger bra cup size, and smoking [5, 8, 12, 14–16, 18, 25, 32]. The increased acute skin reactions observed in larger breasted women have been attributed to dose inhomogeneity and self-bolus in the axilla and inframammary fold region [33].

There have been no studies to date which have examined differences in acute skin toxicity based on race in women treated with breast-conserving surgery and radiation. Two studies have reported worse cosmesis in African-American women [26, 34], while one has not [35]. None of these studies commented on acute reactions. Ulff et al. [36] reported a more pronounced acute dermatitis in patients with fair or Fitzpatrick type 1 skin [37]. However, Herst et al. [38] found no association between Fitzpatrick skin type and the incidence of moist desquamation.

The role of common genetic variants (single nucleotide polymorphisms) in predicting acute radiation skin reactions has been the focus of several recent studies in breast cancer patients. De Langhe et al. [18] reported increased acute skin toxicity in women with a genetic variation in MLH1 rs1800734. Acute radiation dermatitis has not been associated with SNPs in the DNA repair genes of *XRCC1*, *APE1*, and *XPD* [39] or polymorphisms in the *TP53* or *p21* genes [40]. *ATM* SNPs have more commonly been associated with late toxicity [41–44]. However, Iannuzzi et al. [43] also reported an increased incidence of ATM mutations in women who developed moist desquamation. To date there has been no correlation with BRCA 1/2 mutations and acute radiation skin toxicity in breast cancer patients [45–48].

Treatment-related factors that have diminished the frequency of grade 2 or higher acute skin reactions include the use of intensity-modulated radiation therapy (IMRT) [5, 12, 18, 25], the use of higher energy photons [5], the prone position [18, 49], and the use of moderately hypofractionated regimens [50–54].

The use of antiperspirants and deodorants during breast cancer radiation in the past was contraindicated due to concern for a possible bolus or irritant effect resulting in increased axillary acute skin toxicity. Five randomized trials have now demonstrated that the use of nonaluminum- [55–57] and aluminum-containing deodorants [58, 59] does not increase acute axillary skin reactions with conventionally or hypofractionated regimens. Guidelines developed by the Oncology Nursing Society [60] for the treatment and prevention of radiation dermatitis include allowing patients to use nonaluminum-based deodorants during treatment. The recommendation can now include the use of aluminum-containing antiperspirants.

7.2.2 Postmastectomy

Moist desquamation is the most clinically relevant acute skin toxicity in patients receiving postmastectomy radiation given the frequent use of bolus to increase skin dose. Patient-related factors that have been associated with an increased frequency of moist desquamation in women receiving postmastectomy radiation include African-American ethnicity [13], postmenopausal status, higher BMI or larger chest wall separation, and smoking [6, 8, 13].

Treatment-related factors associated with moist desquamation include the use and frequency of bolus [6, 13]. Pignol et al. [6] reported moist desquamation in 22 % of the women who received alternate day bolus compared to 41 % for daily bolus. Wright et al. [13] reported small or moderate areas of moist desquamation in 45 % of 110 patients and confluent moist desquamation in 8 % at the end of treatment with the use of daily 0.5 cm bolus in addition to a scar boost.

7.2.3 Interactions with Systemic Therapy

The concurrent use of tamoxifen or an aromatase inhibitor has been associated with increased acute skin toxicity in women treated with breast-conserving surgery and radiation [12, 18]. Moist desquamation has been reported in 45–50 % of patients treated with breast-conserving surgery, radiation, and concurrent chemotherapy with cyclophosphamide, methotrexate, and 5-fluorouracil [15] even with dose reductions in the whole breast [61].

Preclinical data suggested a radiosensitizing effect of trastuzumab on breast cancer cells [62], but its effect on normal cells was unknown. Belkacemi et al. [63] reported grade 2 or higher radiation dermatitis (CTCAE v3.0 scale) in 51 % of 135 women receiving concurrent trastuzumab on a 3-week schedule. Jacob et al. [64] reported grade 2 toxicity in 21.7 % and grade 3 in 3.9 % (CTCAE v3.0) with concurrent trastuzumab given every 3 weeks, and Caussa et al. [65] reported grade 2–3 toxicity in 15 % with a concurrent 3-week regimen. Bellon et al. [66] reported grade 2–3 skin toxicity in 48 % of women receiving trastuzumab weekly compared to 8 % for the every 3-week schedule. Two additional studies have reported no increase in acute skin toxicity with concurrent trastuzumab [18, 67].

7.3 Late Effects

Late effects are generally considered those that develop 3 months or more after radiation is completed. Late reactions have been correlated with the severity of acute reactions [5, 68–70].

7.3.1 Recall Dermatitis

Radiation recall dermatitis is uncommon and typically is confined to the site(s) of radiation. It occurs after the acute skin changes from radiation have resolved. It has been reported in patients taking tamoxifen [71–75] and nonsteroidal aromatase inhibitors [76, 77]. The most common chemotherapy agents reported to precipitate radiation recall include the anthracyclines (doxorubicin), taxanes (docetaxel, paclitaxel), and antimetabolites (gemcitabine and capecitabine) [78]. Haffty et al. [79] reported radiation recall in 18 % of women treated with MammoSite brachytherapy and chemotherapy initiated within 3 weeks compared to 7 % when chemotherapy was delayed for more than 3 weeks. Ioannidis et al. [80] reported recall dermatitis with everolimus and exemestane in a single patient 10 years after whole breast radiation. Radiation recall dermatitis has also been reported with trastuzumab [81–83].

7.3.2 Telangiectasias

Telangiectasias are dilated superficial blood vessels. Their appearance has been correlated with the extent and severity of acute reactions, with an increased incidence in areas of prior moist desquamation [69, 70]. They are permanent and tend to increase with time [25, 84]. Vicini et al. [26] reported a lower incidence of telangiectasia in African-American women when compared to Caucasian women (3 % vs. 10 %). Older age, large breast size, postoperative infection, and tumor bed boost were associated with an increased incidence of telangiectasia in the Cambridge randomized trial of IMRT [85]. This trial [85] and other single institution studies have reported a decreased incidence of telangiectasia with IMRT [25, 86]. Freedman et al. [25] reported telangiectasia in 8.2 % of women at 3 years treated with IMRT. Mukesh et al. [85] reported telangiectasia in 15 % of women treated with IMRT compared to 24 % treated with wedged tangential fields at 6 years. The concurrent administration of chemotherapy with radiation resulted in a significant increase in telangiectasia in the ARCOSEIN randomized trial of concurrent versus sequential chemotherapy [84]. Telangiectasias have been reported in women receiving ado-trastuzumab emtansine (T-DM1) for breast cancer [87]. However, to date there have been no reports of increased telangiectasias in women receiving breast radiation. Laser therapy has been used to remove telangiectasias, but multiple sessions are often required, and the telangiectasias may reappear.

7.3.3 Morphea

Morphea is a localized form of scleroderma. It can be characterized by circumscribed patches or plaques of sclerosis with induration or more diffuse areas. The areas may be erythematous or hypopigmented. Radiation-induced morphea has been reported in women with breast cancer treated with breast-conserving surgery and whole breast radiation [88–90] or partial breast radiation [91]. The changes may appear outside of the area of radiation [90]. It is reported to occur in 1/500 women treated for breast cancer [92, 93]. The interval from radiation to the appearance of morphea ranges from 1 month to 32 years [92, 94, 95]. It is not a precursor to systemic sclerosis, and it should not be confused with a recall reaction.

7.3.4 Fibrosis

Radiation can induce fibrosis in the skin and subcutaneous tissues which results in loss of parenchymal cells with the increased formation of fibrous tissue. In the skin and soft tissues, the affected area(s) becomes firmer, indurated, and tighter and at times painful. There may be shrinkage of the irradiated breast (intact or autologous reconstruction) and pericapsular fibrosis and contracture in the tissue expander/implant-reconstructed breast. Both patient- and treatment-related factors contribute to the risk of fibrosis.

Patient-related factors that contribute to the risk of radiation fibrosis in women with breast cancer include the collagen vascular diseases of scleroderma and lupus erythematosus. A review of eight observational studies demonstrated increased late effects from radiation in patients with connective tissue diseases [96]. Marked subcutaneous fibrosis has been reported in women with collagen vascular disease who received radiation [97–101]. African-American women have not been reported to have an increased incidence of breast fibrosis when compared to Caucasian women (19 % vs. 15 %) [26].

Individual genetic variations have been associated with adverse radiation responses in women with breast cancer. ATM heterozygosity occurs in 1 % of the general population [102]. Increased late ≥2 grade fibrosis (RTOG)) has been reported in women with DNA sequence alterations in the ATM gene [41–44]. Iannuzzi et al. [43] reported an increased incidence of grade 3–4 subcutaneous fibrosis/necrosis in women with two ATM mutations. Variations in the *TGFB1*, *XRCC1*, *XRCC3*, *SOD2*, and *RAD21* genes have also been reported to be associated with radiation-induced fibrosis in breast cancer patients [42, 103–105]. In contrast, women with *BRCA 1/2* or *CHEK2* mutations have not been reported to have increased late reactions when treated with breast-conserving surgery and radiation [45, 46, 106] and compared to sporadic controls.

Various radiation treatment-related factors may affect the incidence of subcutaneous fibrosis in women with breast cancer. These include higher total dose, greater dose inhomogeneity, the use of a boost, brachytherapy, and overlapping radiation fields (tangents with supraclavicular field and/or internal mammary field) [25, 107–110]. Rates of fibrosis are low with contemporary treatment using intensity-modulated radiation therapy (IMRT) in women undergoing breast-conserving surgery [25, 111]. Freedman et al. [25] reported a 6.8 % incidence of fibrosis in women who received IMRT following breast-conserving surgery. In contrast, grade 3–4 contracture has been reported in 22 % of women with tissue expander/implant reconstruction receiving postmastectomy radiation [112].

The correlation between radiation-induced fibrosis and tamoxifen has been evaluated in several studies. Tamoxifen induces transforming growth factor-B (TGF-B) secretion which is associated with fibrosis. The concurrent administration of tamoxifen with radiation has been reported to be a factor in radiation-induced breast fibrosis in some studies [25, 109, 113] but not others [30, 31]. Subcutaneous fibrosis was not increased with concurrent letrozole in a phase 2 randomized trial of concurrent versus sequential therapy [114]. Similarly concurrent anastrozole with whole breast radiation did not increase late toxicity [115]. In contrast, the ACOSEIN randomized trial reported grade ≥2 (LENT-SOMA) subcutaneous fibrosis in 19 % of women receiving concurrent chemotherapy compared to 5 % receiving sequential chemotherapy [84].

Fibrotic changes were previously thought to be irreversible but preclinical models, and limited success with clinical interventions suggests some degree of reversibility [116, 117]. Regression of superficial subcutaneous fibrosis with a combination of pentoxifylline and vitamin E was reported by Delanian et al. [118] However, sustained benefit required long-term treatment. Symptoms of severe breast fibrosis were improved with partial mastectomy and latissimus flap reconstruction in one study [119].

7.4 Interventions for Breast Cancer Patients with Acute Radiation Dermatitis

Interventions are divided into prevention and treatment strategies.

7.4.1 Prevention

Topical agents used to prevent or decrease the severity of the acute skin reactions are divided into steroid and nonsteroidal agents. Nonsteroidal creams/gels may be categorized as emollients, humectants, or occlusive agents. Skin emollients provide lubrication and moisture in areas where sebaceous glands are depleted. They vary in their ability to penetrate the skin. The use of oil-based emulsions has generally been discouraged due to concern for a residue that could act as bolus. However, two recent studies have reported no increased acute skin toxicity with a natural oil-based emulsion [120] or emu oil [121]. Topical agents which have not been shown to diminish the acute skin reaction in breast cancer patients include aloe vera [8, 122–124] and trolamine [14, 125]. A single randomized trial demonstrated the superiority of *Calendula officinalis* when compared to trolamine for preventing of ≥2 grade (RTOG) scale) dermatitis [126]. Topical hyaluronic acid-based gel resulted in a significantly higher incidence of ≥2 grade (CTCAE v3.0) dermatitis when compared to petrolatum-based ointment in a randomized trial from MD Anderson Cancer Center [127]. A randomized trial from the Institut Curie [128] reported no difference in the severity of the acute skin reaction (RTOG scale) when comparing hyaluronic acid or an emollient-containing urea 2 % and glycerol 9.5 %.

A systematic review of the randomized trials of topical prophylactic steroid creams concluded that their use significantly decreased the incidence of acute dermatitis, especially moist desquamation [129]. Three randomized trials in breast cancer patients [7, 36, 130] demonstrated a beneficial effect of daily application of high-potency steroid creams in decreasing the severity of acute radiation dermatitis. The North Central

Cancer Treatment Group trial [131] reported no difference in the maximum grade of CTCAE v3.0 toxicity (provider assessed) or incidence of grade 3 toxicity when comparing 0.1 % mometasone furoate with a placebo cream. However, the use of the steroid cream significantly decreased the patient-reported symptoms of pruritus and skin irritation. The potency of the steroid cream which best achieves maximum benefit is unknown. Prolonged use of high-potency creams should be avoided to decrease the risk of skin atrophy.

Barrier-forming products include Cavillon No Sting Barrier (spray on), Mepilex Lite dressings, and Mepitel Film. These products provide protection from friction and rubbing of the skin. The film formulation of the Cavillon No Sting Barrier was shown in a small trial to reduce the severity of acute radiation dermatitis in breast cancer patients [132]. However, the cream formulation, which also contained emollients and dimethicone, did not produce similar results in a randomized trial of 333 postmastectomy patients [21]. Mepitel Film (Safetac-based soft silicone) was reported to completely prevent moist desquamation in a small trial of 78 women receiving postmastectomy radiation [38]. Bolus was used in only 18 % of the patients. It was estimated that the film had a 0.12 mm bolus effect. In contrast, Mepilex Lite dressings have been reported to decrease the severity of the acute reactions but not significantly decrease the incidence of moist desquamation [133]. Their bolus effect is reported to be 0.5 mm [38]. Mepitel Film is worn continuously even in the shower and during the radiation treatment. Mepilex Lite dressings cannot be worn in the shower and should not be worn during treatment.

7.4.2 Treatment

Dry desquamation is characterized by hyperpigmented or erythematous, peeling, dry flaky, and pruritic skin. The goal of treatment for dry desquamation is to minimize patient discomfort and maintain the moisture balance of the skin. We start with a mild enzymatic wound cleanser such as Skintegrity. The wound cleanser is mild, does not irritate the skin, and promotes gentle exfoliation. This allows moisturizers to better penetrate the skin. Moisturization can then be achieved by the use of emollient, occlusive, or humectant moisturizers such as calendula, A&D Ointment, white petroleum, or Medihoney with a hydrogel base or secondary dressing. Topical steroids can be used to treat the associated pruritus if the skin remains intact.

Dressings such as Mepilex Lite, hydrogel colloidal sheets with or without Medihoney, can be applied to the areas such as the inframammary fold or axilla to reduce friction, and irritation, and to assist in maintaining the skin's hydration. Medihoney works well with dry desquamation as it is soothing, is healing, and promotes hydration. Care should be taken when removing the hydrogel sheets that are self-adhering as they can cause a skin tear upon removal. Patients are instructed to remove these dressings in the shower if they do not easily lift off.

Maintaining adherence of the soft silicone dressing (Mepilex) can be difficult once the skin is moisturized. Patients are advised to wait 30–60 min to apply the dressing or spray the area with Cavillon No Sting Barrier to promote adherence of the dressing.

Moist desquamation is characterized by a loss of the integrity of the epidermis with weeping of the tissues. Secondary *Staphylococcus aureus* infections have occurred in patients with untreated or prolonged moist desquamation. Hydrocolloid and or hydrogel dressings have been used and suggested in the management of moist desquamation. The dressings maintain a moist environment for skin reepithelialization. Moist environments have been found to promote wound healing. However, a study by Mcmillan et al. [134], comparing the effects of hydrogel to a dry dressing on the healing time of moist desquamation, reported that healing time in the hydrogel dressing group was significantly prolonged. It is possible that the prolonged moisture in this patient population can lead to increased maceration.

We have seen this anecdotally in some of our patients with moist desquamation. Our approach to moist desquamation is to promote drying, healing, and patient comfort during this time. We have used a combination of therapies including topical anti-infectives such as zinc and bacitracin, in a one-to-one mixture, with a secondary cover dressing of Telfa to minimize skin trauma and a cover dressing such as soft absorbent silicone (Mepilex Lite or Mepilex). Following the wound care literature, we leave the dressing in place for 24 h to minimize trauma to the wound. The dressing is removed daily and cleansed with a 0.5 % Hibiclens solution or Skintegrity. The area is redressed and left in place for another 24 h. Healing usually occurs over 3–4 days.

Silver ion dressings such as Aquacel Ag or Mepilex Ag have been applied directly to the wound that has been cleansed with Skintegrity or 0.5 % Hibiclens solution. This has been effective in prevention of infection and promotion of healing through maintenance of adequate moisture balance, allowing wound healing and preventing maceration. The dressing is left in place for 24–48 h. Healing usually occurs over 3–4 days. All of these dressings provide immediate comfort for the patients' wounds and promote healing of moist desquamation.

7.5 Photographs and Recommendations

Below are general skin care recommendations (Table 7.2), week-by-week treatment instructions, and photographs that demonstrate typical skin reactions over time for patients undergoing breast-conserving surgery (Table 7.3), mastectomy with autologous reconstruction (Table 7.4), mastectomy with implant-based reconstruction (Table 7.5), and mastectomy without reconstruction (Table 7.6). Photographs of skin reactions varying by ethnicity are provided in Table 7.7, and photographs of special cases and reactions, with treatment instructions, are provided in Table 7.8 [135]. Figure 7.1 is a suggested general treatment algorithm for skin care for breast cancer patients.

Table 7.2 General principles of skin care for breast cancer patients

Patient should:
• Cleanse daily with mild soap and water
• Use lotions and creams recommended by provider
• Continue to wear garments that provide support to the breast such as bras, tube tops, and tank tops
Patient should not:
• Rub, put pressure on, or scratch radiated area
• Take hot water showers or baths, use wash cloths, or use loofahs
• Apply any lotion, cream, or ointment within the 3 hours prior to radiation treatment
• Wash off lotion, cream, or ointments if applied three or more hours before radiation treatment
• Apply drying agents to the skin unless instructed to do so

Table 7.3 Examples of typical acute skin reactions and recommended interventions for women undergoing breast-conserving surgery and whole breast radiation are provided below

Week	Skin reaction	Reaction type	Intervention
1	48-year-old Filipino, S/P breast-conserving surgery 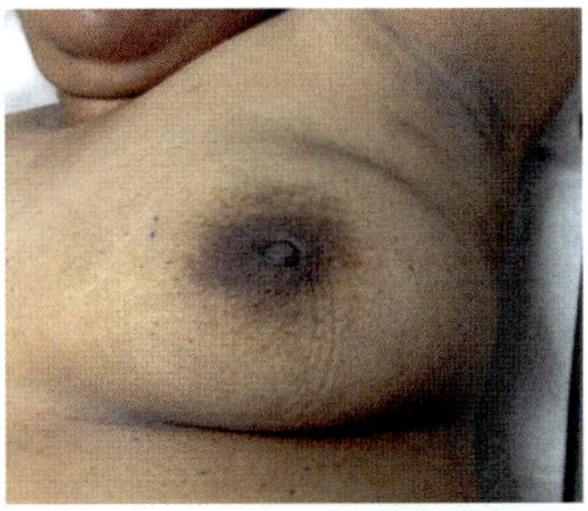	No reaction	• Cleanse daily with mild soap and water • Apply Lotion Soft twice a day
2	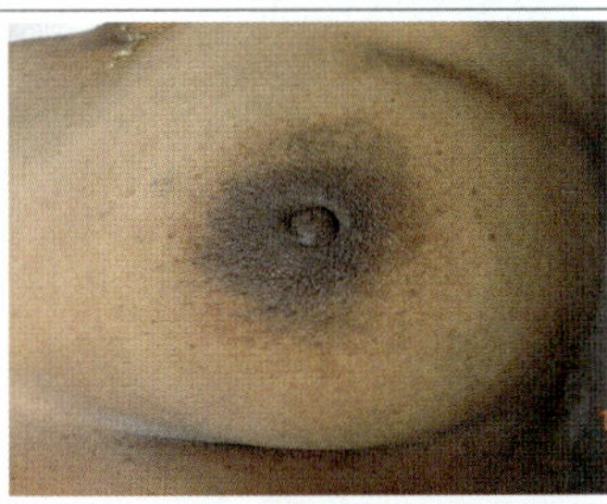	No reaction	• Cleanse daily with mild soap and water • Apply Lotion Soft twice a day
3	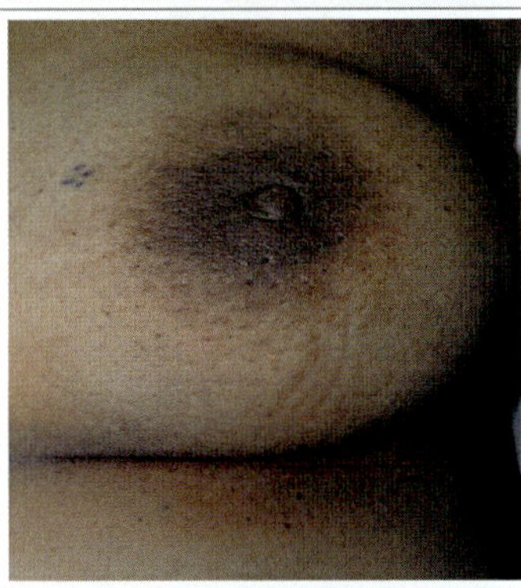	Hyperpigmentation and early erythema in the inframammary fold	• Cleanse daily with mild soap and water • Switch to calendula cream and apply twice a day • Avoid application 3 h prior to receiving radiation
4	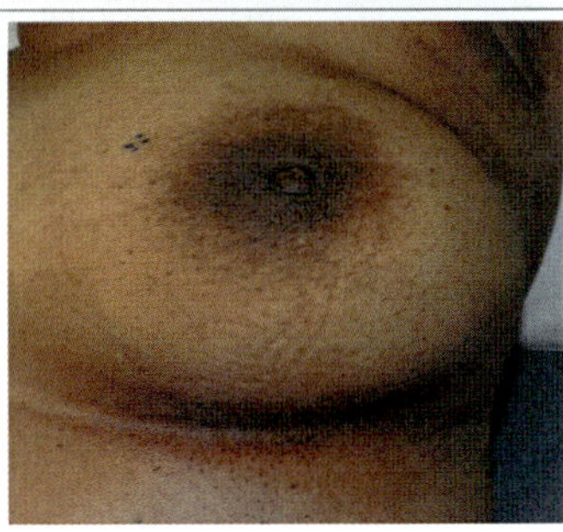	Erythema most prominent in the inframammary fold and axilla with hyperpigmentation	• Apply Skintegrity spray once a day to skin before shower and rinse off after 1–2 min • Continue calendula twice a day • Liberally apply A&D Ointment to radiated site once a day at bedtime. It does not need to be washed off in the morning. Patient can wear an old cotton tee shirt as the ointment has a faint yellow tinge and can stain sheets and undergarments

(continued)

Table 7.3 (continued)

Week	Skin reaction	Reaction type	Intervention
5	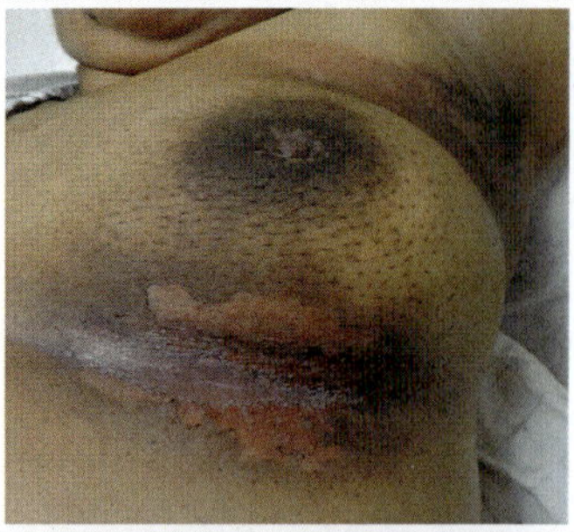	On treatment; combination of early moist desquamation, dry desquamation, and hyperpigmentation	• Continue Skintegrity once a day to the entire radiation site • Manually debride areas of dry desquamation • Continue calendula once to twice a day
5	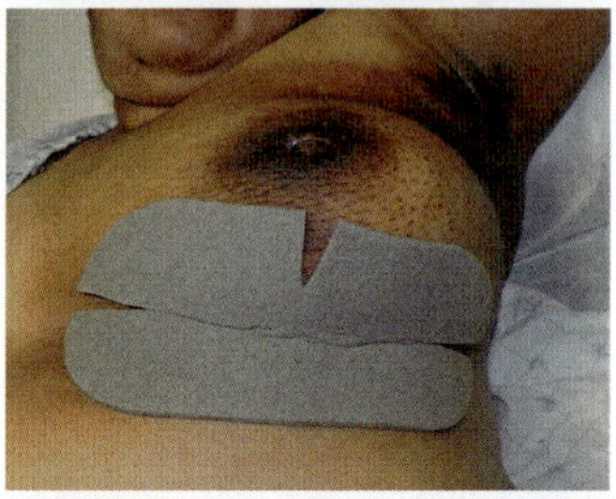	Moist desquamation with Mepilex Ag	• Apply Mepilex Ag to areas of moist desquamation to protect and allow healing • Ensure dressings are completely removed from skin prior to radiation treatment • Continue A&D Ointment, to the undressed area, once a day before bed
1 week post radiation	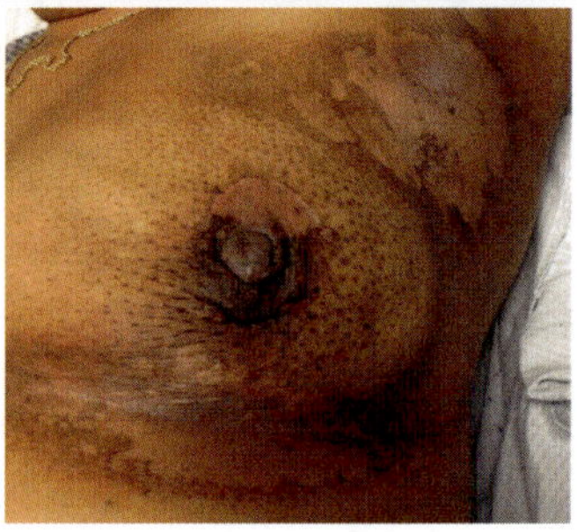	Dry desquamation; evidence of peeling has occurred	• Continue Skintegrity once a day • Manually debride peeling skin with tweezers or gently with clean gauze • Continue calendula twice a day • Continue A&D Ointment once a day at bedtime • Avoid agents that will dry the skin (Domeboro, aloe vera) as this will cause discomfort to the patient • Mepilex Lite to the inframammary fold and axilla as needed to reduce skin friction and promote comfort
2 weeks post radiation	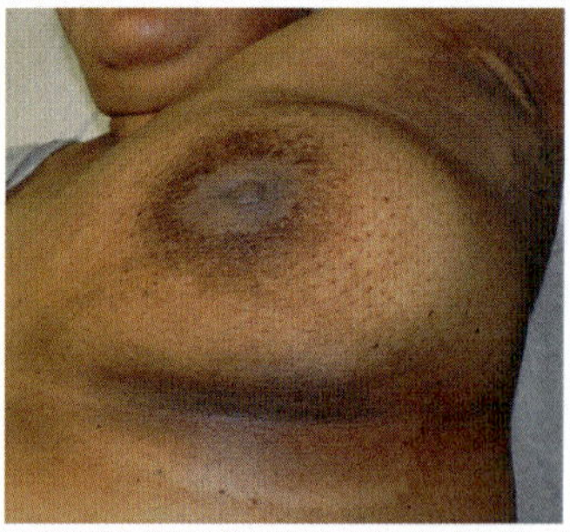	Resolution of desquamation and resolving of hyperpigmentation	• Cleanse daily with mild soap and water • Moisturize daily with an agent of patient's choice • May continue or discontinue Skintegrity

Table 7.4 Examples of typical acute skin reactions and recommended interventions for women undergoing mastectomy with autologous reconstruction and postmastectomy radiation are provided below

Week	Skin reaction	Reaction type	Intervention
1–2	58-year-old Caucasian female with stage III right breast cancer S/P deep inferior epigastric perforator (DIEP) reconstruction. Custom bolus used every other day 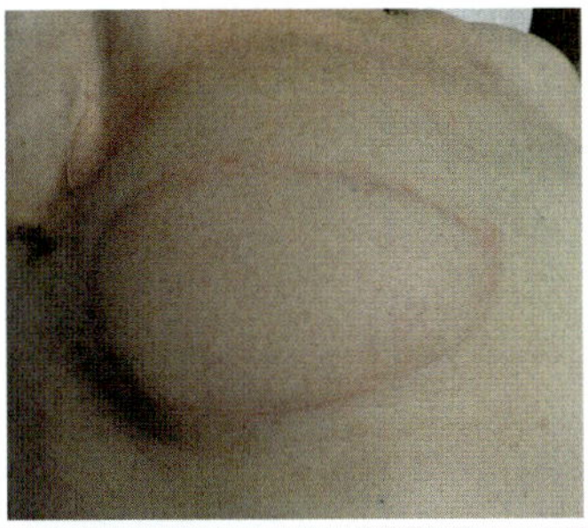	No reaction	• Cleanse daily with mild soap and water • Apply a thin coat of 1 % hydrocortisone cream twice a day • Apply Lotion Soft twice a day • Avoid application 3 h prior to receiving radiation
3	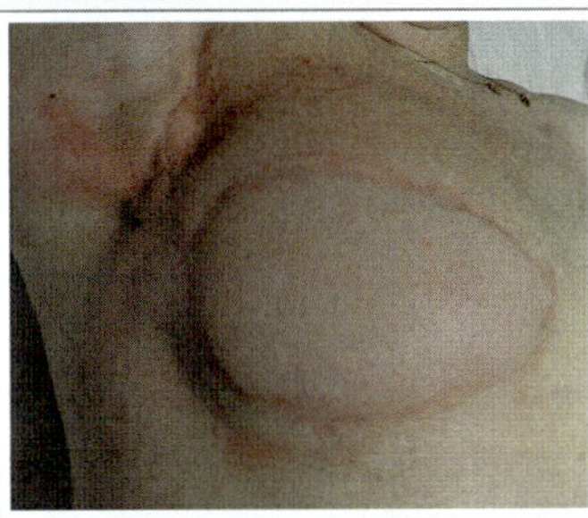	Diffuse mild erythema	• Cleanse with Skintegrity spray once a day. Allow to remain on the skin for 1–2 min and then rinse off • Continue to apply a thin coat of 1 % hydrocortisone cream twice a day • Switch to calendula cream and apply twice a day • Avoid application 3 h prior to receiving radiation
4	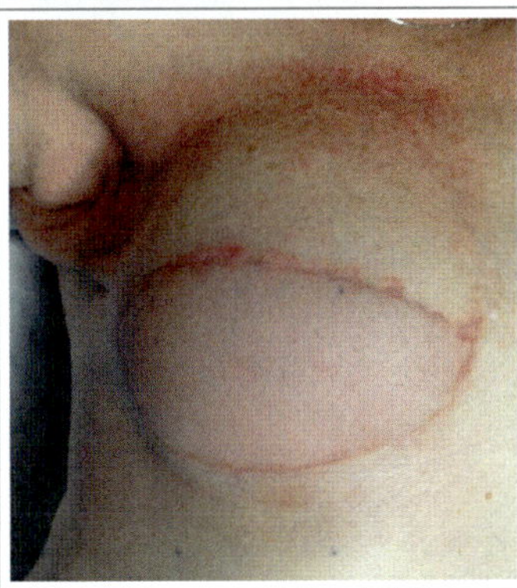	Erythema and follicular reaction on upper inner quadrant	• Continue to cleanse with Skintegrity spray once a day • Continue hydrocortisone twice a day • Continue to apply calendula cream once or twice a day • Liberally apply A&D Ointment to radiated site once a day at bedtime. It does not need to be washed off in the morning. Patient can wear an old cotton tee shirt as the ointment has a faint yellow tinge and can stain sheets and undergarments

(continued)

Table 7.4 (continued)

Week	Skin reaction	Reaction type	Intervention
5	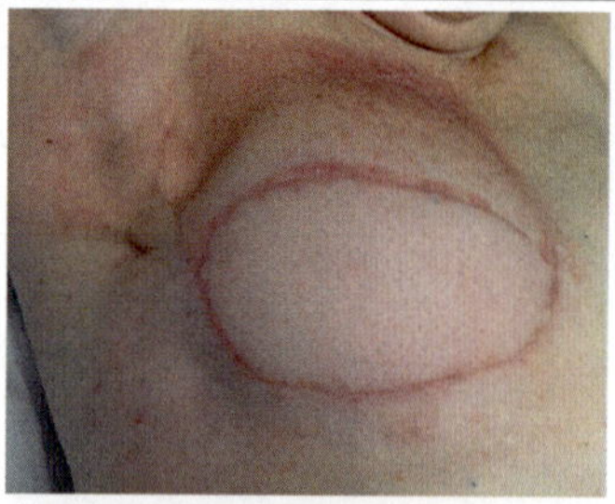 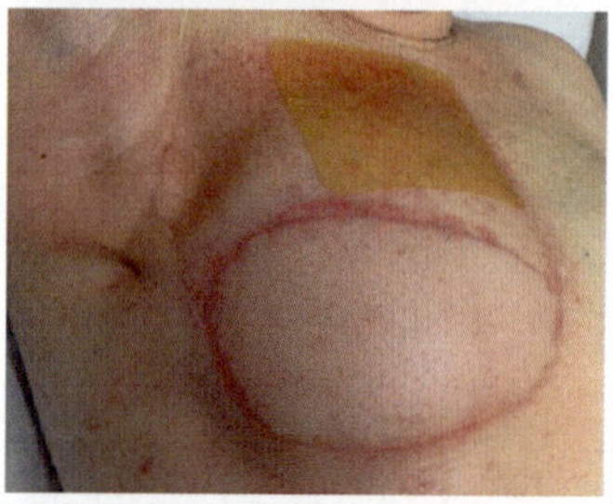	Erythema with pruritic follicular reaction	• Continue to cleanse with Skintegrity spray once a day • Medihoney HFC pad to follicular reaction. Leave in place for 24–48 h (remove prior to treatment) • Continue hydrocortisone twice a day to remaining skin • Continue to apply calendula cream and A&D ointment once a day to the uncovered skin
6 months post radiation	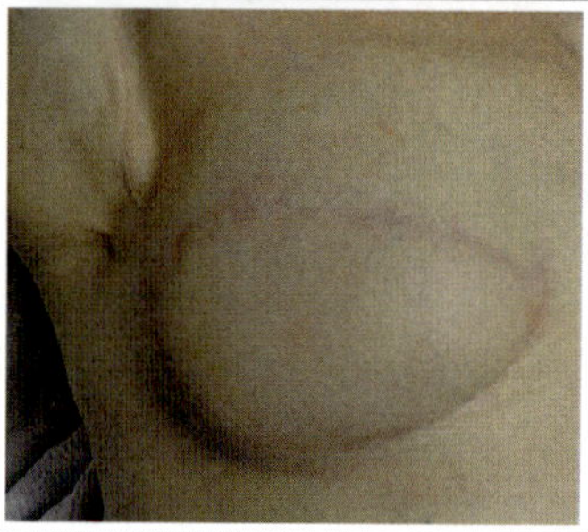		• Continue to moisturize the skin daily with a moisturizing agent of the patient's choice

Table 7.5 Examples of typical acute skin reactions and recommended interventions for women undergoing total skin-sparing mastectomy with implant-based reconstruction and postmastectomy radiation are provided below

Week	Skin reaction	Reaction type	Intervention
1–2	47-year-old Caucasian female with Stage III breast cancer S/P total skin-sparing mastectomy (TSSM). Custom bolus used every other day 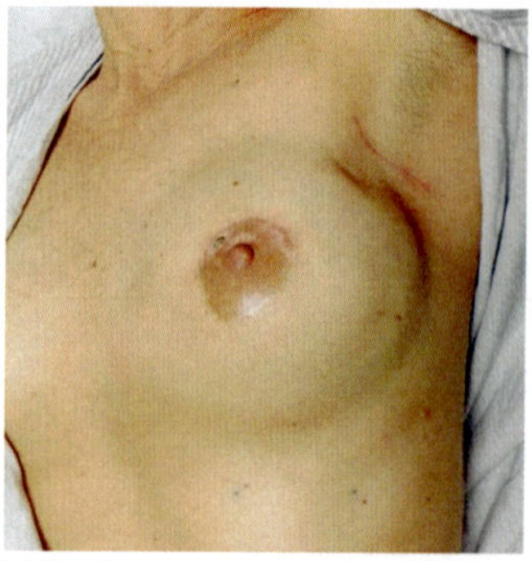	No reaction	• Cleanse daily with mild soap and water • Apply a light moisturizer such as Lotion Soft twice a day

(continued)

Table 7.5 (continued)

Week	Skin reaction	Reaction type	Intervention
3	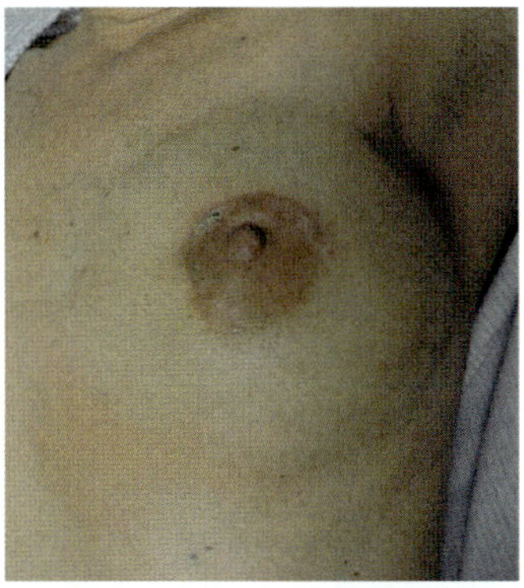	Mild hyperpigmentation	• Cleanse daily with mild soap and water • Continue light moisturizer twice a day • Avoid application 3 h prior to receiving radiation
4	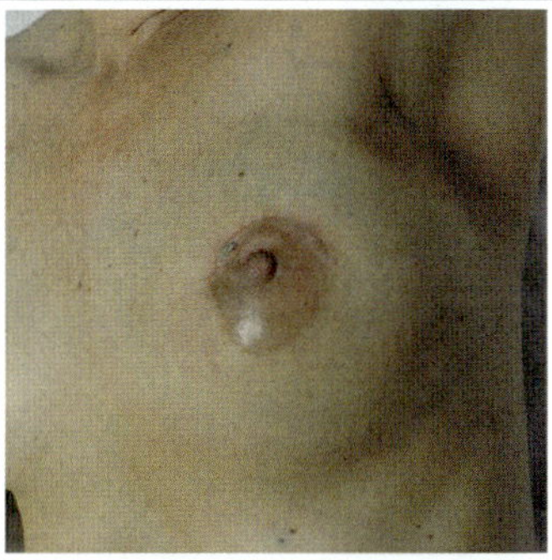	Early erythema	• Cleanse with Skintegrity spray once a day. Allow to remain on the skin for 1–2 min and then rinse off • Switch to calendula cream and apply twice a day • Avoid application 3 h prior to receiving radiation
5	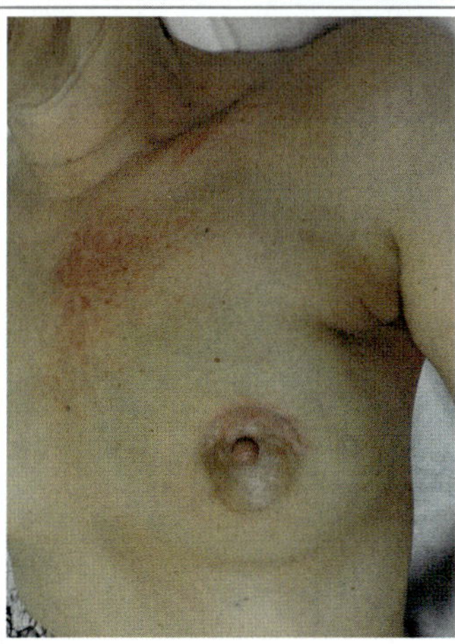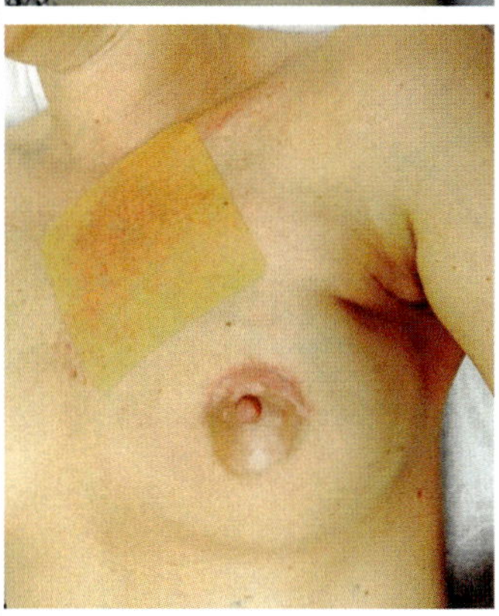	Follicular reaction and mild erythema Medihoney HFC pad applied to follicular reaction	• Continue to cleanse with Skintegrity spray once a day • Continue calendula twice a day • Apply 1 % hydrocortisone cream to the follicular reaction, twice a day, or apply Medihoney HFC pad to the area and leave in place till next radiation treatment • Liberally apply A&D Ointment to radiated site once a day at bedtime. It does not need to be washed off in the morning. Patient can wear an old cotton tee shirt as the ointment has a faint yellow tinge and can stain sheets and undergarments

(continued)

Table 7.5 (continued)

Week	Skin reaction	Reaction type	Intervention
1 week post radiation	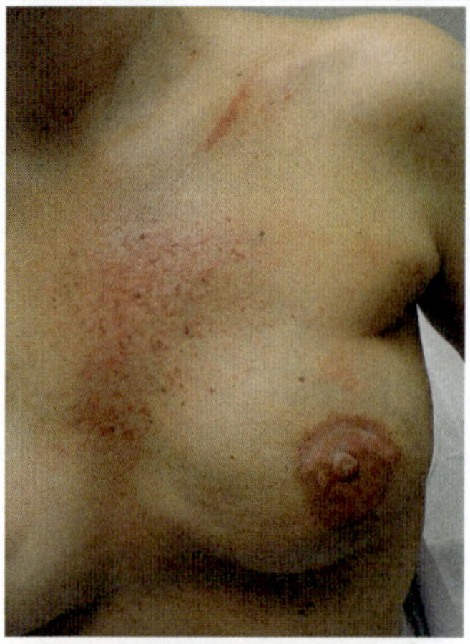	Brisk erythema with continued follicular reaction	• Manually debride areas of dry desquamation • Continue treatment as above
2 weeks post radiation	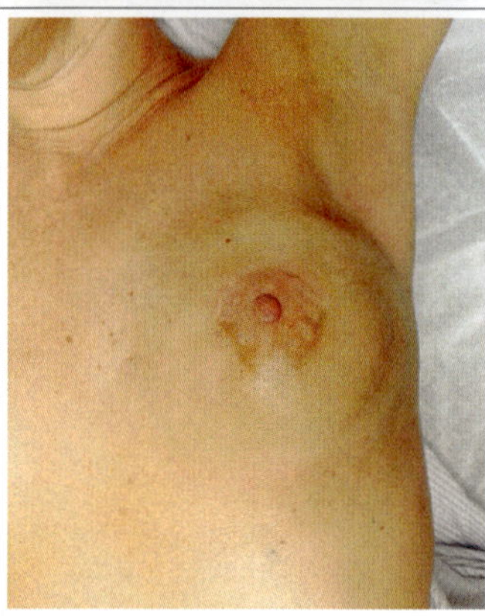		• Continue to cleanse with Skintegrity spray once a day • Continue to apply calendula twice a day • Apply Mepilex Ag to moist desquamation to allow healing and prevent infection • Cleanse daily with mild soap and water. Moisturize area with agent of choice
1 week post radiation	43-year-old Asian female with chest wall recurrence. S/P total skin-sparing mastectomy and permanent implant. Treated with custom bolus every other day 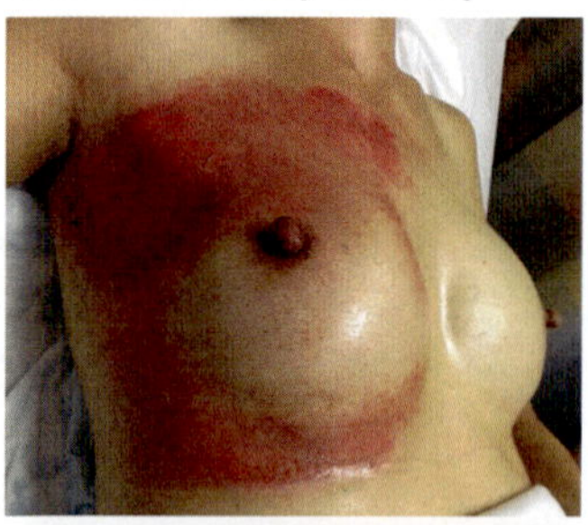 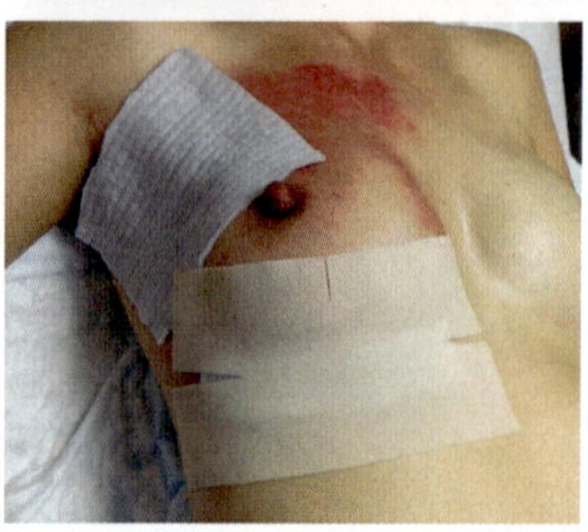	Moist desquamation and marked erythema	• Cleanse with diluted 0.5 % Hibiclens wash or Skintegrity spray once a day. Allow to remain on the skin for 1–2 min to and then rinse off • Apply Aquacel Ag (or similar dressing) cut to fit over the area of moist desquamation. Cover this with a secondary dressing, such as Mepilex Lite • May apply Cavillon No Sting Barrier under the edges of the Mepilex to help it adhere to the skin better • Do not use tape or adhesives on the radiated skin • Continue calendula cream to undressed skin • Change dressing every 24 h • Wet the primary dressing thoroughly if it does not come off easily to avoid traumatizing new skin with dressing removal

(continued)

Table 7.5 (continued)

Week	Skin reaction	Reaction type	Intervention
2–3 weeks post radiation	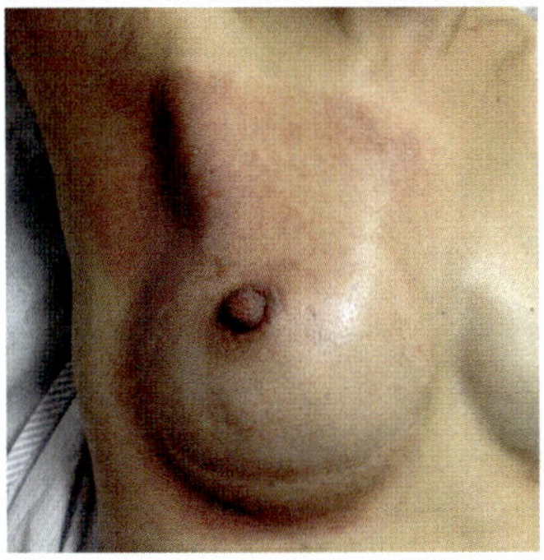	Resolved moist desquamation with residual hyperpigmentation	• Continue to moisturize the skin daily with calendula or a moisturizing agent of the patient's choice

Table 7.6 Examples of typical acute skin reactions and recommended interventions for women undergoing mastectomy without reconstruction. Bolus used every other day

Week	Skin reaction	Reaction type	Intervention
3–4	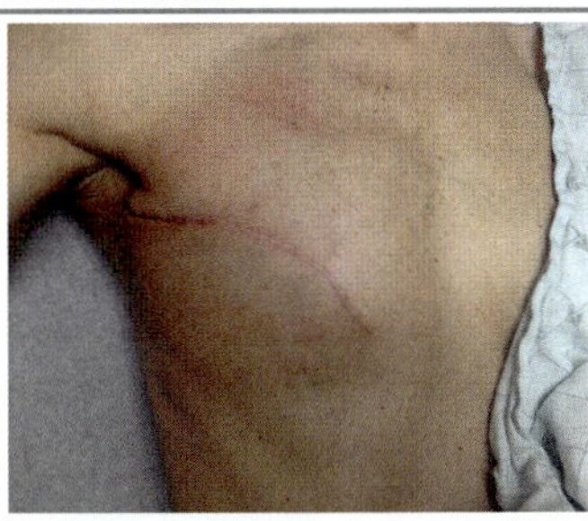	Hyperpigmentation and mild erythema	• Cleanse the site daily with Skintegrity. Spray once a day to the skin and rinse off after 1–2 min in shower • Discontinue Lotion Soft • Switch to calendula cream and apply twice a day • Avoid application 3 h prior to receiving radiation
4–5	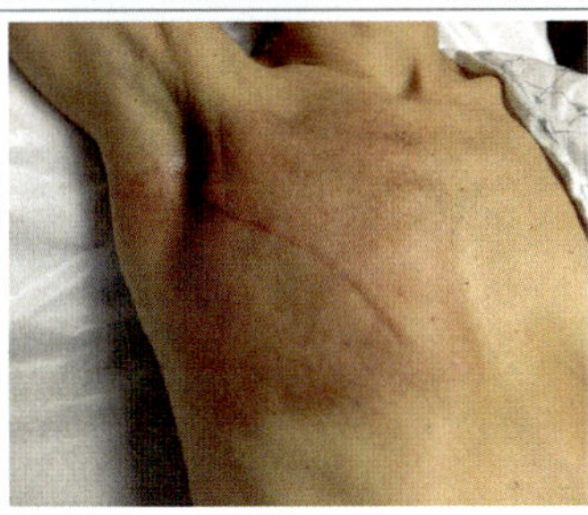	Moderate erythema, hyperpigmentation, and dry desquamation in the axilla	• Cleanse the site daily with Skintegrity spray once a day to the skin, allow it to sit for 1–2 min, and then rinse it off in the shower • Continue calendula twice a day • Liberally apply A&D Ointment to radiated site once a day before bed. It does not need to be washed off in the morning. Patient should wear an old cotton tee shirt as the ointment has a faint yellow tinge and can stain sheets and undergarments • Continue A&D Ointment for 1 week post radiation and then discontinue • Manually debride peeling skin with tweezers or gently wipe the area with clean gauze if tolerated by the patient • Avoid agents that will dry the skin (Domeboro, aloe vera) as this will cause discomfort to the patient • Mepilex Lite can be applied to the axilla as needed to reduce friction • Ensure dressings are completely removed from the skin prior to radiation treatment

(continued)

Table 7.6 (continued)

Week	Skin reaction	Reaction type	Intervention
2 weeks post radiation	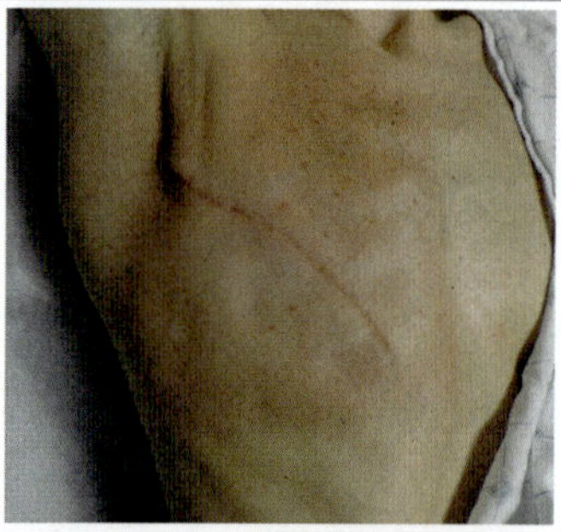	Resolution of desquamation and reduction of hyperpigmentation	• Cleanse daily with mild soap and water • Discontinue Skintegrity • Discontinue A&D Ointment • Avoid agents that will dry the skin • Moisturize daily with calendula or an agent of patient's choice
6 months post radiation	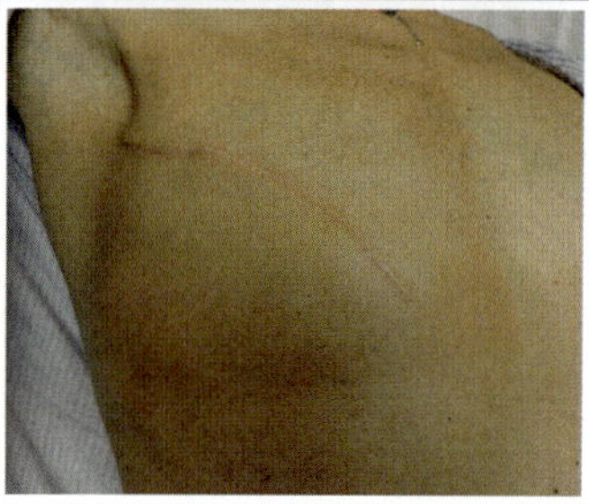	Mild residual hyperpigmentation	• Moisturize daily with agent of patient's choice

Table 7.7 Skin reaction by ethnicity: week five, breast-conserving surgery plus radiation

Asian	Caucasian	African American	Filipino	Hispanic
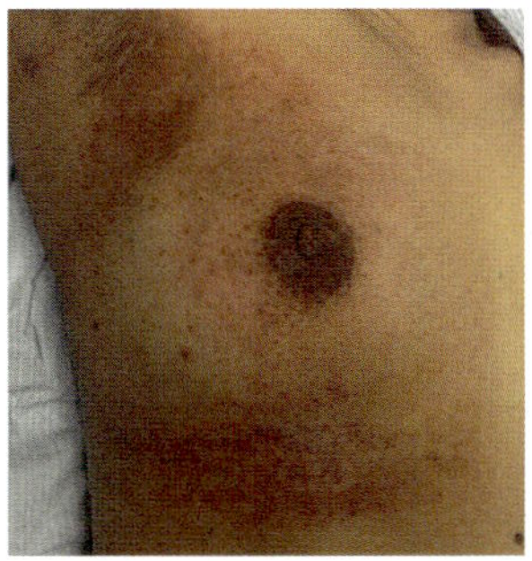	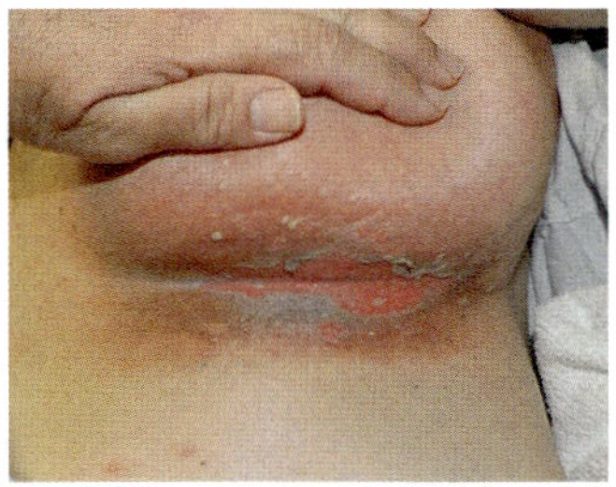	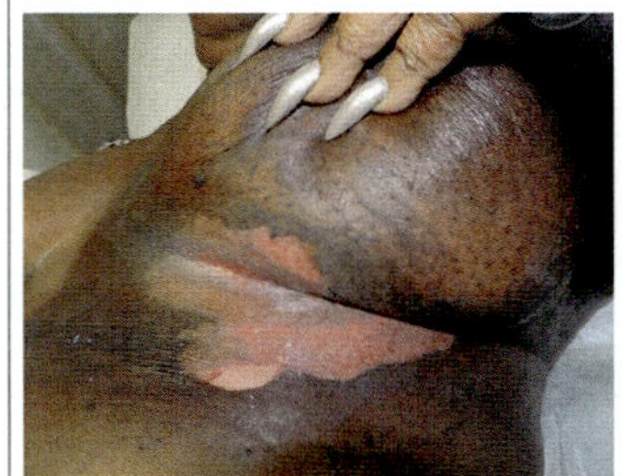	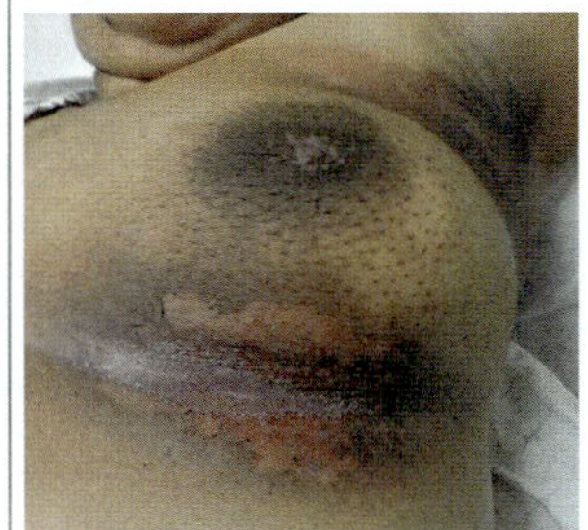	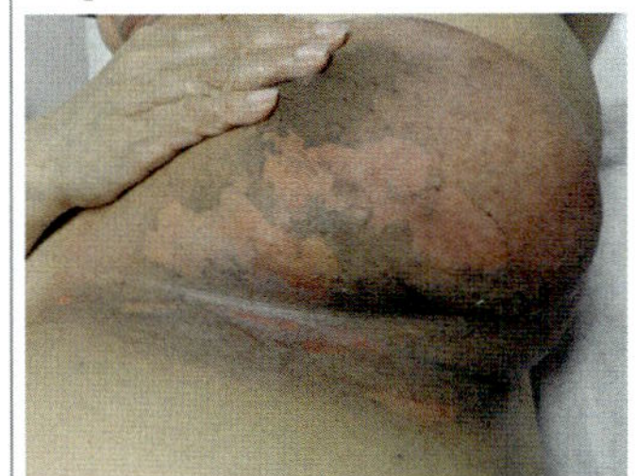

Table 7.8 Special cases and reactions

Special cases and reactions	Reaction type	Treatment and intervention
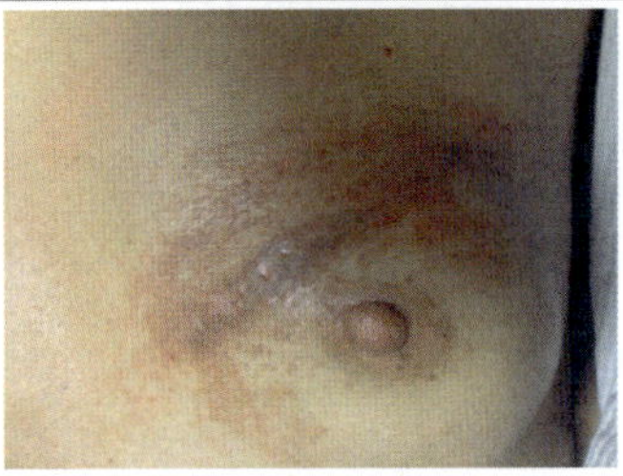 Caucasian female with development of cutaneous candidiasis along incision site that had been sealed with glue	Cutaneous candidiasis	• Cleanse daily with mild soap and water • Hold or discontinue the moisturizing agents over the affected site • Apply clotrimazole cream and 1 % HC cream in equal amounts to the area three times daily for 7–10 days • If no improvement in 72 h, switch to Miconazole cream
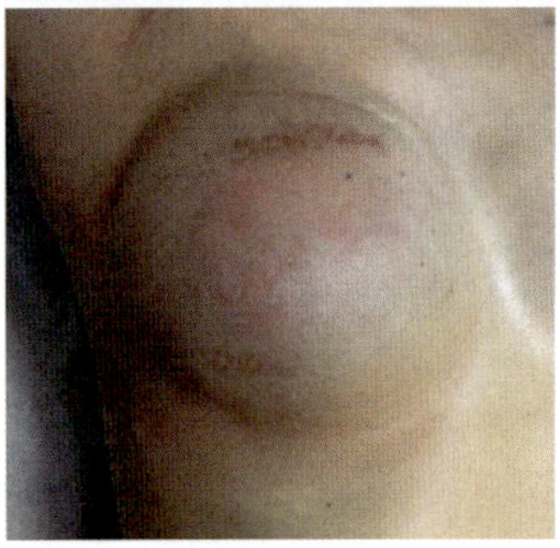 2 weeks post radiation to reconstructed breast Caucasian female with cellulitis, reconstructed breast following upper respiratory tract infection	Cellulitis in reconstructed breast	• Cleanse daily with mild soap and water • Moisturize lightly • Oral antibiotics (Septra DS, doxycycline, clindamycin) • Communicate findings with plastic surgeon • Follow up in 48–72 h to ensure improvement
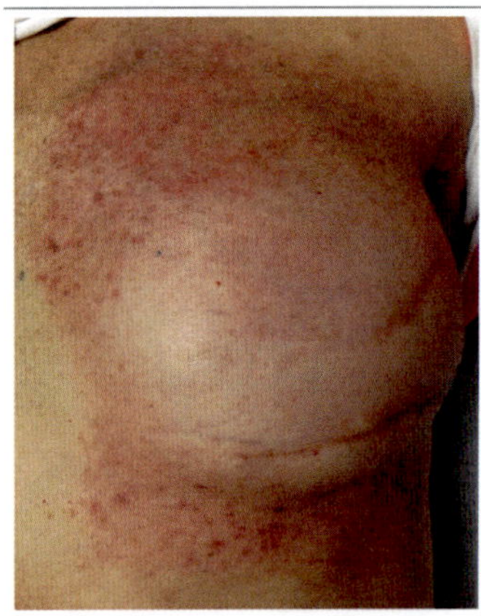 Caucasian female 1 week post radiation to her reconstructed breast	Folliculitis upper inner aspect and inframammary fold	• Cleanse daily with Skintegrity spray or mild soap and water • Apply Medihoney hydrogel pad to affected area. Leave in place for 24 h. Reapply daily as needed

(continued)

Table 7.8 (continued)

<table>
<tr><th>Special cases and reactions</th><th>Reaction type</th><th>Treatment and intervention</th></tr>
<tr><td>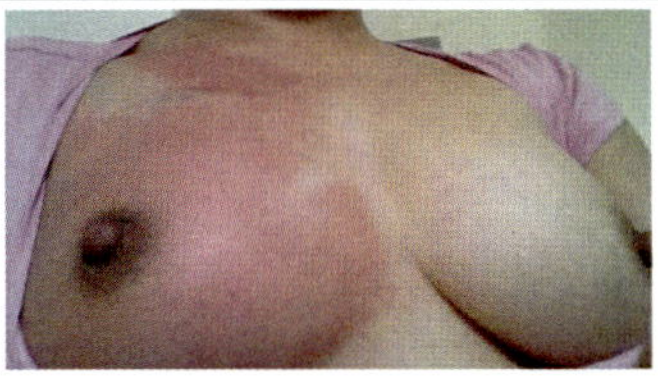
Asian female 1 year post radiation</td><td>Radiation recall with initiation of chemotherapy</td><td>• Cleanse daily with mild soap and water
• Keep skin clean and dry
• Moisturize twice daily with calendula or a light moisturizer
• Consider topical or oral steroids
• No antibiotics or antimicrobials needed unless infection occurs
• Usually self-limiting</td></tr>
<tr><td>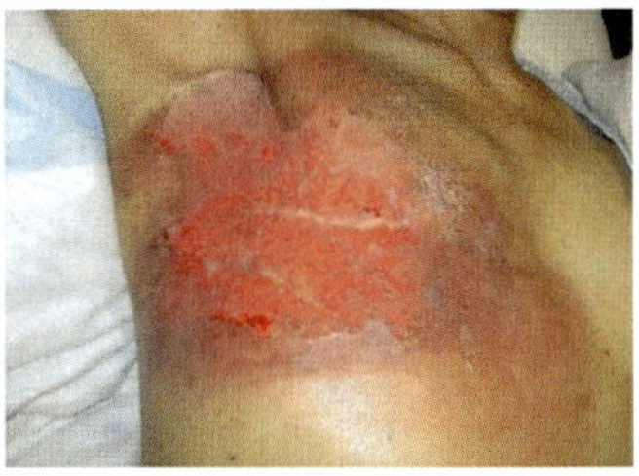
Vietnamese female 6 weeks post radiation for chest wall recurrence with new onset of moist desquamation</td><td>Radiation recall with moist desquamation following liposomal doxorubicin transarterial chemoembolization for hepatocellular cancer</td><td>• Cleanse daily with diluted Hibiclens 0.5 %. Rinse this away
• Apply Aquacel Ag or Mepilex Ag to the desquamated area. Ensure that the Aquacel Ag covers the wound
• Cover with Mepilex Lite
• Secure in place with an abdominal binder or snug fitting tunic</td></tr>
<tr><td>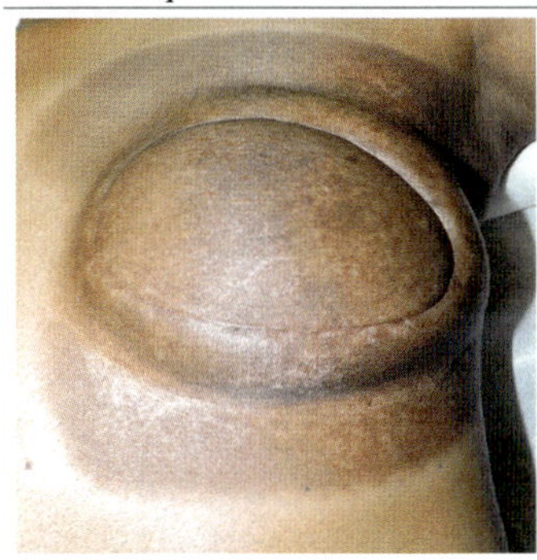
Indian female with locally recurrent inflammatory breast cancer. Bolus daily with concurrent Xeloda and chest wall boost</td><td>Continued hyperpigmentation 6 months post radiation</td><td>• Cleanse daily with mild soap and water
• Moisturize daily with calendula or agent of the patient's choice
• This may take months to years to fade
• Consider dermatology referral for application of tretinoin gel 0.01 %</td></tr>
<tr><td>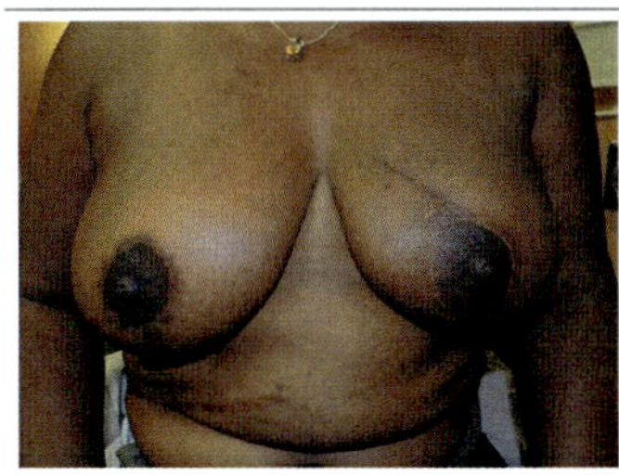
56-year-old African-American female 5 years post completion of radiation for T1aNi+left breast cancer</td><td>Complete resolution</td><td>• Tretinoin gel was applied to the left breast daily for a 1-month period to diminish persistent moderate to marked hyperpigmentation. Skin pigmentation left breast now almost identical to right
• Per personal communication from Dr. William Keith, Los Angeles, California</td></tr>
</table>

(continued)

Table 7.8 (continued)

Special cases and reactions	Reaction type	Treatment and intervention
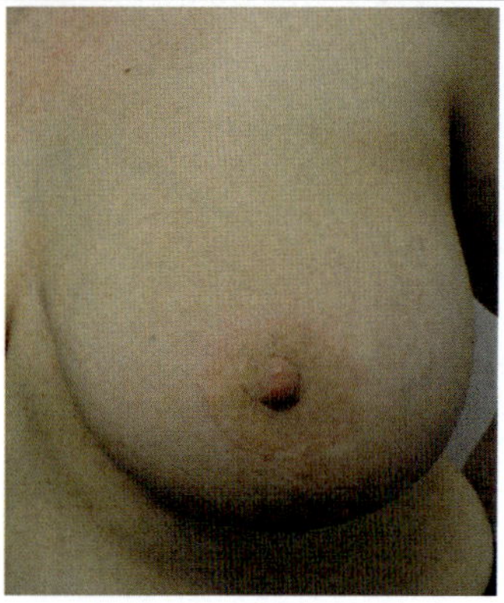 Caucasian female with breast-conserving therapy and mastopexy 6 months post radiation	Mild residual hyperpigmentation as a result of radiation and tamoxifen	• Cleanse daily with mild soap and water • Moisturize daily with calendula or agent of the patient's choice • Hyperpigmentation will continue to resolve, but reaction may be prolonged with patients on endocrine therapy
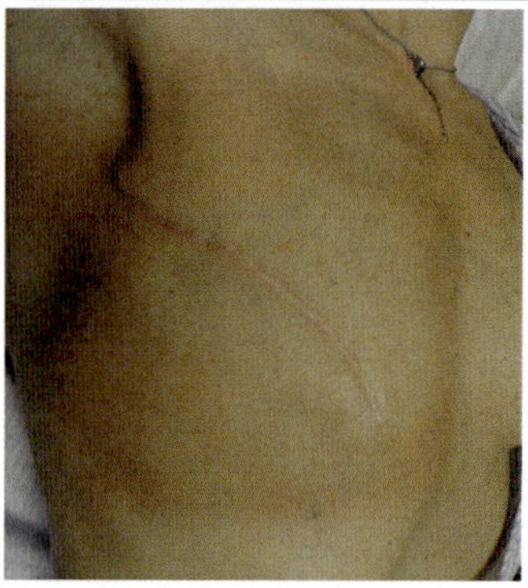 Caucasian female with mastectomy 6 months post radiation	Residual hyperpigmentation as a result of radiation and tamoxifen	• Cleanse daily with mild soap and water • Moisturize daily with calendula or agent of the patient's choice • Hyperpigmentation will continue to resolve, but reaction may be prolonged with patients on endocrine therapy
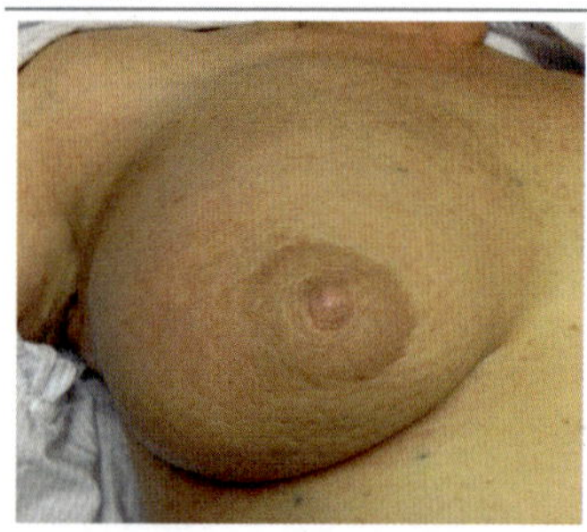 Caucasian female 4 months post radiation	Breast edema 4 months post radiation therapy	• Cleanse daily with mild soap and water • Moisturize daily with calendula or agent of the patient's choice • Advised to wear a well-fitting sport bra for comfort and compression • Physical therapy with manual lymph massage

(continued)

Table 7.8 (continued)

Special cases and reactions	Reaction type	Treatment and intervention
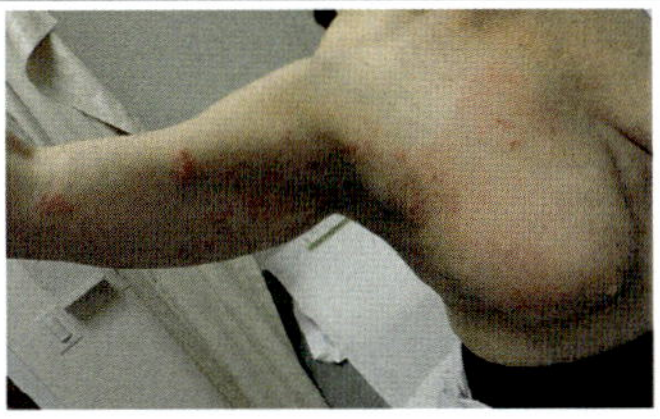 Same Caucasian female as above 6 months post radiation	Zoster and continued breast edema 6 months post radiation	• Cleanse daily with mild soap and water • Moisturize daily with calendula or agent of the patient's choice • Apply Domeboro soaks twice a day as needed for comfort and drying of the lesions • Acyclovir or Valtrex for outbreak with 48–72 h
Patient 16 weeks pregnant post radiation 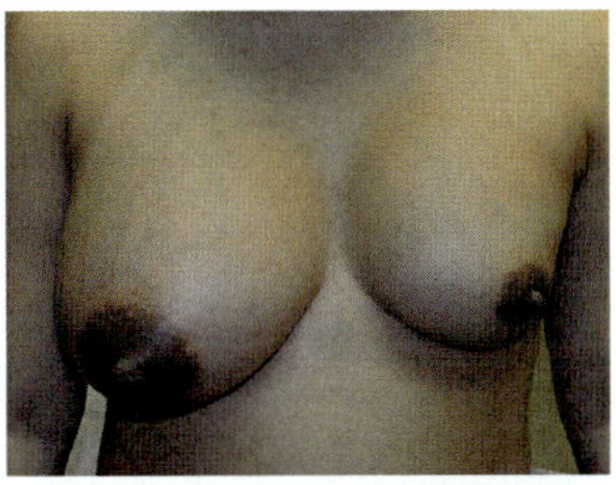		• Left breast post radiation does not enlarge during pregnancy • Prothesis can be added to bra for symmetry
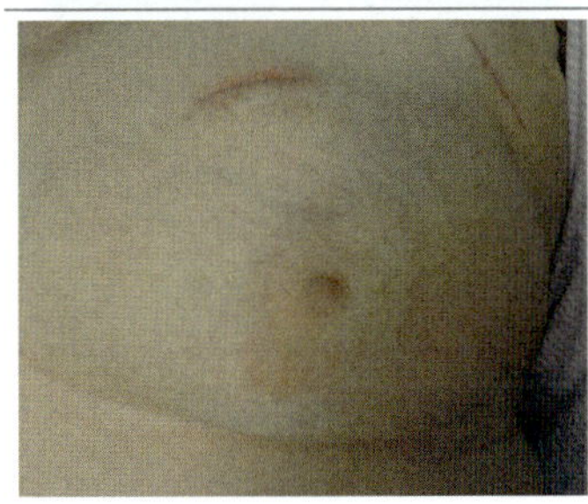 1 month post intraoperative radiation with Intrabeam	Induration, mild erythema, surgical scar	• Moisturize area daily following bath or shower • Gentle manual massage when applying lotion
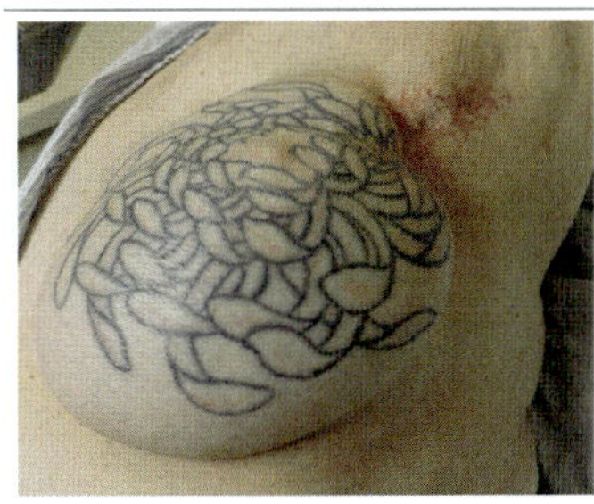 68-year-old female with local recurrence in transverse rectus abdominus myocutaneous flap following mastectomy	Radiation for recurrence was completed in 2008, and patient has continued to develop telangiectasias in the area of the boost field. Chrysanthemum tattoo was added to improve cosmetic appearance	• Pulse laser therapy if desired to remove telangiectasias. No treatment or intervention needed if appearance is not bothersome

(continued)

Table 7.8 (continued)

Special cases and reactions	Reaction type	Treatment and intervention
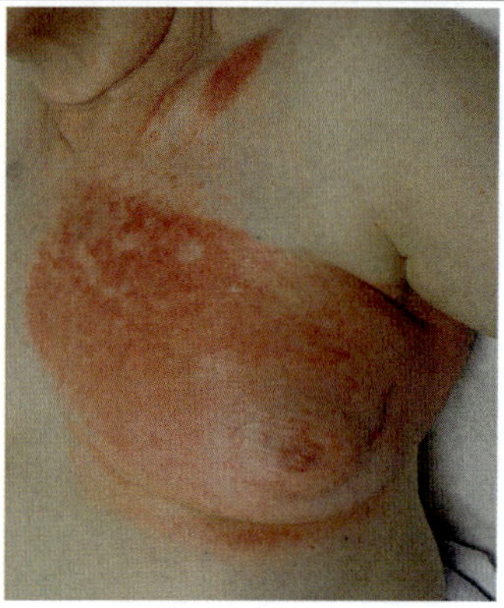 66-year-old female with inflammatory breast cancer and drug-induced cutaneous lupus erythematosus receiving preoperative radiation. Custom bolus used every third day	Patient received trastuzumab and pertuzumab during radiation as well as hydroxychloroquine (for cutaneous lupus) 10 days post radiation	• Cleanse the site daily with Skintegrity. Spray once a day to the skin and rinse off after 1–2 min in shower • Liberally apply GlucanPro 3000 ointment two to three times a day to the radiation site • Patient wore a cotton tee shirt, no other dressing applied
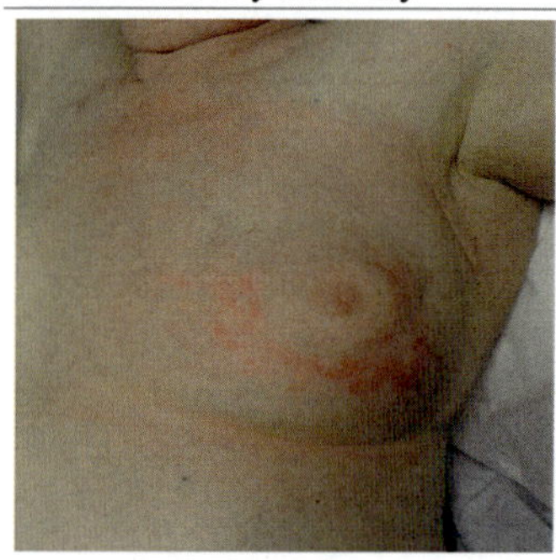	Resolution of erythema 3 weeks post radiation	• Cleanse the site daily with Skintegrity. Spray once a day to the skin and rinse off after 1–2 min in shower • Continue GlucanPro 3000 cream twice daily or switch to calendula cream for an additional 1–2 weeks • Patient wore a cotton tee shirt, no other dressing applied *GlucanPro 3000 ointment and cream are emollients containing oat beta-glucan and were effective for decreasing her pruritus, desquamation, and residual hyperpigmentation
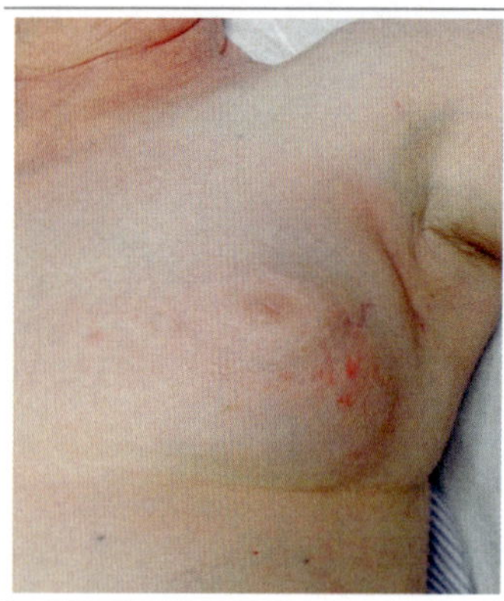	Resolution of erythema 4 weeks post radiation	• Patient was instructed to cleanse the site daily with mild soap and water • Moisturize daily with remaining glucan cream or a light moisturizer

Table 7.8 (continued)

<table>
<tr><th>Special cases and reactions</th><th>Reaction type</th><th>Treatment and intervention</th></tr>
<tr><td>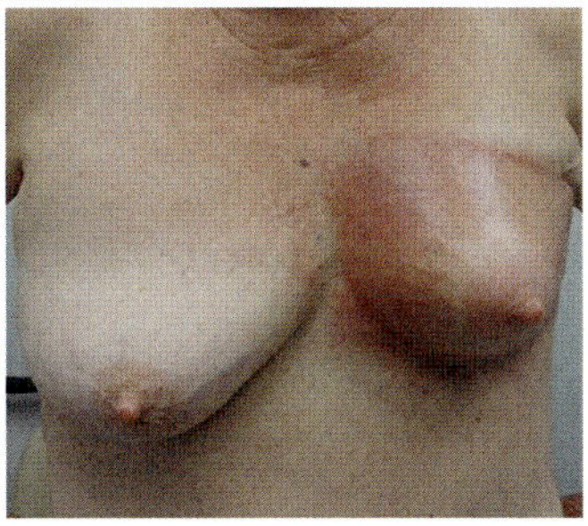
Photo courtesy of Jyoti Mayadev, MD
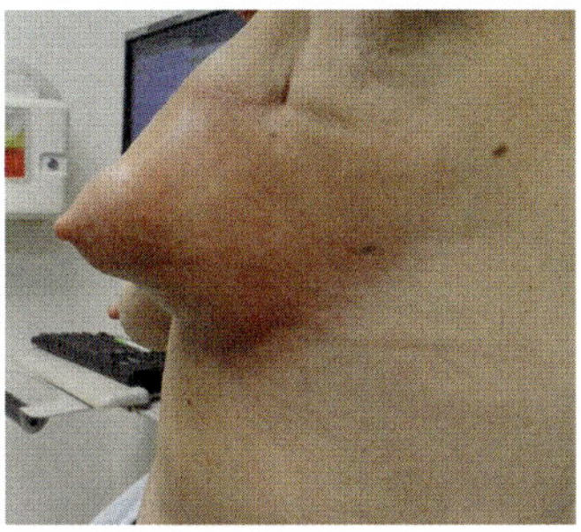
70-year-old female with pT2N0 luminal A cancer S/P lumpectomy and radiation
Photo courtesy of Jyoti Mayadev, MD</td><td>Radiation-induced morphea presenting 7 months post treatment</td><td>• Improvement may occur spontaneously but is unlikely. Treatment may include topical steroids, systemic immunosuppressants, phototherapy, topical tacrolimus, imiquimod, calcipotriol cream with topical steroid. Success is limited. Mastectomy has rarely been employed [135]</td></tr>
</table>

Week	Apply to Radiated Area	Notes
1-2	Lotion Soft → Apply 2x/day	Lotion Soft is a thin moisturizing lotion that is quickly absorbed.
3	Switch to calendula → Apply 2x/day	Calendula is a thicker cream used to help maintain moisture. Continue for at least 1- 2 weeks post radiation.
4-6 (Without Moist Desquamation)	Calendula → Apply 1-2x/day A&D Ointment → Apply 1x/day at night. Skintegrity → Spray 1x/day on affected area and wash off in shower or bath after 1-2 minutes.	Important to apply this combination as erythema progresses and moisture loss becomes apparent. Apply calendula 1-2 times a day. Apply A&D at night. Spray Skintegrity daily before bathing and rinse off to prevent build up residue on the skin.
4-6 (With Moist Desquamation)	Cleanser: Skintegrity OR 0.5% Hibiclens Solution Dressing: Aquacel AG OR Mepilex Ag Antibiotic: Topical Bacitracin and Zinc oxide OR Mupirocin; Oral (Bactrim, doxycycline, clindamycin) if . . .	Cleanser Cleanse with 0.5% Hibiclens solution or Skintegrity and wash off after 1-2 minutes. 3 Dressings Options 1. Apply Aquacel Ag and cover with Mepilex lite. 2. Apply zinc and bacitracin in a 1:1 mixture. Cover with Mepilex lite and leave in place for 24 hours. 3. Apply Mepilex Ag alone over desquamated area.
1-3 Weeks Post Radiation	Calendula → Apply 2x/day + A&D Ointment → Apply 1x/day at night. + Skintegrity → Spray 1x/day on affected area and wash off in shower after 1-2 minutes.	Apply calendula twice a day until normal skin color returns. Apply A&D for 1-2 weeks post radiation. Continue Skintegrity until dry desquamation is resolved.

Fig. 7.1 Suggested treatment algorithm for skin care

References

1. Cancer Facts and Figures 2015. American Cancer Society. 2015. http://www.cancer.org/research/cancerfactsstatistics/cancerfactsfigures2015/index. Accessed 16 Apr 2015
2. Albornoz CR, Cordeiro PG, Pusic AL, McCarthy CM, Mehrara BJ, Disa JJ, et al. Diminishing relative contraindications for immediate breast reconstruction: a multicenter study. J Am Coll Surg. 2014;219:788–95. doi:10.1016/j.jamcollsurg.2014.05.012.
3. Kummerow KL, Du L, Penson DF, Shyr Y, Hooks MA. Nationwide trends in mastectomy for early-stage breast cancer. JAMA Surg. 2015;150:9–16. doi:10.1001/jamasurg.2014.2895.
4. Jagsi R, Abrahamse P, Morrow M, Hawley ST, Griggs JJ, Graff JJ, et al. Patterns and correlates of adjuvant radiotherapy receipt after lumpectomy and after mastectomy for breast cancer. J Clin Oncol. 2010;28:2396–403. doi:10.1200/JCO.2009.26.8433.
5. Pignol JP, Olivotto I, Rakovitch E, Gardner S, Sixel K, Beckham W, et al. A multicenter randomized trial of breast intensity-modulated radiation therapy to

reduce acute radiation dermatitis. J Clin Oncol. 2008;26:2085–92. doi:10.1200/JCO.2007.15.2488.
6. Pignol JP, Vu TT, Mitera G, Bosnic S, Verkooijen HM, Truong P. Prospective evaluation of severe skin toxicity and pain during postmastectomy radiation therapy. Int J Radiat Oncol Biol Phys. 2015;91:157–64. doi:10.1016/j.ijrobp.2014.09.022.
7. Hindley A, Zain Z, Wood L, Whitehead A, Sanneh A, Barber D, et al. Mometasone furoate cream reduces acute radiation dermatitis in patients receiving breast radiation therapy: results of a randomized trial. Int J Radiat Oncol Biol Phys. 2014;90:748–55. doi:10.1016/j.ijrobp.2014.06.033.
8. Hoopfer D, Holloway C, Gabos Z, Alidrisi M, Chafe S, Krause B, et al. Three-arm randomized phase iii trial: quality aloe and placebo cream versus powder as skin treatment during breast cancer radiation therapy. Clin Breast Cancer. 2014. doi:10.1016/j.clbc.2014.12.006.
9. RTOG Acute Radiation Morbidity Scoring Criteria. Radiation Therapy Oncology Group. 2015. http://www.rtog.org/ResearchAssociates/AdverseEventReporting/AcuteRadiationMorbidityScoringCriteria.aspx. Accessed 4 May 2015.
10. Common Terminology Criteria for Adverse Events (CTCAE) Version 4.0. In: Cancer Therapy Evaluation Program. National Cancer Institute, National Institutes of Health, U.S. Department of Health and Human Services. 2010. http://evs.nci.nih.gov/ftp1/CTCAE/CTCAE_4.03_2010–06–14_QuickReference_8.5x11.pdf. Accessed 16 Apr 2015.
11. Porock D, Kristjanson L, Nikoletti S, Cameron F, Pedler P. Predicting the severity of radiation skin reactions in women with breast cancer. Oncol Nurs Forum. 1998;25:1019–29.
12. Freedman GM, Li T, Nicolaou N, Chen Y, Ma CC, Anderson PR. Breast intensity-modulated radiation therapy reduces time spent with acute dermatitis for women of all breast sizes during radiation. Int J Radiat Oncol Biol Phys. 2009;74:689–94. doi:10.1016/j.ijrobp.2008.08.071.
13. Wright JL, Takita C, Reis IM, Zhao W, Lee E, Hu JJ. Racial variations in radiation-induced skin toxicity severity: data from a prospective cohort receiving postmastectomy radiation. Int J Radiat Oncol Biol Phys. 2014;90:335–43. doi:10.1016/j.ijrobp.2014.06.042.
14. Fisher J, Scott C, Stevens R, Marconi B, Champion L, Freedman GM, et al. Randomized phase III study comparing Best Supportive Care to Biafine as a prophylactic agent for radiation-induced skin toxicity for women undergoing breast irradiation: Radiation Therapy Oncology Group (RTOG) 97–13. Int J Radiat Oncol Biol Phys. 2000;48:1307–10.
15. Back M, Guerrieri M, Wratten C, Steigler A. Impact of radiation therapy on acute toxicity in breast conservation therapy for early breast cancer. Clin Oncol (R Coll Radiol). 2004;16:12–6.
16. Rutter C, Qin L, Higgins S, Moran M, Evans S. Dosimetric and clinical predictors of the development of moist desquamation in breast cancer irradiation. J Radiat Oncol. 2014;3:147–52. doi:10.1007/s13566-013-0129-0.
17. Freedman GM, Anderson PR, Goldstein LJ, Ma CM, Li J, Swaby RF, et al. Four-week course of radiation for breast cancer using hypofractionated intensity modulated radiation therapy with an incorporated boost. Int J Radiat Oncol Biol Phys. 2007;68:347–53. doi:10.1016/j.ijrobp.2006.12.035.
18. De Langhe S, Mulliez T, Veldeman L, Remouchamps V, van Greveling A, Gilsoul M, et al. Factors modifying the risk for developing acute skin toxicity after whole-breast intensity modulated radiotherapy. BMC Cancer. 2014;14:711. doi:10.1186/1471-2407-14-711.
19. McDonald MW, Godette KD, Butker EK, Davis LW, Johnstone PA. Long-term outcomes of IMRT for breast cancer: a single-institution cohort analysis. Int J Radiat Oncol Biol Phys. 2008;72:1031–40. doi:10.1016/j.ijrobp.2008.02.053.
20. Harsolia A, Kestin L, Grills I, Wallace M, Jolly S, Jones C, et al. Intensity-modulated radiotherapy results in significant decrease in clinical toxicities compared with conventional wedge-based breast radiotherapy. Int J Radiat Oncol Biol Phys. 2007;68:1375–80. doi:10.1016/j.ijrobp.2007.02.044.
21. Graham PH, Plant N, Graham JL, Browne L, Borg M, Capp A, et al. A paired, double-blind, randomized comparison of a moisturizing durable barrier cream to 10% glycerine cream in the prophylactic management of postmastectomy irradiation skin care: trans Tasman Radiation Oncology Group (TROG) 04.01. Int J Radiat Oncol Biol Phys. 2013;86:45–50. doi:10.1016/j.ijrobp.2012.12.009.
22. Ma J, Li J, Xie J, Chen J, Zhu C, Cai G, et al. Post mastectomy linac IMRT irradiation of chest wall and regional nodes: dosimetry data and acute toxicities. Radiat Oncol. 2013;8:81. doi:10.1186/1748-717X-8-81.
23. Spierer MM, Hong LX, Wagman RT, Katz MS, Spierer RL, McCormick B. Postmastectomy CT-based electron beam radiotherapy: dosimetry, efficacy, and toxicity in 118 patients. Int J Radiat Oncol Biol Phys. 2004;60:1182–9. doi:10.1016/j.ijrobp.2004.04.044.
24. Cuaron JJ, Chon B, Tsai H, Goenka A, DeBlois D, Ho A, et al. Early toxicity in patients treated with postoperative proton therapy for locally advanced breast cancer. Int J Radiat Oncol Biol Phys. 2015;92:284–91. doi:10.1016/j.ijrobp.2015.01.005.
25. Freedman GM, Anderson PR, Bleicher RJ, Litwin S, Li T, Swaby RF, et al. Five-year local control in a phase II study of hypofractionated intensity modulated radiation therapy with an incorporated boost for early stage breast cancer. Int J Radiat Oncol Biol Phys. 2012;84:888–93. doi:10.1016/j.ijrobp.2012.01.091.

26. Vicini F, Jones P, Rivers A, Wallace M, Mitchell C, Kestin L, et al. Differences in disease presentation, management techniques, treatment outcome, and toxicities in African-American women with early stage breast cancer treated with breast-conserving therapy. Cancer. 2010;116:3485–92. doi:10.1002/cncr.25088.
27. Verbelen H, Gebruers N, Beyers T, De Monie AC, Tjalma W. Breast edema in breast cancer patients following breast-conserving surgery and radiotherapy: a systematic review. Breast Cancer Res Treat. 2014;147:463–71. doi:10.1007/s10549-014-3110-8.
28. Adriaenssens N, Verbelen H, Lievens P, Lamote J. Lymphedema of the operated and irradiated breast in breast cancer patients following breast conserving surgery and radiotherapy. Lymphology. 2012;45:154–64.
29. Barnett GC, Wilkinson JS, Moody AM, Wilson CB, Twyman N, Wishart GC, et al. The Cambridge Breast Intensity-modulated Radiotherapy Trial: patient- and treatment-related factors that influence late toxicity. Clin Oncol (R Coll Radiol). 2011;23:662–73. doi:10.1016/j.clon.2011.04.011.
30. Fowble B, Fein DA, Hanlon AL, Eisenberg BL, Hoffman JP, Sigurdson ER, et al. The impact of tamoxifen on breast recurrence, cosmesis, complications, and survival in estrogen receptor-positive early-stage breast cancer. Int J Radiat Oncol Biol Phys. 1996;35:669–77.
31. Harris EE, Christensen VJ, Hwang WT, Fox K, Solin LJ. Impact of concurrent versus sequential tamoxifen with radiation therapy in early-stage breast cancer patients undergoing breast conservation treatment. J Clin Oncol. 2005;23:11–6. doi:10.1200/JCO.2005.09.056.
32. Twardella D, Popanda O, Helmbold I, Ebbeler R, Benner A, von Fournier D, et al. Personal characteristics, therapy modalities and individual DNA repair capacity as predictive factors of acute skin toxicity in an unselected cohort of breast cancer patients receiving radiotherapy. Radiother Oncol. 2003;69:145–53.
33. Moody AM, Mayles WP, Bliss JM, A'Hern RP, Owen JR, Regan J, et al. The influence of breast size on late radiation effects and association with radiotherapy dose inhomogeneity. Radiother Oncol. 1994;33:106–12.
34. Tuamokumo NL, Haffty BG. Clinical outcome and cosmesis in African-American patients treated with conservative surgery and radiation therapy. Cancer J. 2003;9:313–20.
35. Pierce L, Fowble B, Solin LJ, Schultz DJ, Rosser C, Goodman RL. Conservative surgery and radiation therapy in black women with early stage breast cancer. Patterns of failure and analysis of outcome. Cancer. 1992;69:2831–41.
36. Ulff E, Maroti M, Serup J, Falkmer U. A potent steroid cream is superior to emollients in reducing acute radiation dermatitis in breast cancer patients treated with adjuvant radiotherapy. A randomised study of betamethasone versus two moisturizing creams. Radiother Oncol. 2013;108:287–92. doi:10.1016/j.radonc.2013.05.033.
37. Fitzpatrick TB. The validity and practicality of sun-reactive skin types I through VI. Arch Dermatol. 1988;124:869–71.
38. Herst PM, Bennett NC, Sutherland AE, Peszynski RI, Paterson DB, Jasperse ML. Prophylactic use of Mepitel Film prevents radiation-induced moist desquamation in an intra-patient randomised controlled clinical trial of 78 breast cancer patients. Radiother Oncol. 2014;110:137–43. doi:10.1016/j.radonc.2014.01.005.
39. Chang-Claude J, Popanda O, Tan XL, Kropp S, Helmbold I, von Fournier D, et al. Association between polymorphisms in the DNA repair genes, XRCC1, APE1, and XPD and acute side effects of radiotherapy in breast cancer patients. Clin Cancer Res. 2005;11:4802–9. doi:10.1158/1078-0432.CCR-04-2657.
40. Tan XL, Popanda O, Ambrosone CB, Kropp S, Helmbold I, von Fournier D, et al. Association between TP53 and p21 genetic polymorphisms and acute side effects of radiotherapy in breast cancer patients. Breast Cancer Res Treat. 2006;97:255–62. doi:10.1007/s10549-005-9119-2.
41. Ho AY, Fan G, Atencio DP, Green S, Formenti SC, Haffty BG, et al. Possession of ATM sequence variants as predictor for late normal tissue responses in breast cancer patients treated with radiotherapy. Int J Radiat Oncol Biol Phys. 2007;69:677–84. doi:10.1016/j.ijrobp.2007.04.012.
42. Andreassen CN, Overgaard J, Alsner J, Overgaard M, Herskind C, Cesaretti JA, et al. ATM sequence variants and risk of radiation-induced subcutaneous fibrosis after postmastectomy radiotherapy. Int J Radiat Oncol Biol Phys. 2006;64:776–83. doi:10.1016/j.ijrobp.2005.09.014.
43. Iannuzzi CM, Atencio DP, Green S, Stock RG, Rosenstein BS. ATM mutations in female breast cancer patients predict for an increase in radiation-induced late effects. Int J Radiat Oncol Biol Phys. 2002;52:606–13.
44. Edvardsen H, Tefre T, Jansen L, Vu P, Haffty BG, Fossa SD, et al. Linkage disequilibrium pattern of the ATM gene in breast cancer patients and controls; association of SNPs and haplotypes to radio-sensitivity and post-lumpectomy local recurrence. Radiat Oncol. 2007;2:25. doi:10.1186/1748-717X-2-25.
45. Pierce LJ, Strawderman M, Narod SA, Oliviotto I, Eisen A, Dawson L, et al. Effect of radiotherapy after breast-conserving treatment in women with breast cancer and germline BRCA1/2 mutations. J Clin Oncol. 2000;18:3360–9.
46. Shanley S, McReynolds K, Ardern-Jones A, Ahern R, Fernando I, Yarnold J, et al. Late toxicity is not increased in BRCA1/BRCA2 mutation carriers undergoing breast radiotherapy in the United

Kingdom. Clin Cancer Res. 2006;12:7025–32. doi:10.1158/1078-0432.CCR-06-1244.

47. Huszno J, Budryk M, Kolosza Z, Nowara E. The influence of BRCA1/BRCA2 mutations on toxicity related to chemotherapy and radiotherapy in early breast cancer patients. Oncology. 2013;85:278–82. doi:10.1159/000354834.
48. Park H, Choi DH, Noh JM, Huh SJ, Park W, Nam SJ, et al. Acute skin toxicity in Korean breast cancer patients carrying BRCA mutations. Int J Radiat Biol. 2014;90:90–4. doi:10.3109/09553002.2013.835504.
49. Mulliez T, Veldeman L, van Greveling A, Speleers B, Sadeghi S, Berwouts D, et al. Hypofractionated whole breast irradiation for patients with large breasts: a randomized trial comparing prone and supine positions. Radiother Oncol. 2013;108:203–8. doi:10.1016/j.radonc.2013.08.040.
50. Chadha M, Woode R, Sillanpaa J, Lucido D, Boolbol SK, Kirstein L, et al. Early-stage breast cancer treated with 3-week accelerated whole-breast radiation therapy and concomitant boost. Int J Radiat Oncol Biol Phys. 2013;86:40–4. doi:10.1016/j.ijrobp.2012.11.010.
51. Corbin KS, Dorn PL, Jain SK, Al-Hallaq HA, Hasan Y, Chmura SJ. Hypofractionated radiotherapy does not increase acute toxicity in large-breasted women: results from a prospectively collected series. Am J Clin Oncol. 2014;37:322–6. doi:10.1097/COC.0b013e31827b45b7.
52. Hannan R, Thompson RF, Chen Y, Bernstein K, Kabarriti R, Skinner W, et al. Hypofractionated whole-breast radiation therapy: does breast size matter? Int J Radiat Oncol Biol Phys. 2012;84:894–901. doi:10.1016/j.ijrobp.2012.01.093.
53. Tortorelli G, Di Murro L, Barbarino R, Cicchetti S, di Cristino D, Falco MD, et al. Standard or hypofractionated radiotherapy in the postoperative treatment of breast cancer: a retrospective analysis of acute skin toxicity and dose inhomogeneities. BMC Cancer. 2013;13:230. doi:10.1186/1471-2407-13-230.
54. Chen MF, Chen WC, Lai CH, Hung CH, Liu KC, Cheng YH. Predictive factors of radiation-induced skin toxicity in breast cancer patients. BMC Cancer. 2010;10:508. doi:10.1186/1471-2407-10-508.
55. Theberge V, Harel F, Dagnault A. Use of axillary deodorant and effect on acute skin toxicity during radiotherapy for breast cancer: a prospective randomized noninferiority trial. Int J Radiat Oncol Biol Phys. 2009;75:1048–52. doi:10.1016/j.ijrobp.2008.12.046.
56. Gee A, Moffitt D, Churn M, Errington R. A randomised controlled trial to test a non-metallic deodorant used during a course of radiotherapy. J Radiother Pract. 2000;1:205–12. doi:10.1017/S1460396999000321.
57. Bennett C. An investigation into the use of a non-metallic deodorant during radiotherapy treatment: a randomised controlled trial. J Radiother Pract. 2009;8:3–9. doi:10.1017/S146039690800647X.
58. Watson LC, Gies D, Thompson E, Thomas B. Randomized control trial: evaluating aluminum-based antiperspirant use, axilla skin toxicity, and reported quality of life in women receiving external beam radiotherapy for treatment of Stage 0, I, and II breast cancer. Int J Radiat Oncol Biol Phys. 2012;83:e29–34. doi:10.1016/j.ijrobp.2011.12.006.
59. Lewis L, Carson S, Bydder S, Athifa M, Williams AM, Bremner A. Evaluating the effects of aluminum-containing and non-aluminum containing deodorants on axillary skin toxicity during radiation therapy for breast cancer: a 3-armed randomized controlled trial. Int J Radiat Oncol Biol Phys. 2014;90:765–71. doi:10.1016/j.ijrobp.2014.06.054.
60. Feight D, Baney T, Bruce S, McQuestion M. Putting evidence into practice. Clin J Oncol Nurs. 2011;15:481–92. doi:10.1188/11.CJON.481-492.
61. Dubey A, Recht A, Come SE, Gelman RS, Silver B, Harris JR, et al. Concurrent CMF and radiation therapy for early stage breast cancer: results of a pilot study. Int J Radiat Oncol Biol Phys. 1999;45:877–84.
62. Pietras RJ, Poen JC, Gallardo D, Wongvipat PN, Lee HJ, Slamon DJ. Monoclonal antibody to HER-2/neureceptor modulates repair of radiation-induced DNA damage and enhances radiosensitivity of human breast cancer cells overexpressing this oncogene. Cancer Res. 1999;59:1347–55.
63. Belkacemi Y, Gligorov J, Ozsahin M, Marsiglia H, De Lafontan B, Laharie-Mineur H, et al. Concurrent trastuzumab with adjuvant radiotherapy in HER2-positive breast cancer patients: acute toxicity analyses from the French multicentric study. Ann Oncol. 2008;19:1110–6. doi:10.1093/annonc/mdn029.
64. Jacob J, Belin L, Pierga JY, Gobillion A, Vincent-Salomon A, Dendale R, et al. Concurrent administration of trastuzumab with locoregional breast radiotherapy: long-term results of a prospective study. Breast Cancer Res Treat. 2014;148:345–53. doi:10.1007/s10549-014-3166-5.
65. Caussa L, Kirova YM, Gault N, Pierga JY, Savignoni A, Campana F, et al. The acute skin and heart toxicity of a concurrent association of trastuzumab and locoregional breast radiotherapy including internal mammary chain: a single-institution study. Eur J Cancer. 2011;47:65–73. doi:10.1016/j.ejca.2010.08.013.
66. Bellon JR, Gover MT, Burstein HJ, Harris JR, Harris LN. Concurrent trastuzumab and radiation therapy (RT) in the adjuvant treatment of breast cancer. Int J Radiat Oncol Biol Phys. 2005;63:S55–6. doi:10.1016/j.ijrobp.2005.07.097.
67. Halyard MY, Pisansky TM, Dueck AC, Suman V, Pierce L, Solin L, et al. Radiotherapy and adjuvant trastuzumab in operable breast cancer: tolerability and adverse event data from the NCCTG Phase III Trial N9831. J Clin Oncol. 2009;27:2638–44. doi:10.1200/JCO.2008.17.9549.

68. Fernando IN, Ford HT, Powles TJ, Ashley S, Glees JP, Torr M, et al. Factors affecting acute skin toxicity in patients having breast irradiation after conservative surgery: a prospective study of treatment practice at the Royal Marsden Hospital. Clin Oncol (R Coll Radiol). 1996;8:226–33.
69. Bentzen SM, Overgaard M. Relationship between early and late normal-tissue injury after postmastectomy radiotherapy. Radiother Oncol. 1991;20:159–65.
70. Lilla C, Ambrosone CB, Kropp S, Helmbold I, Schmezer P, von Fournier D, et al. Predictive factors for late normal tissue complications following radiotherapy for breast cancer. Breast Cancer Res Treat. 2007;106:143–50. doi:10.1007/s10549-006-9480-9.
71. Bostrom A, Sjolin-Forsberg G, Wilking N, Bergh J. Radiation recall—another call with tamoxifen. Acta Oncol. 1999;38:955–9.
72. Kundranda MN, Daw HA. Tamoxifen-induced radiation recall dermatitis. Am J Clin Oncol. 2006;29:637–8. doi:10.1097/01.coc.0000189693.23157.8d.
73. Singer EA, Warren RD, Pennanen MF, Collins BT, Hayes DF. Tamoxifen-induced radiation recall dermatitis. Breast J. 2004;10:170–1.
74. Parry BR. Radiation recall induced by tamoxifen. Lancet. 1992;340:49.
75. Rhee J, Kim GE, Lee CH, Kwon JM, Han SH, Kim YS, et al. Radiation recall dermatitis induced by tamoxifen during adjuvant breast cancer treatment. Radiat Oncol J. 2014;32:262–5. doi:10.3857/roj.2014.32.4.262.
76. Haydaroglu A, Sert F, Kazandi AC, Unal I. Radiation recall reaction with anastrozole treatment in breast cancer. Pract Radiat Oncol. 2012;2:e65–8. doi:10.1016/j.prro.2012.03.001.
77. Foster LM, Mahoney ME, Harmon MW, Allen JW, Luh JY. Radiation recall reaction with letrozole therapy in breast cancer. Clin Breast Cancer. 2014;14:e95–7. doi:10.1016/j.clbc.2013.12.011.
78. Burris 3rd HA, Hurtig J. Radiation recall with anticancer agents. Oncologist. 2010;15:1227–37. doi:10.1634/theoncologist.2009-0090.
79. Haffty BG, Vicini FA, Beitsch P, Quiet C, Keleher A, Garcia D, et al. Timing of Chemotherapy after MammoSite radiation therapy system breast brachytherapy: analysis of the American Society of Breast Surgeons MammoSite breast brachytherapy registry trial. Int J Radiat Oncol Biol Phys. 2008;72:1441–8. doi:10.1016/j.ijrobp.2008.02.070.
80. Ioannidis G, Gkogkou P, Charalampous P, Diamandi M, Ioannou R. Radiation-recall dermatitis with the everolimus/exemestane combination ten years after adjuvant whole-breast radiotherapy. Radiother Oncol. 2014;112:449–50. doi:10.1016/j.radonc.2014.08.030.
81. Lee HE, Jeong NJ, Lee Y, Seo YJ, Kim CD, Lee JH, et al. Radiation recall dermatitis and pneumonitis induced by trastuzumab (Herceptin(R)). Int J Dermatol. 2014;53:e159–60.
82. Chung C, Stuart D, Keyes M. Radiation recall reaction induced by adjuvant trastuzumab (herceptin). Case Rep Med. 2009;2009:307894. doi:10.1155/2009/307894.
83. Shrimali RK, McPhail NJ, Correa PD, Fraser J, Rizwanullah M. Trastuzumab-induced radiation recall dermatitis—first reported case. Clin Oncol (R Coll Radiol). 2009;21:634–5. doi:10.1016/j.clon.2009.03.003.
84. Toledano A, Garaud P, Serin D, Fourquet A, Bosset JF, Breteau N, et al. Concurrent administration of adjuvant chemotherapy and radiotherapy after breast-conserving surgery enhances late toxicities: long-term results of the ARCOSEIN multicenter randomized study. Int J Radiat Oncol Biol Phys. 2006;65:324–32. doi:10.1016/j.ijrobp.2005.12.020.
85. Mukesh MB, Barnett GC, Wilkinson JS, Moody AM, Wilson C, Dorling L, et al. Randomized controlled trial of intensity-modulated radiotherapy for early breast cancer: 5-year results confirm superior overall cosmesis. J Clin Oncol. 2013;31:4488–95. doi:10.1200/JCO.2013.49.7842.
86. Barnett GC, Wilkinson JS, Moody AM, Wilson CB, Twyman N, Wishart GC, et al. Randomized controlled trial of forward-planned intensity modulated radiotherapy for early breast cancer: interim results at 2 years. Int J Radiat Oncol Biol Phys. 2012;82:715–23. doi:10.1016/j.ijrobp.2010.10.068.
87. Sibaud V, Niec RE, Schindler K, Busam KJ, Roche H, Modi S, et al. Ado-trastuzumab emtansine-associated telangiectasias in metastatic breast cancer: a case series. Breast Cancer Res Treat. 2014;146:451–6. doi:10.1007/s10549-014-3001-z.
88. Dancey AL, Waters RA. Morphea of the breast. Two case reports and discussion of the literature. J Plast Reconstr Aesthet Surg. 2006;59:1114–7. doi:10.1016/j.bjps.2006.01.018.
89. Cheah NL, Wong DW, Chetiyawardana AD. Radiation-induced morphea of the breast: a case report. J Med Case Rep. 2008;2:136. doi:10.1186/1752-1947-2-136.
90. Ardern-Jones MR, Black MM. Widespread morphoea following radiotherapy for carcinoma of the breast. Clin Exp Dermatol. 2003;28:160–2.
91. Wernicke AG, Goltser Y, Trichter S, Sabbas A, Gaan J, Swistel AJ, et al. Morphea as a consequence of accelerated partial breast irradiation. Clin Breast Cancer. 2011;11:67–70. doi:10.3816/CBC.2011.n.012.
92. Bleasel NR, Stapleton KM, Commens C, Ahern VA. Radiation-induced localized scleroderma in breast cancer patients. Australas J Dermatol. 1999;40:99–102.
93. Davis DA, Cohen PR, McNeese MD, Duvic M. Localized scleroderma in breast cancer patients treated with supervoltage external beam radiation: radiation port scleroderma. J Am Acad Dermatol. 1996;35:923–7.
94. Walsh N, Rheaume D, Barnes P, Tremaine R, Reardon M. Postirradiation morphea: an underrecognized complication of treatment for breast cancer.

Hum Pathol. 2008;39:1680–8. doi:10.1016/j.humpath.2008.04.010.
95. Schaffer JV, Carroll C, Dvoretsky I, Huether MJ, Girardi M. Postirradiation morphea of the breast presentation of two cases and review of the literature. Dermatology. 2000;200:67–71.
96. Holscher T, Bentzen SM, Baumann M. Influence of connective tissue diseases on the expression of radiation side effects: a systematic review. Radiother Oncol. 2006;78:123–30. doi:10.1016/j.radonc.2005.12.013.
97. Robertson JM, Clarke DH, Pevzner MM, Matter RC. Breast conservation therapy. Severe breast fibrosis after radiation therapy in patients with collagen vascular disease. Cancer. 1991;68:502–8.
98. Fleck R, McNeese MD, Ellerbroek NA, Hunter TA, Holmes FA. Consequences of breast irradiation in patients with pre-existing collagen vascular diseases. Int J Radiat Oncol Biol Phys. 1989; 17:829–33.
99. Mayr NA, Riggs Jr CE, Saag KG, Wen BC, Pennington EC, Hussey DH. Mixed connective tissue disease and radiation toxicity. A case report. Cancer. 1997;79:612–8.
100. Chen AM, Obedian E, Haffty BG. Breast-conserving therapy in the setting of collagen vascular disease. Cancer J. 2001;7:480–91.
101. Hernandez S, Evans SB, Wazer DE. Severe acute toxicity from whole breast radiotherapy in the setting of collagen vascular disease. Am J Clin Oncol. 2006;29:647–8. doi:10.1097/01.coc.0000239164.01855.50.
102. Swift M, Morrell D, Cromartie E, Chamberlin AR, Skolnick MH, Bishop DT. The incidence and gene frequency of ataxia-telangiectasia in the United States. Am J Hum Genet. 1986;39:573–83.
103. Andreassen CN, Alsner J, Overgaard M, Overgaard J. Prediction of normal tissue radiosensitivity from polymorphisms in candidate genes. Radiother Oncol. 2003;69:127–35.
104. Quarmby S, Fakhoury H, Levine E, Barber J, Wylie J, Hajeer AH, et al. Association of transforming growth factor beta-1 single nucleotide polymorphisms with radiation-induced damage to normal tissues in breast cancer patients. Int J Radiat Biol. 2003;79:137–43.
105. Moullan N, Cox DG, Angele S, Romestaing P, Gerard JP, Hall J. Polymorphisms in the DNA repair gene XRCC1, breast cancer risk, and response to radiotherapy. Cancer Epidemiol Biomarkers Prev. 2003;12:1168–74.
106. Meyer A, Dork T, Sohn C, Karstens JH, Bremer M. Breast cancer in patients carrying a germ-line CHEK2 mutation: Outcome after breast conserving surgery and adjuvant radiotherapy. Radiother Oncol. 2007;82:349–53. doi:10.1016/j.radonc.2006.12.002.
107. Delanian S, Porcher R, Balla-Mekias S, Lefaix JL. Randomized, placebo-controlled trial of combined pentoxifylline and tocopherol for regression of superficial radiation-induced fibrosis. J Clin Oncol. 2003;21:2545–50. doi:10.1200/JCO.2003.06.064.
108. Cuttino LW, Heffernan J, Vera R, Rosu M, Ramakrishnan VR, Arthur DW. Association between maximal skin dose and breast brachytherapy outcome: a proposal for more rigorous dosimetric constraints. Int J Radiat Oncol Biol Phys. 2011;81:e173–7. doi:10.1016/j.ijrobp.2010.12.023.
109. Bartelink H, Horiot JC, Poortmans PM, Struikmans H, Van den Bogaert W, Fourquet A, et al. Impact of a higher radiation dose on local control and survival in breast-conserving therapy of early breast cancer: 10-year results of the randomized boost versus no boost EORTC 22881–10882 trial. J Clin Oncol. 2007;25:3259–65. doi:10.1200/JCO.2007.11.4991.
110. Collette S, Collette L, Budiharto T, Horiot JC, Poortmans PM, Struikmans H, et al. Predictors of the risk of fibrosis at 10 years after breast conserving therapy for early breast cancer: a study based on the EORTC Trial 22881–10882 'boost versus no boost'. Eur J Cancer. 2008;44:2587–99. doi:10.1016/j.ejca.2008.07.032.
111. Donovan E, Bleakley N, Denholm E, Evans P, Gothard L, Hanson J, et al. Randomised trial of standard 2D radiotherapy (RT) versus intensity modulated radiotherapy (IMRT) in patients prescribed breast radiotherapy. Radiother Oncol. 2007;82:254–64. doi:10.1016/j.radonc.2006.12.008.
112. Ho AL, Bovill ES, Macadam SA, Tyldesley S, Giang J, Lennox PA. Postmastectomy radiation therapy after immediate two-stage tissue expander/implant breast reconstruction: a University of British Columbia perspective. Plast Reconstr Surg. 2014; 134:1–10. doi:10.1097/PRS.0000000000000292.
113. Azria D, Gourgou S, Sozzi WJ, Zouhair A, Mirimanoff RO, Kramar A, et al. Concomitant use of tamoxifen with radiotherapy enhances subcutaneous breast fibrosis in hypersensitive patients. Br J Cancer. 2004;91:1251–60. doi:10.1038/sj.bjc.6602146.
114. Azria D, Belkacemi Y, Romieu G, Gourgou S, Gutowski M, Zaman K, et al. Concurrent or sequential adjuvant letrozole and radiotherapy after conservative surgery for early-stage breast cancer (CO-HO-RT): a phase 2 randomised trial. Lancet Oncol. 2010;11:258–65. doi:10.1016/S1470-2045(10)70013-9.
115. Valakh V, Trombetta MG, Werts ED, Labban G, Khalid MK, Kaminsky A, et al. Influence of concurrent anastrozole on acute and late side effects of whole breast radiotherapy. Am J Clin Oncol. 2011; 34:245–8. doi:10.1097/COC.0b013e3181df4b62.
116. Westbury CB, Yarnold JR. Radiation fibrosis—current clinical and therapeutic perspectives. Clin Oncol (R Coll Radiol). 2012;24:657–72. doi:10.1016/j.clon.2012.04.001.
117. Delanian S, Balla-Mekias S, Lefaix JL. Striking regression of chronic radiotherapy damage in a clinical trial of combined pentoxifylline and tocopherol. J Clin Oncol. 1999;17:3283–90.

118. Delanian S, Porcher R, Rudant J, Lefaix JL. Kinetics of response to long-term treatment combining pentoxifylline and tocopherol in patients with superficial radiation-induced fibrosis. J Clin Oncol. 2005; 23:8570–9. doi:10.1200/JCO.2005.02.4729.
119. van Geel AN, Lans TE, Haen R, Tjong Joe Wai R, Menke-Pluijmers MB. Partial mastectomy and m latissimus dorsi reconstruction for radiation-induced fibrosis after breast-conserving cancer therapy. World J Surg. 2011;35:568–72. doi:10.1007/s00268-010-0911-8.
120. Chan RJ, Mann J, Tripcony L, Keller J, Cheuk R, Blades R, et al. Natural oil-based emulsion containing allantoin versus aqueous cream for managing radiation-induced skin reactions in patients with cancer: a phase 3, double-blind, randomized, controlled trial. Int J Radiat Oncol Biol Phys. 2014;90:756–64. doi:10.1016/j.ijrobp.2014.06.034.
121. Rollmann DC, Novotny PJ, Petersen IA, Garces YI, Bauer HJ, Yan ES, et al. Double-blind, placebo-controlled pilot study of processed ultra emu oil versus placebo in the prevention of radiation dermatitis. Int J Radiat Oncol Biol Phys. 2015. doi:10.1016/j.ijrobp.2015.02.028.
122. Heggie S, Bryant GP, Tripcony L, Keller J, Rose P, Glendenning M, et al. A Phase III study on the efficacy of topical aloe vera gel on irradiated breast tissue. Cancer Nurs. 2002;25:442–51.
123. Williams MS, Burk M, Loprinzi CL, Hill M, Schomberg PJ, Nearhood K, et al. Phase III double-blind evaluation of an aloe vera gel as a prophylactic agent for radiation-induced skin toxicity. Int J Radiat Oncol Biol Phys. 1996;36:345–9.
124. Richardson J, Smith JE, McIntyre M, Thomas R, Pilkington K. Aloe vera for preventing radiation-induced skin reactions: a systematic literature review. Clin Oncol (R Coll Radiol). 2005;17:478–84.
125. Gosselin TK, Schneider SM, Plambeck MA, Rowe K. A prospective randomized, placebo-controlled skin care study in women diagnosed with breast cancer undergoing radiation therapy. Oncol Nurs Forum. 2010;37:619–26. doi:10.1188/10.ONF.619-626.
126. Pommier P, Gomez F, Sunyach MP, D'Hombres A, Carrie C, Montbarbon X. Phase III randomized trial of Calendula officinalis compared with trolamine for the prevention of acute dermatitis during irradiation for breast cancer. J Clin Oncol. 2004;22:1447–53. doi:10.1200/JCO.2004.07.063.
127. Pinnix C, Perkins GH, Strom EA, Tereffe W, Woodward W, Oh JL, et al. Topical hyaluronic acid vs. standard of care for the prevention of radiation dermatitis after adjuvant radiotherapy for breast cancer: single-blind randomized phase III clinical trial. Int J Radiat Oncol Biol Phys. 2012;83:1089–94. doi:10.1016/j.ijrobp.2011.09.021.
128. Kirova YM, Fromantin I, De Rycke Y, Fourquet A, Morvan E, Padiglione S, et al. Can we decrease the skin reaction in breast cancer patients using hyaluronic acid during radiation therapy? Results of phase III randomised trial. Radiother Oncol. 2011;100:205–9. doi:10.1016/j.radonc.2011.05.014.
129. Meghrajani CF, Co HC, Ang-Tiu CM, Roa FC. Topical corticosteroid therapy for the prevention of acute radiation dermatitis: a systematic review of randomized controlled trials. Expert Rev Clin Pharmacol. 2013;6:641–9. doi:10.1586/17512433.2013.841079.
130. Bostrom A, Lindman H, Swartling C, Berne B, Bergh J. Potent corticosteroid cream (mometasone furoate) significantly reduces acute radiation dermatitis: results from a double-blind, randomized study. Radiother Oncol. 2001;59:257–65.
131. Miller RC, Schwartz DJ, Sloan JA, Griffin PC, Deming RL, Anders JC, et al. Mometasone furoate effect on acute skin toxicity in breast cancer patients receiving radiotherapy: a phase III double-blind, randomized trial from the North Central Cancer Treatment Group N06C4. Int J Radiat Oncol Biol Phys. 2011;79:1460–6. doi:10.1016/j.ijrobp.2010.01.031.
132. Graham P, Browne L, Capp A, Fox C, Graham J, Hollis J, et al. Randomized, paired comparison of No-Sting Barrier Film versus sorbolene cream (10% glycerine) skin care during postmastectomy irradiation. Int J Radiat Oncol Biol Phys. 2004;58:241–6.
133. Paterson D, Poonam P, Bennett N, Peszynski R, Van Beekhuizen M, Jasperse M, et al. Randomized intra-patient controlled trial of mepilex lite dressings versus aqueous cream in managing radiation-induced skin reactions post-mastectomy. J Cancer Sci Ther. 2012;4:347–56.
134. Mcmillan MS, Wells M, MacBride S, Raab GM, Munro A, MacDougall H. Randomized comparison of dry dressings versus hydrogel in management of radiation-induced moist desquamation. Int J Radiat Oncol Biol Phys. 2007;68:864–72. doi:10.1016/j.ijrobp.2006.12.049.
135. Spalek M, Jonska-Gmyrek J, Galecki J. Radiation-induced morphea—a literature review. J Eur Acad Dermatol Venereol. 2015;29:197–202. doi:10.1111/jdv.12704.

8 Gastrointestinal Cancer

Mekhail Anwar and Jennifer Bohm

Cancers of the gastrointestinal tract include those arising in the esophagus, stomach, pancreas, gallbladder, biliary tree, liver, small and large bowel, and anus. There are an estimated 291,150 gastrointestinal cancers in the United States in 2015 with 163,050 cases in men and 128,100 in women [1]. Many of these cancers employ dual or trimodality therapy, integrating chemotherapy, radiation, and surgery. Chemotherapy, when combined with radiation, is used as a radiation sensitizer amplifying both the therapeutic effect and, unfortunately, the toxicity. While hematologic and gastrointestinal toxicities are notable in this group, of particular importance is the management of the skin toxicity, since the locations of some of the tumors require radiation to the perianal skin. There are 7,270 and 39,610 annual cases of anal and rectal cancer, respectively, diagnosed in the United States. Therefore, this chapter focuses on these two disease entities and the management of the associated skin toxicity. Nonetheless, these methods can be extended to other areas in the management of gastrointestinal malignancies where skin reactions may occur, such as the neck in cervical esophageal tumors.

M. Anwar, MD, PhD (✉) • J. Bohm, RN, BSN
Department of Radiation Oncology, University of California, San Francisco, 1600 Divisadero, Cancer Cntr Room 1031, Box 1708, San Francisco, CA 94115, USA
e-mail: Mekhail.Anwar@ucsf.edu

8.1 Anal Cancer

Anal cancer is a relatively rare entity, with an expected incidence of 7270 cases and 1010 deaths in 2015 [2, 3]. Almost 90 % of cases are attributed to human papillomavirus (HPV) [4], and similar to cervical cancer, anal cancer often begins as high-grade anal dysplasia. Patients who are immunocompromised are particularly susceptible. HIV-positive patients represent a special category of anal cancer patients, and anal cancer is twice as common in these patients as compared to HIV-negative patients. Anal-receptive intercourse is a risk factor in males.

Despite multiple attempts to modify and improve treatment, the fundamental treatment paradigm dates to 1980. Prior to this, the standard of care was an abdominal perineal resection (APR), resulting in a permanent colostomy. Dr. Nigro [5] at Wayne State University pioneered the use of neoadjuvant chemotherapy with radiation followed by surgery. The majority of patients treated with chemotherapy and radiation had no residual tumor at the time of surgery, and subsequently surgery was reserved for salvage. Overall 24 of 28 patients had a clinical complete response to chemoradiation, and thus was born the era of definitive chemoradiation for anal cancer. Since that time, the use of 5-fluorouracil (5-FU) and mitomycin C (MMC) has remained unchanged. This regimen can cause significant skin toxicity (in addition to hematologic toxicity).

B. Fowble et al. (eds.), *Skin Care in Radiation Oncology*, DOI 10.1007/978-3-319-31460-0_8

While multiple trials have endeavored to eliminate or replace MMC, the colostomy-free survivals without MMC have been inferior to combination regimens that include it.

8.1.1 Frequency of Acute Dermatologic Toxicity and Factors Affecting Acute Toxicity

Table 8.1 [6–11] presents the frequency of acute grade 3 or greater skin toxicity in patients with anal cancer. The high rate of skin toxicity is due to both radiation and concurrent chemotherapy. Therefore, in an effort to mitigate toxicity, studies focusing both on the modification of chemotherapy (both eliminating the components of the regimen, as well as replacing them) and radiotherapy were done.

The benefit of adding chemotherapy to radiation was evaluated in the UKCCCR Anal Cancer Trial (ACT 1) [6, 12] where 585 patients were randomized to radiation with or without MMC and 5-FU chemotherapy. Severe acute dermatologic toxicity was 14 % with radiation and 17 % with radiation and chemotherapy, but local control was compromised with radiation alone. An EORTC trial randomized 110 patients with anal cancer to radiation or chemoradiation with 5-FU and MMC [7]. Grade 3–4 dermatologic toxicity was reported in 50 % of the radiation patients compared to 57 % of the chemoradiation patients. However, an increased incidence of anal canal ulcers was observed in the chemoradiation arm. The addition of MMC to 5-FU did not increase the frequency of acute skin toxicity in the RTOG 87–04 trial [8]. With the evidence for increased local control with the inclusion of chemotherapy, subsequent studies investigated whether the chemotherapy regimen could be modified for an improved therapeutic ratio. A landmark trial, RTOG 9811 [9, 13], addressed two questions: can cisplatin replace MMC, with the hopes of reducing toxicity, and does adding neoadjuvant chemotherapy to chemoradiation improve outcomes? In this trial, where the standard arm of 5-FU and MMC with radiation was compared against induction 5-FU and cisplatin, followed by 5-FU, cisplatin, and radiation, combined grade 3 and 4 skin toxicity was 48 and 41 % by the treatment arm, respectively. The UNICANCER ACCORD 03 phase 3 trial evaluated induction chemotherapy with 5-FU and cisplatin and dose escalation of the radiation boost. Grade 3–4 nonhematologic toxicity was similar among the treatment arms.

Anti-*EGFR-1* targeted therapies have been evaluated in the treatment of anal cancer. Olivatto et al. [14] reported 52 % grade 3–4 acute radiation dermatitis in a phase 1 study of 23 patients treated with 5-FU, cisplatin, and cetuximab. A phase 2 trial evaluating concurrent chemoradiation with cetuximab was closed due to excessive toxicity [15].

HIV-positive patients require special attention. Patients with CD4 counts above 200 can be considered for treatment according to standard therapy on a case-by-case basis, and their outcomes with ongoing antiretroviral therapy can be on par with HIV-negative patients [16–21]. However, patients with CD4 counts approaching and below 200 must be managed with extreme caution. The low CD4 counts make them particularly susceptible to skin toxicity, infection, and poor healing. A study from UCSF [20] reported that of eight patients with CD4 < 200, four required hospitalization for the management of toxicities including moist desquamation. At our institution we consider radiotherapy alone or a less intensive chemotherapy regimen for these patients, depending on their comorbidities.

In an effort to mitigate toxicity, more modern techniques of radiation delivery, targeting the tumor while sparing normal tissue, have been extensively investigated. Radiation was traditionally done with two opposing anterior–posterior and posterior–anterior fields. While this was effective in targeting the tumor at areas of at-risk disease, it also encompassed significant amounts of normal tissue, including the skin not at risk for tumor involvement. The effects of this can be seen in studies reporting grade 3 or greater toxicity ranging from 32 to 65 % of patients receiving conventional or 3D conformal radiation.

The ability to conformally shape radiation therapy has significantly improved over the last

Table 8.1 Acute toxicity

Trial	Notes	Treatment	RT dose	Grade 1	Grade 2	Grade 3	Grade 4	Grade 5
RTOG 87–04 [8]	To study the effect of removal of MMC from standard regimen. The colostomy rate increased from 9 to 22 % with the loss of MMC (DFS* 73–51 %)	RT/5-FU						
		RT/5-FU/MMC				55 % (G3 or greater)		
RTOG 92–08 [10]	RT Dose escalation to 59.6 Gy to improve CFS with a mandatory 2 week break. The colostomy rate at 2 years increased from 7 to 30 % with a break, despite dose escalation					34 % (G3 or greater)		
UKCCR [6]	Local failure was reduced from approximately 60–40 % at 5 years with the addition of chemotherapy; late morbidity was similar between arms	RT (N = 279)	45 Gy (±15–20 Gy boost)			14 %		
		RT/5-FU/MMC (*N* = 283)				17 %		
EORTC [7]	The addition of chemotherapy increased complete remission rate from 54 to 80 %, and the local control was improved by 18 % at 5 years. The CFS was improved by 32 %, and the cause-specific survival (although not OS) was improved with CMT	RT (*N* = 52)	45 Gy (±15–20 Gy boost)			50 % (G3/4)		
		RT/5-FU/MMC (*N* = 51)				57 % (G3/4)		
RTOG 9811 [9]	This study asked if the toxicity and outcomes of SOC RT/5-FU/MMC can be improved with neoadjuvant and concurrent 5-FU/Cis. The outcomes in terms of CFS were worse, likely due to the longer treatment time with neoadjuvant chemotherapy	RT/5-FU/Cis (*N* = 320)	45–50.5 Gy (± 5–9 Gy boost)	9 % (30)	38 % (122)	39 % (126)	2 % [6]	
		RT/5-FU/MMC (*N* = 324)		9 % (28)	35 % (113)	43 % (140)	5 % [15]	
ACT 2 [11]	This study had 2 randomizations to study the questions [1]: can cisplatin replace MMC, and [2] does adjuvant 5-FU/Cis improve outcomes? Outcomes were similar to the SOC arm, and RT/5-FU/MMC remains the SOC	RT/5FT/ Cis ± 5-FU/Cis	50.4 Gy			61 % (NHT)		
		RT/5FT/ MMC ± 5-FU/Cis				65 % (NHT)		

NHT Non-hematologic toxicity (skin toxicity not broken out), *DFS* disease-free survival

Table 8.2 IMRT for anal cancer

Trial	Notes	Treatment	RT Dose	Grade 1	Grade 2	Grade 3	Grade 4	Grade 5
Chicago [22]	Retrospective, $N=17$	RT/5-FU/MMC				No G3 or greater toxicity		
Duke [23]	Retrospective, $N=47$	RT/5-FU/MMC	54 Gy		93 %	0		
RTOG 0529 [24]	Single-arm comparison of IMRT versus historical 3D	RT/5-FU/MMC	50–54 Gy	RT/5-FU/MMC	50–54 Gy			23 % (≥G3)

two decades, and the use of intensity-modulated radiation therapy (IMRT) has been incorporated into many cancer subsites, including GI tumors. The use of IMRT allows for the reduction of dose to normal tissues including the skin.

Due to the toxicity associated with anal cancer treatments, incorporation of IMRT into the treatment of this disease was investigated by several institutions. Table 8.2 [22–24] shows the results of IMRT series and includes a single-arm prospective trial, RTOG 0529, testing the hypothesis that delivery of radiation with IMRT could preserve historical outcomes in terms of overall survival and colostomy-free survival, but reduce skin toxicity [25]. As expected, the rates of grade 3 or higher skin toxicity, in comparison with the control arm of RTOG 9811, demonstrated improved outcomes with less skin toxicity using IMRT. Therefore, IMRT with 5-FU and MMC now represent the standard of care.

8.2 Rectal Cancer

Rectal cancer patients also undergo chemoradiation, but the location of the tumor is often deeper within the pelvis, reducing the radiation dose to the perianal area, where toxicity is the greatest. The treatment paradigm for rectal cancer consists of preoperative radiation and chemotherapy, with radiation to the whole pelvis and concurrent 5-FU. Unlike anal cancer patients, rectal cancer patients undergo resection with a total mesorectal excision (TME), often followed by adjuvant chemotherapy. Several factors contribute to lower toxicity in rectal cancer patients compared to anal cancer patients: (1) chemotherapy is single-agent 5-FU, and MMC is not used, (2), the radiation dose is lower since patients will be getting surgery after to remove the tumor, and (3) due to the location within the deep pelvis, radiation fields do not typically extend to the skin. Nonetheless, these patients can also exhibit skin toxicities, and management of these skin toxicities is similar.

The incorporation of IMRT into rectal cancer treatment has also been investigated. RTOG 0822 was designed in a similar fashion to RTOG 0529 discussed above: a single-arm trial using IMRT, with toxicity outcomes to be compared with historical controls. This study did not show a reduction in toxicity with IMRT, but utilized a nonstandard regimen of capecitabine and oxaliplatin, as opposed to the standard of care, capecitabine alone. Therefore, it is difficult to say if IMRT will result in a significantly lower toxicity if used with the standard of care regimen. A retrospective study [26] at the Mayo Clinic (Arizona) showed improved grade 2 and greater toxicity outcomes with IMRT compared to conventional techniques, but the reported toxicity outcomes did not include skin toxicity and were mainly attributed to the reduction in GI toxicity.

Table 8.3 Long-term toxicity

Trial	Treatment	RT Dose	Grade 1	Grade 2	Grade 3	Grade 4	Grade 5
RTOG 9811 [13]	RT/5-FU/Cis (N=324)				1 %	1 %	
	RT/5-FU/MMC (N=325)				2 %	2 %	
Bujko (Rectal Cancer) [27]	Short-course RT → surgery	25 Gy (5 fractions)			Non-healing perineal wound 0 %		
	Chemoradiation → surgery	50.4 Gy			Non-healing perineal wound 2.8 %		

8.3 Long-Term Toxicity

Long-term toxicities can be significant and patients must be adequately counseled. The rates of long-term grade 3 and greater skin toxicity is low, as shown in Table 8.3 [13, 27]. Common long-term side effects include sterility, as well as rectal and urinary urgency. The function of the anal sphincter can be compromised, resulting in less control over bowel movements. Less common long-term toxicities include erectile dysfunction, decreased vaginal secretions, menopause, and vaginal stenosis (requiring vaginal dilators). Damage to the bones of the hip and pelvis makes patients more susceptible to fracture. Rarely, bowel complications such as ulcers, small bowel obstruction (SBO), or perforation require surgical intervention. As with all diseases treated with radiation, there is a small risk of secondary malignancies.

8.4 Management Strategies

Due to the high rates of skin toxicity, anticipation and planning for skin toxicity must be incorporated into treatment at each phase. In the treatment planning stage, particularly when IMRT is used, we recommend examining the skin dose closely and placing film dosimeters at first treatment. Doses should not exceed the anticipated dosage by more than 10 %. Patients should be extensively counseled both prior to treatment and on treatment for skin toxicity. Strategies for skin management as a function of time on treatment are listed below. Furthermore, management of gastrointestinal toxicity is also important as diarrhea can cause significant irritation of the skin (in addition to dehydration). We recommend instituting antidiarrheal medications when the patient exceeds three loose bowel movements per day. All patients also undergo nutrition consult prior to starting therapy, both to ensure adequate oral intake and to learn which foods can mitigate diarrhea.

Below are general skin care recommendations (Table 8.4), week by week treatment instructions with examples of acute and late skin reactions for anal cancer patients undergoing IMRT (Table 8.5), and photographs that demonstrate how skin reactions in anal cancer patients may vary by ethnicity (Table 8.6). Photographs of special reactions and instructions on how to treat these more uncommon cases are also provided (Table 8.7). Figure 8.1 is a general suggested treatment algorithm for skin care for gastrointestinal cancer patients.

Table 8.4 General principles of skin care for gastrointestinal cancer patients

Patient should:
• Cleanse daily with mild soap and water
• Perform a sitz bath with diluted 0.5 % Hibiclens added twice daily
• Rinse the area with water or perform a sitz bath following each bowel movement and urination (females)
• Use lotions and creams recommended and instructed
• Wear soft undergarments that provide support and control moisture. (Boxers, cotton underwear, mesh underpants, Depends, etc.)
• Receive treatment for fungal infections in perineal and groin folds
• When sitting or lying down, use donut seat pillows if perianal region is being treated
• If incontinent of urine or stools, keep area clean and dry with frequent pad and undergarment changes and use moisture barrier cream to protect the tissues around the vagina and anus
• Remove zinc-containing products, silver ion hydrogels, and dressings prior to daily radiation treatment
Patient should not:
• Rub, put pressure on, or scratch radiated area
• Wear tight-fitting clothes or underwear
• Take hot water showers/hot baths and use wash cloths, or anything other than hands to cleanse the area
• Apply any lotion, cream, or ointment within 3 hours prior to radiation treatment
• Wash off lotion, cream, or ointments if applied three or more hours before radiation treatment
• Apply drying agents to the skin unless instructed to do so
• Use any tape or adhesives on the radiated skin

Table 8.5 Examples of acute and late skin reactions for anal cancer patients undergoing IMRT

Week	Skin reaction	Reaction type	Treatment and intervention
1–3	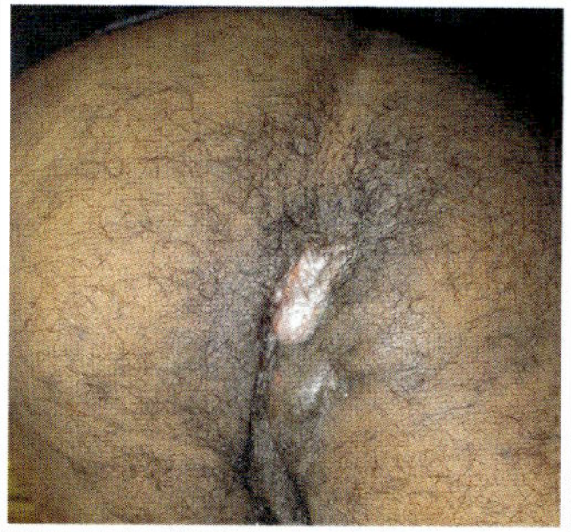	Mild erythema and mild hyperpigmentation	• Cleanse daily with mild soap and water (or similar cleanser such as peri wash) • Perform sitz bath twice a day. Pour 15 ml of diluted 0.5 % Hibiclens into the sitz • Apply calendula cream twice daily to groins, perineum, and gluteal folds • May apply A & D ointment or Aquaphor twice a day to the tumor site • May apply 5 % Lidocaine cream to the rectum prior to bowel movements • After each bowel movement, cleanse the area with water in a peri bottle or perform a sitz bath containing diluted Hibiclens • Remove all dressings and rinse away all products if applied within 3 h prior to treatment
4	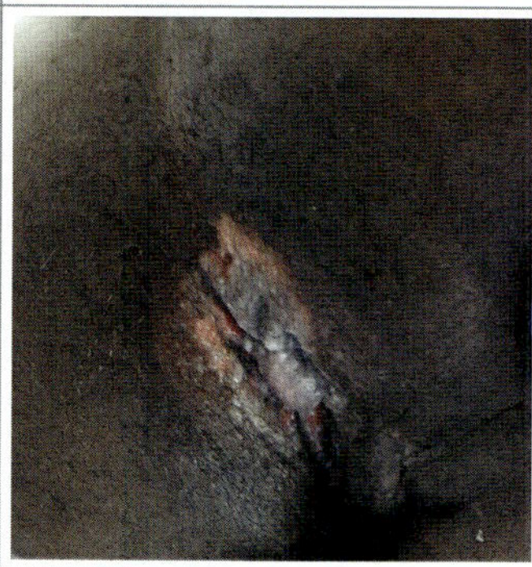	Onset of moist desquamation in the perineum and increased hyperpigmentation	• Add Skintegrity wound cleanser spray (or similar). Liberally spray the site with Skintegrity, allow it to remain on the skin for 1–2 min, then rinse • Continue calendula use twice daily to intact the skin in the radiation field • Apply A+D ointment or Aquaphor twice a day to erythematous or dry areas • Continue sitz baths with diluted Hibiclens twice daily and more often if diarrhea develops • If diarrhea develops apply a skin barrier cream to the perianal skin for protection • Apply Aquacel Ag to areas of moist desquamation and cover with Mepilex Lite or mesh pants • Apply 5 % Lidocaine cream to the anal area for pain. May apply topically up to four times a day
5	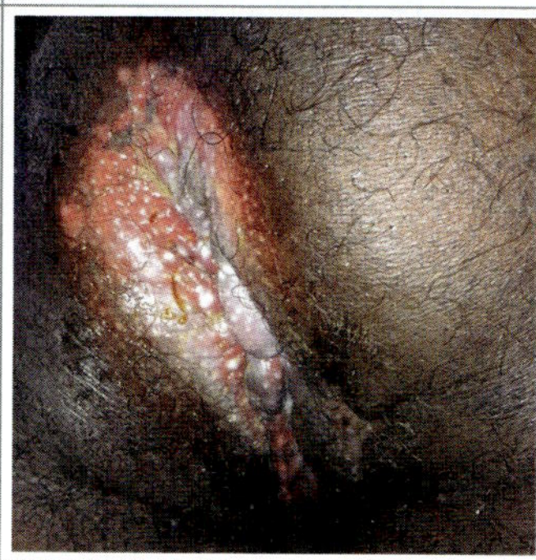	Dry desquamation and moderate to severe moist desquamation with islands of re-epithelialization (white patches)	• Continue as above • Apply Aquacel Ag (or similar) or Mepilex Ag; transfer directly to the moist desquamation. Use care when removing these dressings; ensure they are moistened with water or normal saline for trauma and pain-free removal. May keep in place with Mepilex Lite, mesh pants, or similar • Remove all dressings and rinse away all products if applied within 3 h prior to treatment

(continued)

Table 8.5 (continued)

Week	Skin reaction	Reaction type	Treatment and intervention
2 week break due to the severe reactions	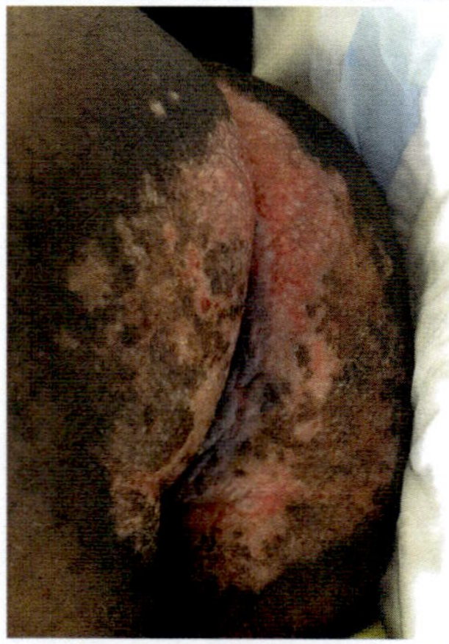	Beginning resolution of severe and widespread moist desquamation in the perineum, anus, and surrounding tissue	• Continue care as above
7–8	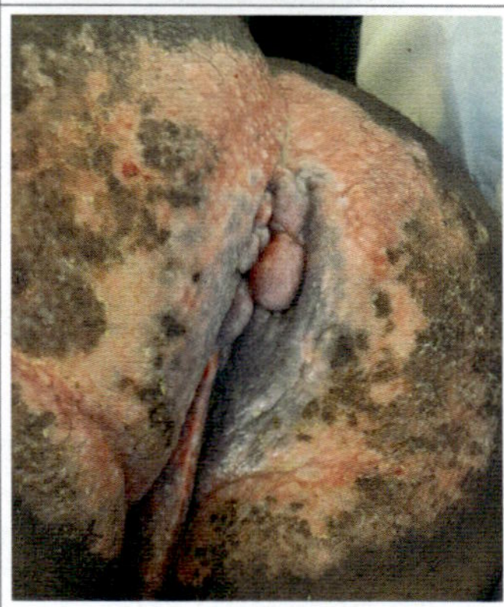	Healing of moist desquamation; residual dry desquamation remaining Resumption of treatment	• Dressings may be adjusted for patient comfort, i.e., Aquacel Ag, Mepilex Transfer Ag, Zinc/Bacitracin (does not need to be completely cleansed away if patient is on a treatment break) • Moisturize the site with Aquaphor or A + D ointment twice a day

1 week post radiation	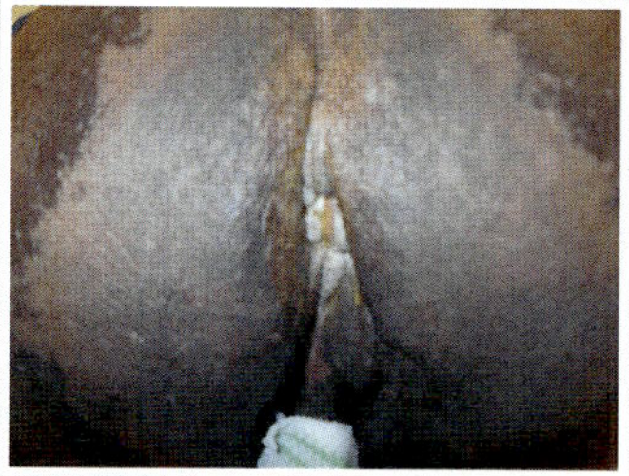	Completion of final week of radiation. Healing of desquamation and hypopigmentation around the anus	• Continue to cleanse the skin daily with Skintegrity spray • Moisturize the skin with calendula twice a day • Apply A+D or Aquaphor in the evening prior to bed
12 days post radiation	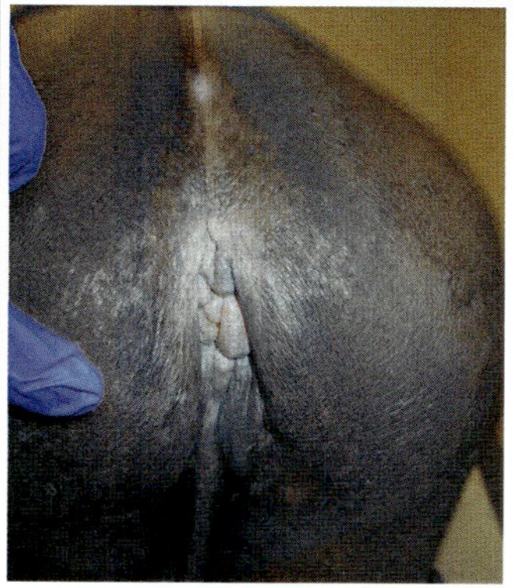	Dry skin with areas of mixed hypo- and hyperpigmentation	• May discontinue Skintegrity. Cleanse daily with mild soap and water • Moisturize the skin daily with calendula or a moisturizer of the patient's choice
1 month post radiation	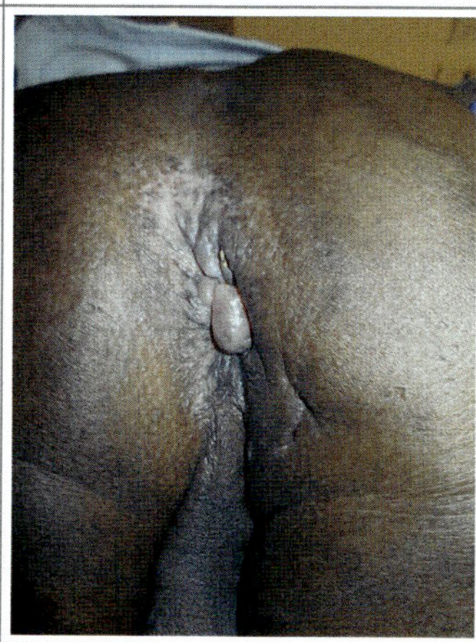	Slight hypopigmentation around the immediate anus with most skin returning to normal color	• Moisturize daily with an agent of patient's choice

Table 8.6 How skin reactions in anal cancer patients may vary by ethnicity

Caucasian	African American
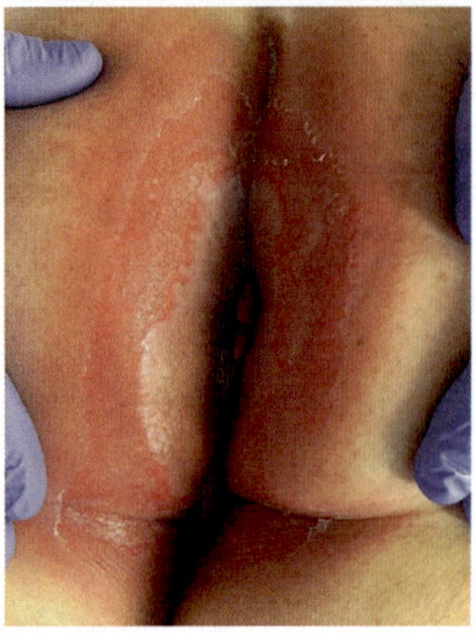	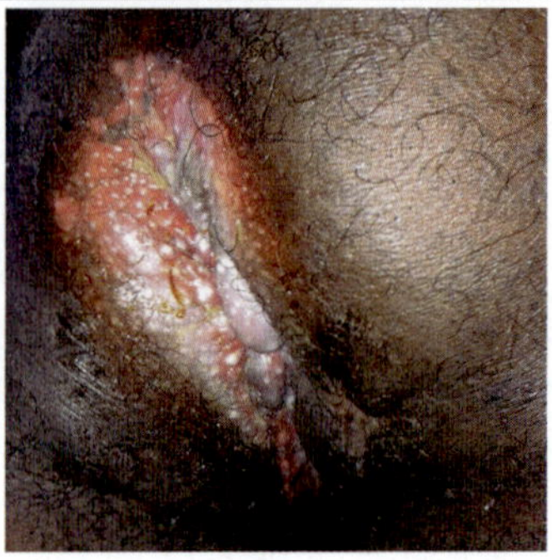
Week 5	Week 5

Table 8.7 Special cases and skin reactions

Case	Reaction type	Treatment and intervention
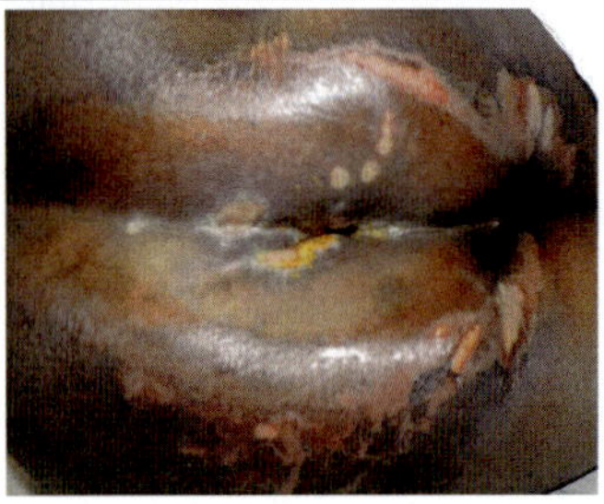	Mixture of focal moist and diffuse dry desquamation undergoing healing process	• Cleanse daily with Skintegrity wound cleanser. Spray liberally to the skin in the radiation field. Allow it to remain on the skin for 1–2 min and rinse off • Apply A & D ointment liberally twice a day • Apply topical Lidocaine 5 % cream for pain (up to four times a day) • Sitz baths with 15 ml of 0.5 % diluted Hibiclens added, twice a day and after stools • Aquacel Ag, Mepitel Transfer Ag, (or similar) may be placed over the rectal wound. The buttocks (cheeks) will assist in holding it in place
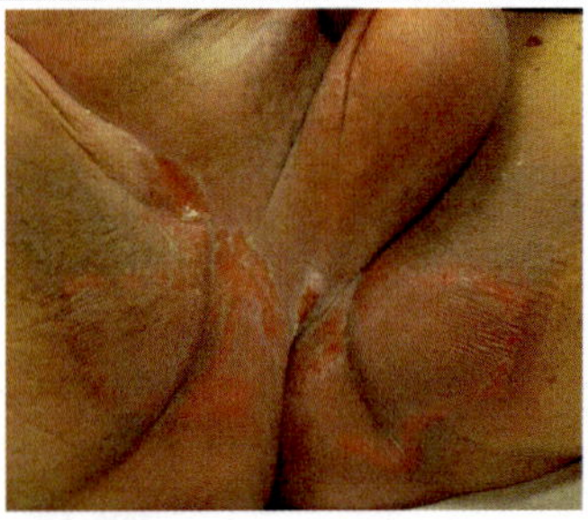	Moist desquamation in perineum folds	• Cleanse daily with Skintegrity wound cleanser. Spray liberally to the skin in the radiation field. Allow it to remain on the skin for 1–2 min and rinse off • Sitz baths with 15 ml of 0.5 % diluted Hibiclens added, twice a day and after stools • Gently debride nonviable tissue with tweezers • Aquacel Ag, Mepitel Transfer Ag, (or similar) may be placed over the moist desquamated site. Use care when removing the dressing. Ensure it is moist enough to lift off without causing tissue trauma. If the dressing sticks, moisten with water or normal saline or have the patient remove it while showering. This is a difficult site to maintain a dressing

(continued)

Table 8.7 (continued)

Case	Reaction type	Treatment and intervention
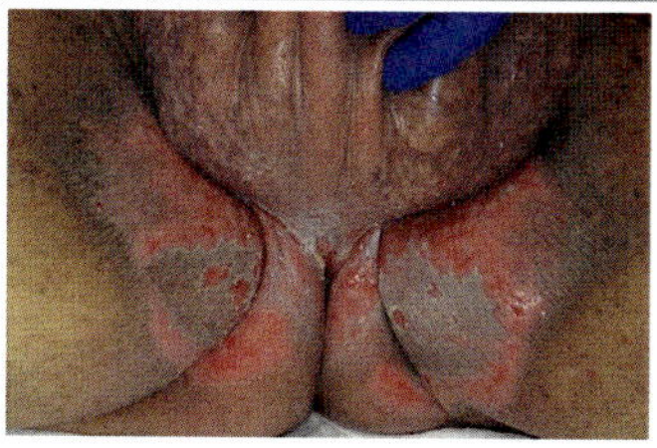 Week 6	Increased moist desquamation and peeling	• Alternative if the patient is on a treatment break: Apply a 1:1 mixture of Zinc and Bacitracin to areas of moist desquamation and nearby skin. Leave this in place for 12–24 h. This can be gently cleansed off with mineral oil followed by Skintegrity or soap and water or Baza cleanser, then reapplied. The paste is soothing and assists in drying and healing the moist desquamation • Apply Aquaphor or A+D to undressed sites twice a day
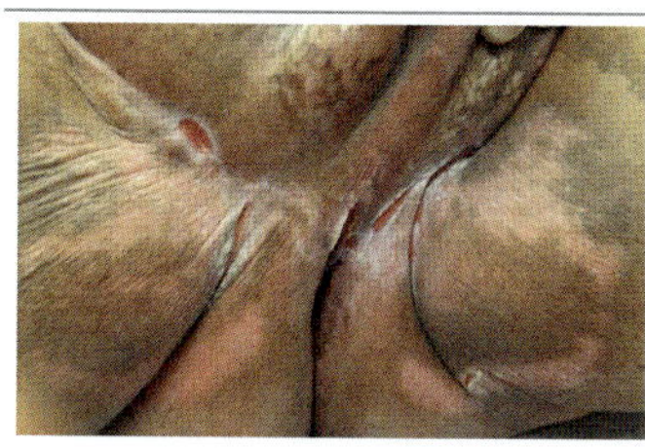 6 days post XRT	Moist desquamation beginning to heal along with areas of dry desquamation at wound edges	
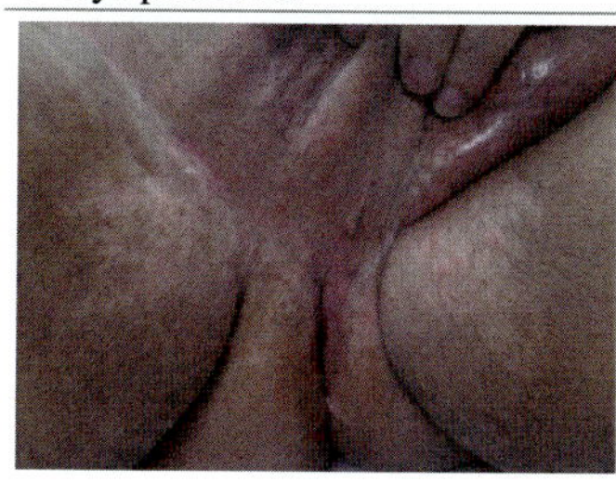 3 months post XRT	Resolution of skin with persistent pigmentation changes	

(continued)

Table 8.7 (continued)

Case	Reaction type	Treatment and intervention
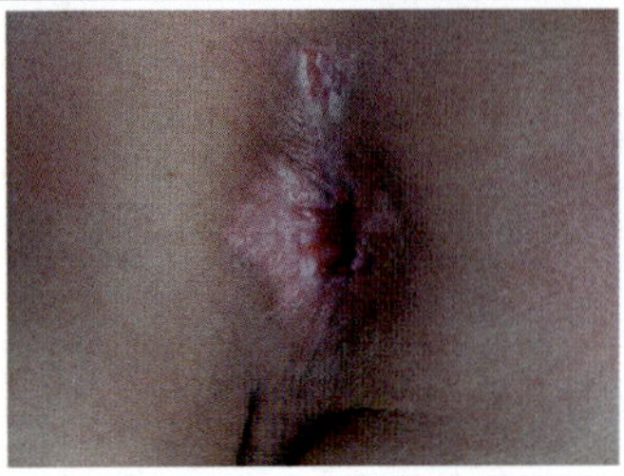 2700 cGY—early Week 3	Onset of moist desquamation around the anus	• Cleanse daily with mild soap and water or Skintegrity • Following a bowel movement, patient should thoroughly cleanse the site with soap and water (i.e., peri bottle or sitz bath) • Apply calendula twice a day to outer gluteal folds • Aquaphor, Medihoney gel, or Silvasorb Ag can be applied to the small focal area of moist desquamation. Alternatively a small piece of Mepilex Transfer Ag, Aquacel Ag, Medihoney foam, or similar can be tucked into the fold for comfort, moisture control, and healing
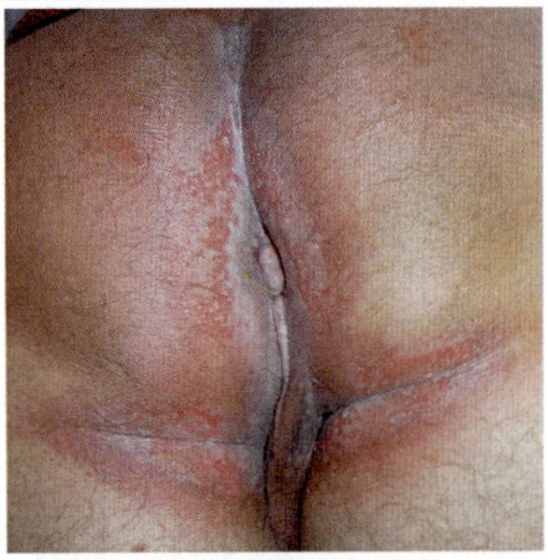	Healing of moist desquamation and formation of new skin islands	• Apply Skintegrity, leave in place for 2–3 min, and rinse off in shower • Apply A+D ointment or Aquaphor twice a day to the undressed skin in the radiation field • Place a sheet of Aquacel Ag or similar between the gluteal folds once a day or as needed if it gets soiled to areas of moist desquamation
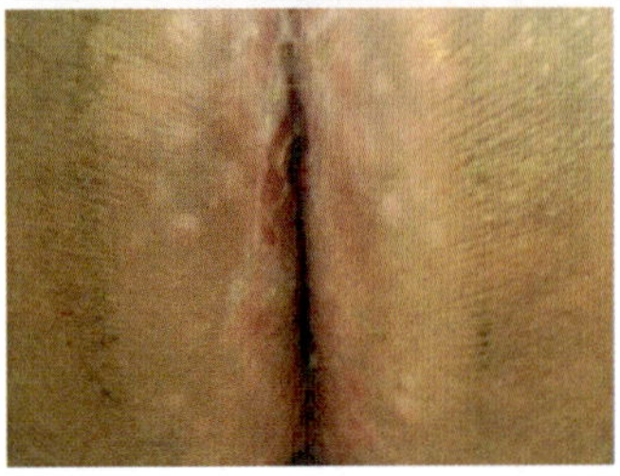	Hypopigmentation	• As above

Fig. 8.1 Suggested treatment algorithm for skin care

Week	Apply to Radiated Area	Notes
1-3	Calendula → Apply 2x/day Lidocaine cream → Use with bowel movements Sitz Baths → Use 2x/day and after bowel movements	Thicker cream to help maintain moisture. Can continue until skin erythema resolves, typically 2 weeks post radiation. Use lidocaine cream as needed for bowel movements and/or urination for women. Continue for duration of treatment.
3+	Calendula → Apply 2x/day Lidocaine cream → Use with bowel movements A+D Ointment OR Aquaphor → Apply 2x/day Sitz Baths → Use 2x/day and after bowel movements	Add A+D Ointment in combination with calendula. Liberally apply over radiated site twice a day. Aquaphor may be used rather than A+D Ointment. Continue to utilize the ointments for 2 - 3 weeks post radiation.
4-6 (without moist desquamation)	Skintegrity → Apply 1x/day A+D Ointment OR Aquaphor → Apply 2x/day Silvasorb OR Medihoney Gel → Apply 1x/day at night (Optional) Sitz Baths → Use 2x/day	Continue as above. Add Skintegrity. Spray Skintegrity onto radiated site and surrounding skin, leave in place for 1 - 2 minutes, and then rinse. Optional: For soothing and healing, may apply Silvasorb or Medihoney gel at bedtime and rinse away in the morning.
4-6 (with moist desquamation) Moist desquamation should be monitored closely and managed with the oncology team as patients are at high risk for anerobic infection and possible sepsis. Patients may require concurrent hydration, pain and nutritional support during this time. If severe a break may be indicated to allow skin healing.	Calendula → Apply 2x/day A+D Ointment OR Aquaphor → Apply 2x/day Skintegrity → Apply 1x/day Sitz Baths → Use 2x/day Dressing Choices → Use 1x/day, replace if it becomes soiled. Aquacel AG (or similar dressing) and cover with Mepilex lite (or similar secondary covering) OR Mepilex Transfer Ag OR Bacitracin with zinc oxide (1:1)	Continue as above. Add a dressing to the desquamated skin, either: Aquacel Ag with or without Mepilex lite (the Aquacel Ag may be tucked into perianal, buttocks or groin folds to hold in place). Aquacel may need to be reapplied throughout the day if it becomes soiled with urine or stool. OR Mepilex transfer Ag may be applied on the moist desquamation, use care when removing. OR Mixture of bacitracin/zinc oxide can be slathered on the desquamated area to promote comfort and healing. May cover with Mepilex, cotton boxers or Depends, etc., as it will be messy. This will need to be cleansed away prior to treatment (mineral oil/baza cleanser, ensure any residual oil residue washed away).

References

1. Surveillance, Epidemiology, and End Results Program, Cancer Statistics Review 1975–2012. National Cancer Institute, National Institutes of Health, U.S. Department of Health and Human Services. 2015. http://seer.cancer.gov/csr/1975_2012/results_single/sect_01_table.01.pdf. Accessed 26 June 2015.
2. Johnson LG, Madeleine MM, Newcomer LM, Schwartz SM, Daling JR. Anal cancer incidence and survival: the surveillance, epidemiology, and end results experience, 1973–2000. Cancer. 2004;101:281–8. doi:10.1002/cncr.20364.
3. Cancer Facts and Figures 2015. American Cancer Society. 2015. http://www.cancer.org/acs/groups/content/@editorial/documents/document/acspc-044552.pdf. Accessed 29 April 2015.
4. Frisch M, Biggar RJ, Goedert JJ. Human papillomavirus-associated cancers in patients with human immunodeficiency virus infection and acquired immunodeficiency syndrome. J Natl Cancer Inst. 2000;92:1500–10.
5. Nigro ND, Seydel HG, Considine B, Vaitkevicius VK, Leichman L, Kinzie JJ. Combined preoperative radiation and chemotherapy for squamous cell carcinoma of the anal canal. Cancer. 1983;51:1826–9.
6. Arnott SJ, Cunningham D, Gallagher J, Gray R, Hardcastle J, Houghton J, et al. Epidermoid anal cancer: Results from the UKCCCR randomised trial of radiotherapy alone versus radiotherapy, 5-fluorouracil, and mitomycin. Lancet. 1996;348:1049–54.
7. Bartelink H, Roelofsen F, Eschwege F, Rougier P, Bosset JF, Gonzalez DG, et al. Concomitant radiotherapy and chemotherapy is superior to radiotherapy alone in the treatment of locally advanced anal cancer: results of a phase III randomized trial of the European Organization for Research and Treatment of Cancer Radiotherapy and Gastrointestinal Cooperative Groups. J Clin Oncol. 1997;15:2040–9.
8. Flam M, John M, Pajak TF, Petrelli N, Myerson R, Doggett S, et al. Role of mitomycin in combination with fluorouracil and radiotherapy, and of salvage chemoradiation in the definitive nonsurgical treatment of epidermoid carcinoma of the anal canal: results of a phase III randomized intergroup study. J Clin Oncol. 1996;14:2527–39.
9. Ajani JA, Winter KA, Gunderson LL, Pedersen J, Benson 3rd AB, Thomas Jr CR, et al. Fluorouracil, mitomycin, and radiotherapy vs fluorouracil, cisplatin, and radiotherapy for carcinoma of the anal canal: a randomized controlled trial. JAMA. 2008;299:1914–21. doi:10.1001/jama.299.16.1914.
10. John M, Pajak T, Flam M, Hoffman J, Markoe A, Wolkov H, et al. Dose escalation in chemoradiation for anal cancer: preliminary results of RTOG 92–08. Cancer J Sci Am. 1996;2:205–11.
11. James R, Wan S, Glynne-Jones R, Sebag-Montefiore D, Kadalayil L, Northover J, et al. A randomized trial of chemoradiation using mitomycin or cisplatin, with or without maintenance cisplatin/5FU in squamous cell carcinoma of the anus (ACT II). J Clin Oncol. 2009;27.
12. Northover J, Glynne-Jones R, Sebag-Montefiore D, James R, Meadows H, Wan S, et al. Chemoradiation for the treatment of epidermoid anal cancer: 13-year follow-up of the first randomised UKCCCR Anal Cancer Trial (ACT I). Br J Cancer. 2010;102:1123–8. doi:10.1038/sj.bjc.6605605.
13. Gunderson LL, Winter KA, Ajani JA, Pedersen JE, Moughan J, Benson 3rd AB, et al. Long-term update of US GI intergroup RTOG 98–11 phase III trial for anal carcinoma: survival, relapse, and colostomy failure with concurrent chemoradiation involving fluorouracil/mitomycin versus fluorouracil/cisplatin. J Clin Oncol. 2012;30:4344–51. doi:10.1200/JCO.2012.43.8085.
14. Olivatto LO, Vieira FM, Pereira BV, Victorino AP, Bezerra M, Araujo CM, et al. Phase 1 study of cetuximab in combination with 5-fluorouracil, cisplatin, and radiotherapy in patients with locally advanced anal canal carcinoma. Cancer. 2013;119:2973–80. doi:10.1002/cncr.28045.
15. Deutsch E, Lemanski C, Paris E, Delarochefordiere A, Martel-Lafay I, Rio E, et al. Cetuximab plus radiochemotherapy in locally advanced anal cancer: Interim results of the French multicenter phase II trial ACCORD16. J Clin Oncol. 2011;29.
16. Chiao EY, Giordano TP, Richardson P, El-Serag HB. Human immunodeficiency virus-associated squamous cell cancer of the anus: epidemiology and outcomes in the highly active antiretroviral therapy era. J Clin Oncol. 2008;26:474–9. doi:10.1200/JCO.2007.14.2810.
17. Seo Y, Kinsella MT, Reynolds HL, Chipman G, Remick SC, Kinsella TJ. Outcomes of chemoradiotherapy with 5-Fluorouracil and mitomycin C for anal cancer in immunocompetent versus immunodeficient patients. Int J Radiat Oncol Biol Phys. 2009;75:143–9. doi:10.1016/j.ijrobp.2008.10.046.
18. Oehler-Janne C, Huguet F, Provencher S, Seifert B, Negretti L, Riener MO, et al. HIV-specific differences in outcome of squamous cell carcinoma of the anal canal: a multicentric cohort study of HIV-positive patients receiving highly active antiretroviral therapy. J Clin Oncol. 2008;26:2550–7. doi:10.1200/JCO.2007.15.2348.
19. Klencke BJ, Palefsky JM. Anal cancer: an HIV-associated cancer. Hematol Oncol Clin North Am. 2003;17:859–72.
20. Hoffman R, Welton ML, Klencke B, Weinberg V, Krieg R. The significance of pretreatment CD4 count on the outcome and treatment tolerance of HIV-positive patients with anal cancer. Int J Radiat Oncol Biol Phys. 1999;44:127–31.
21. Fraunholz I, Weiss C, Eberlein K, Haberl A, Rodel C. Concurrent chemoradiotherapy with 5-fluorouracil and mitomycin C for invasive anal carcinoma in human immunodeficiency virus-positive patients

receiving highly active antiretroviral therapy. Int J Radiat Oncol Biol Phys. 2010;76:1425–32. doi:10.1016/j.ijrobp.2009.03.060.
22. Milano MT, Jani AB, Farrey KJ, Rash C, Heimann R, Chmura SJ. Intensity-modulated radiation therapy (IMRT) in the treatment of anal cancer: toxicity and clinical outcome. Int J Radiat Oncol Biol Phys. 2005;63:354–61. doi:10.1016/j.ijrobp.2005.02.030.
23. Pepek JM, Willett CG, Wu QJ, Yoo S, Clough RW, Czito BG. Intensity-modulated radiation therapy for anal malignancies: a preliminary toxicity and disease outcomes analysis. Int J Radiat Oncol Biol Phys. 2010;78:1413–9. doi:10.1016/j.ijrobp.2009.09.046.
24. Kachnic L, Winter K, Myerson R, Goodyear M, Willins J, Esthappan J, et al. RTOG 0529: A phase II evaluation of dose-painted IMRT in combination with 5-Fluorouracil and Mitomycin-C for reduction of acute morbidity in carcinoma of the anal canal. Int J Radiat Oncol Biol Phys. 2009;75:5. doi:10.1016/j.ijrobp.2009.07.038.
25. Kachnic LA, Winter K, Myerson RJ, Goodyear MD, Willins J, Esthappan J, et al. RTOG 0529: a phase 2 evaluation of dose-painted intensity modulated radiation therapy in combination with 5-fluorouracil and mitomycin-C for the reduction of acute morbidity in carcinoma of the anal canal. Int J Radiat Oncol Biol Phys. 2013;86:27–33. doi:10.1016/j.ijrobp.2012.09.023.
26. Samuelian JM, Callister MD, Ashman JB, Young-Fadok TM, Borad MJ, Gunderson LL. Reduced acute bowel toxicity in patients treated with intensity-modulated radiotherapy for rectal cancer. Int J Radiat Oncol Biol Phys. 2012;82:1981–7. doi:10.1016/j.ijrobp.2011.01.051.
27. Bujko K, Nowacki MP, Nasierowska-Guttmejer A, Michalski W, Bebenek M, Kryj M. Long-term results of a randomized trial comparing preoperative short-course radiotherapy with preoperative conventionally fractionated chemoradiation for rectal cancer. Br J Surg. 2006;93:1215–23. doi:10.1002/bjs.5506.

9 Genitourinary Cancer

Kaveh Maghsoudi, Steve E. Braunstein, and Florence Yuen

Genitourinary cancers include cancers of the kidneys, bladder, and urethra, as well as the prostate, testicle, and penis in men. Local disease is common at presentation, but systemic disease involving bone, lung, or central nervous system sites is not uncommon. Radiation therapy is utilized at various stages in the treatment of all of these conditions. Given the relatively high prevalence of prostate cancer and the relatively high skin toxicity of penile cancer treatment, these two diseases are highlighted in this section.

Of all the GU cancers, prostate cancer is by far the most common, and radiation is a primary treatment modality for both early- and advanced stage, as well as salvage therapy for local recurrence after prostatectomy. The American Cancer Society (ACS) estimates about 220,000 new cases of prostate cancer and approximately 28,000 deaths attributed to prostate cancer in the United States in 2015 [1]. In addition, the ACS estimates that about one in every seven males will be diagnosed with prostate cancer in their lifetime, nearly all over the age of 40 and 60 % older than age 65.

A variety of modalities of radiation therapy are commonly employed in the treatment of prostate cancer including external beam radiation with photons and protons, as well as brachytherapy techniques such as permanent prostate seed implants and high-dose rate brachytherapy. The typical doses used in the treatment of prostate cancer depend on the modality of treatment as well as the clinical setting. In the setting of definitive prostate cancer treatment with external beam radiotherapy using conventional fractionation, doses typically exceed 70 Gy. Since the treatment targets including the prostate, seminal vesicles, and pelvic lymph nodes are well-situated within the pelvis, the resulting dose to the skin, however, is significantly less than the prescribed target dose.

Radiation therapy (including external beam and, increasingly, unsealed sources such as strontium and radium) is also frequently used to palliate sites of bony and soft-tissue metastatic disease, most commonly in prostate, renal, and bladder cancer. In this application, moderate doses of hypofractionated external beam radiotherapy are directed to osseous structures, which may be in proximity to superficial tissues, such as with vertebral metastases, resulting in modest skin dose.

Penile cancer will be diagnosed in nearly 2000 men and will cause about 300 deaths in the United

K. Maghsoudi, MD, PhD • F. Yuen
Department of Radiation Oncology, University of California San Francisco, San Francisco, San Francisco, CA, USA

S.E. Braunstein, MD, PhD (✉)
UCSF Ron Conway Family, Gateway Medical Building, 1825 4th Street, Room M2260, Box 4001, San Francisco, CA 94158, USA

Department of Radiation Oncology, University of California San Francisco, San Francisco, San Francisco, CA, USA
e-mail: Steve.Braunstein@ucsf.edu

B. Fowble et al. (eds.), *Skin Care in Radiation Oncology*, DOI 10.1007/978-3-319-31460-0_9

States in 2015 according to the ACS [1]. The incidence of penile cancer increases with age, ranging from less than 0.1 to greater than 2.5 cases per 100,000 from the age of 20–85 [2]. For patients not undergoing surgical resection, radiation treatment modalities represent organ-sparing and may be psychologically preferable. These include external beam radiation therapy as well as interstitial brachytherapy. The conventionally fractionated doses of external beam radiation therapy typically range from 50 to 65 Gy, with the higher doses corresponding to smaller field boosts. For regional lymphatics such as inguinal nodes that are not removed surgically and are instead treated definitively with radiation therapy, the overall dose to gross disease may be as high as 70–75 Gy.

9.1 Types and Frequency of Skin Reactions

Skin toxicity from modern mega-voltage radiation therapy for prostate cancer is often not as pronounced as in other sites requiring or receiving more superficial dose. The use of more conformal dose deposition techniques, including multiple beam angles, tissue compensators, and intensity-modulated radiation therapy, has enabled increased dose sparing of superficial tissues. Primary nodal sites of prostate cancer spread include pelvic and para-aortic lymph node stations and exclude more superficial inguinal sites, further sparing potential treatment morbidity. Moreover, while acute rectal proctitis is common during prostate radiotherapy, the mucosal reaction is generally limited to regions above the dentate line and does not typically involve the anal or perianal skin region. Thus, acute or late grade ≥2 skin toxicities are not observed or reported in current high-dose prostate cancer treatments [3].

A prospective phase I dose escalation study, RTOG 9406, for the treatment of prostate cancer using 3D-CRT prescribing up to a dose of 79.2 Gy demonstrated relatively minimal skin toxicity including approximately 10 % grade 1 and 2 % grade 2, and 0 % grade 3 or higher early skin toxicities and 1 % grade 2 late skin toxicity [4]. The above skin toxicity includes erythema, irritation, and rarely desquamation of skin along the perineum, addressed by topical creams. The incidence peaks during the final weeks of radiation and typically subsides several weeks following the end of treatment. There can also be regional patchy hair loss corresponding in location to entrance and exit beams and can take on the order of months to grow back.

IMRT has become standard radiation treatment for prostate cancer; however, data on toxicity due to IMRT versus 3D-CRT is mixed. Studies have shown improvement of dose-distribution and urinary/rectal toxicity with IMRT [5, 6]. On the other hand, a phase 3 dose-escalation trial, RTOG 0126, comparing toxicities from IMRT versus 3D-CRT did not appear to show significant difference in patient-reported bowel, bladder, or sexual function [7] even though dose to the corresponding organs at risk was reduced. Skin toxicity was not analyzed in either study, and though the use of IMRT can theoretically limit dose to the skin surface, it is not clear that there is a significant advantage in preventing the already low rates of radiation dermatitis.

In addition, prostate cancer patients treated with brachytherapy can have temporary erythema and inflammation of the underlying perineum. Patients often experience associated soreness of the perineum and are prescribed symptomatic relief with sitz baths and ibuprofen. These symptoms are secondary to skin and soft tissue trauma from catheter placement rather than from radiation exposure, and they typically improve and self-resolve over the course of several days after catheter removal. Patients rarely require narcotic medication for pain relief or antibiotics for infection. No acute or late grade ≥2 skin toxicities have been reported in recent RTOG brachytherapy trials [8, 9].

Unlike prostate cancer, the treatment targets in penile and urethral cancer are much closer to the skin surface, thereby resulting in significantly greater dose and expected increased toxicities. Male penile and both male and female urethral sites have primary lymphatic drainage to the inguinal nodes and thus inguinal sites are included in external beam therapy and may yield significant skin toxicity as is commonly seen in anal and vulvar cancer radiation therapy. As such, the penile and urethral treatments require close surveillance and care during the course of radiation treatment and during follow-up. Toxicities include short-term, brisk, dry, and moist desquamation with possible secondary infections, swelling, and irritation. In addition, long-term effects include fibrosis, telangiectasias, hypo- or hyperpigmentation, meatal-urethral strictures and stenosis, and even ulceration and necrosis.

Treatment and response for short-term skin complications include supportive care outlined in the section on skin cancer. These toxicities typically improve significantly within the first month post-radiation. In one relatively large series involving 49 patients undergoing penile interstitial brachytherapy [10], the rate of soft-tissue necrosis at the implanted site was 16 % (eight men) and the rate of distal urethral stenosis requiring intermittent meatal dilatation was 12 % (six men). The rate of necrosis was significantly associated with the number of needles used in the implant and increased tumor stage. Other studies have reported incidence of soft tissue necrosis as high as nearly one in four patients, peaking in incidence between six and 18 months, and associated with other risk factors including dose of 60 Gy or higher, and volume of implant >30 cm^3 [11, 12].

Treatment of ulceration or soft tissue necrosis includes keeping affected areas clean and applying topical antibiotics and steroid creams. In cases where conservative treatment fails, hyperbaric oxygen treatment and possibly even partial penectomy may be required [13].

9.2 Special Situations

Hypofractionated radiation therapy is increasingly being employed to maximize the intrinsic radiobiologic characteristics of prostate cancer. As with much of the modern prostate literature, initial hypofractionated trial results have not reported skin toxicity [14, 15]. For stereotactic treatments which frequently employ non-coplanar arcs or beamlets, the three-dimensional space occupied by the penis and scrotum is contoured so as to avoid beams passing through this region.

Penile cancer patients who are planning to undergo external beam radiation therapy must undergo circumcision to help better assess tumor response, minimize skin toxicity, and prevent phimosis. Case reports of radiation-induced phimosis have been associated with treatment of rectal cancer [16, 17]. Of note, phimosis has also been described as a risk factor for developing penile cancer, increasing the odds by about 7 [18]. However, since the population risk of developing penile cancer is fairly small, circumcision has not been recommended based on its association with reduced risk of cancer.

Although there are certainly more prevalent causes of scrotal pain and swelling such as testicular torsion and epididymitis, patients may experience these symptoms after radiation therapy. There are reports, particularly in older prostate radiation literature of rare penile lymphedema associated with radiation therapy [19, 20]. However, many patients had prior surgeries including lymph node dissections, making the causation due to radiation controversial. In addition, even lower doses of radiation therapy such as those used in the treatment of testicular cancer have been associated with rare scrotal edema [21]. The etiology is unclear, but could be secondary to spermatic cord obstruction, and the swelling can wax and wane over 2–3 years following radiation therapy. Treatment generally involves ice, elevation, and anti-inflammatory medication such as ibuprofen.

9.3 Photographs and Recommendations

Below are general skin care recommendations (Table 9.1), week by week treatment instructions, and photographs that demonstrate typical skin reactions over time for genitourinary patients (Table 9.2). Photographs of special reactions and instructions on how to treat these more uncommon cases are also provided (Table 9.3). Figure 9.1 is a general suggested treatment algorithm for skin care for genitourinary patients.

Table 9.1 General principles of skin care for genitourinary cancer patients

Patient should:
• Cleanse daily with mild soap and water
• Use recommended lotions and creams
• Wear soft undergarments that control moisture
Patient should not:
• Rub, put pressure on, or scratch radiated area
• Take hot water showers, hot baths, use wash cloth
• Apply any lotion, cream or ointment in the 3 hours prior to radiation treatment
• Apply drying agents to the skin unless instructed to do so
• Use any tape or adhesives on the radiated skin

Table 9.2 Examples of typical acute skin reactions and recommended interventions

Week	Skin reaction	Reaction type	Intervention
1	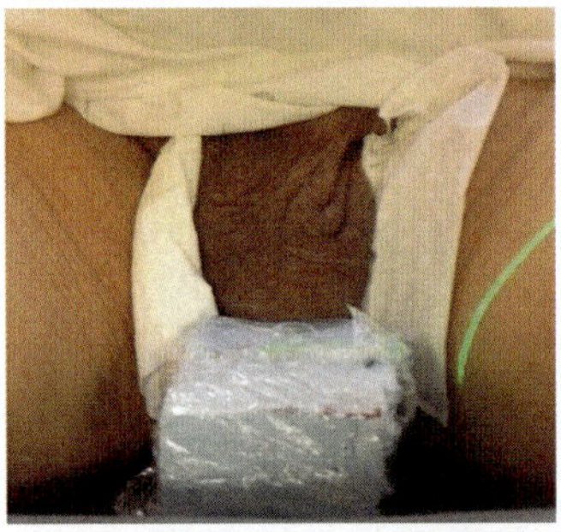	No reaction	• Keep area clean and dry • Wash area with mild soap and water daily • Moisturize twice daily with a light moisturizer such as Lotion Soft or Remedy • Avoid overmoisturizing the skin folds as this could promote fungal overgrowth
2	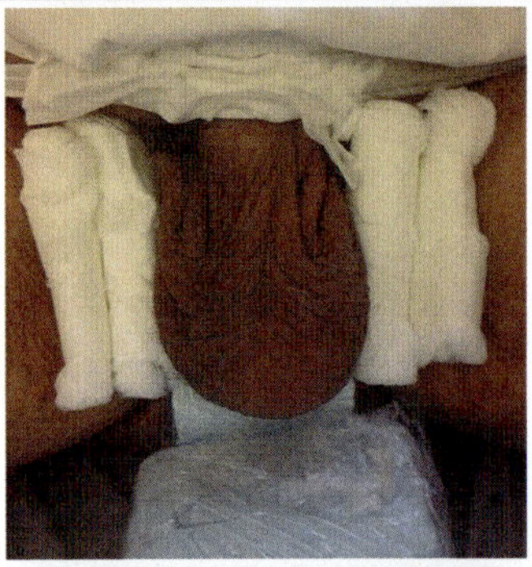	Mild tanning	• Keep area clean and dry • Wash area with mild soap and water daily • Moisturize twice daily with a light moisturizer such as Lotion Soft or Remedy • Avoid overmoisturizing the skin folds as this could promote fungal overgrowth
3	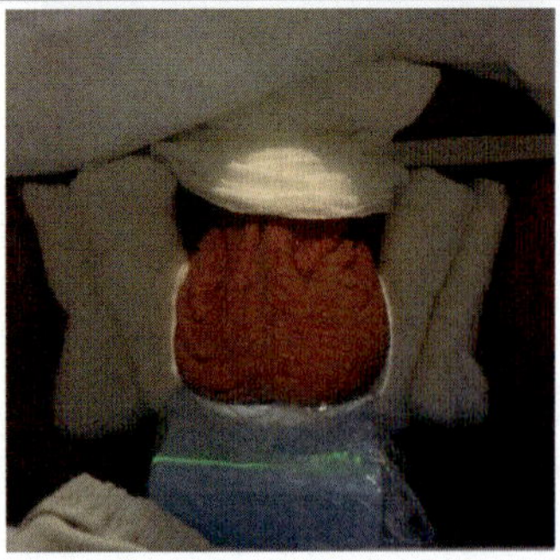	Moderate erythema	• Keep area clean and dry • Wash area with mild soap and water daily • Switch moisturizer to calendula and apply twice daily • Avoid overmoisturizing the skin folds as this could promote fungal overgrowth

77-year-old male with lymphoma with CNS and testicular involvement. Receiving 30 Gy in 15 fractions to the testicles

Table 9.3 Special cases and reactions

High-dose rate brachytherapy for prostate cancer	Reaction type None	Treatment and intervention
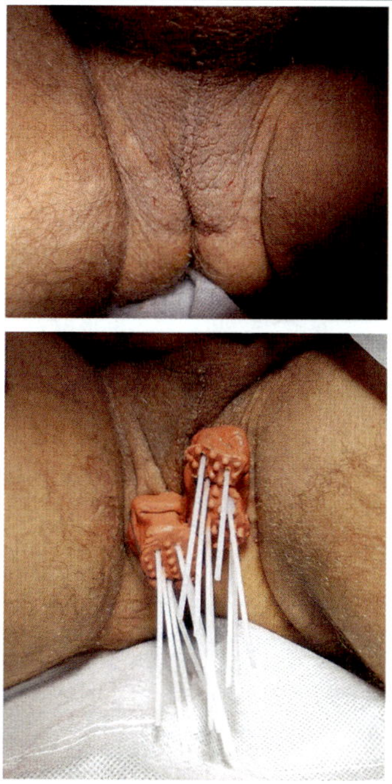	HDR Brachytherapy. 15 Gy in 1 fraction Catheters removed following treatment	• Catheters are inserted under anesthesia • Patient is prepped with betadine solution and 16 catheters are inserted under ultrasound guidance, secured with dental putty and sutured to the perineum • After radiation delivery, the catheters are removed and the area is wiped with an alcohol pad • Use sitz baths daily for up to a week, but otherwise keep the area clean and dry without any topicals • Wear soft absorbent undergarment

Week	Apply to Radiated Area	Notes
1-3	Light moisturizer ↓ Apply 2x/day	Apply thin lotion such as Lotion Soft or Remedy that is quickly absorbed, leaves no residue and is not comedogenic.
3+	Switch to calendula ↓ Apply 2x/day	Thicker cream that can be used to help maintain moisture. Can continue until skin erythema resolves, typically two weeks post radiation. May continue with calendula if the patient does not progress beyond mild to moderate erythema.
4+	Calendula + A&D Ointment/Aquaphor + Skintegrity Calendula ↓ Apply 1x/day A&D Ointment/Aquaphor ↓ Apply 1x/day before bed Skintegrity ↓ Spray 1x/day	Begin applying this combination as erythema progresses and moisture loss becomes apparent Spray Skintegrity and wash off after one to two minutes. Apply A&D or Aquaphor until one week post radiation. Apply calendula until normal skin color returns.

Fig 9.1 Suggested treatment algorithm for skin care. Most of the patients with urologic malignancies will have minimal or no radiation dermatitis. However, those with penile, testicular, or urethral cancers may experience a spectrum of acute radiation skin reactions

References

1. Cancer Facts and Figs. 2015. American Cancer Society. 2015. http://www.cancer.org/acs/groups/content/@editorial/documents/document/acspc-044552.pdf. Accessed 29 April 2015.
2. Surveillance, Epidemiology, and End Results Program, Cancer Statistics Review 1975–2012. National Cancer Institute, National Institutes of Health, U.S. Department of Health and Human Services. 2009. http://seer.cancer.gov/data/. Accessed 26 June 2015.
3. Mohammed N, Kestin L, Ghilezan M, Krauss D, Vicini F, Brabbins D, et al. Comparison of acute and late toxicities for three modern high-dose radiation treatment techniques for localized prostate cancer. Int J Radiat Oncol Biol Phys. 2012;82:204–12. doi:10.1016/j.ijrobp.2010.10.009.
4. Ryu JK, Winter K, Michalski JM, Purdy JA, Markoe AM, Earle JD, et al. Interim report of toxicity from 3D conformal radiation therapy (3D-CRT) for prostate cancer on 3DOG/RTOG 9406, level III (79.2 Gy). Int J Radiat Oncol Biol Phys. 2002;54:1036–46.
5. Zelefsky MJ, Fuks Z, Hunt M, Yamada Y, Marion C, Ling CC, et al. High-dose intensity modulated radiation therapy for prostate cancer: early toxicity and biochemical outcome in 772 patients. Int J Radiat Oncol Biol Phys. 2002;53:1111–6.
6. Wortel RC, Incrocci L, Pos FJ, Lebesque JV, Witte MG, van der Heide UA, et al. Acute toxicity after image-guided intensity modulated radiation therapy compared to 3D conformal radiation therapy in prostate cancer patients. Int J Radiat Oncol Biol Phys. 2015;91:737–44. doi:10.1016/j.ijrobp.2014.12.017.
7. Bruner DW, Hunt D, Michalski JM, Bosch WR, Galvin JM, Amin M, et al. Preliminary patient-reported outcomes analysis of 3-dimensional radiation therapy versus intensity-modulated radiation therapy on the high-dose arm of the Radiation Therapy Oncology Group (RTOG) 0126 prostate cancer trial. Cancer. 2015;121(14):2422–30. doi:10.1002/cncr.29362.
8. Hsu IC, Bae K, Shinohara K, Pouliot J, Purdy J, Ibbott G, et al. Phase II trial of combined high-dose-rate brachytherapy and external beam radiotherapy for adenocarcinoma of the prostate: preliminary results of RTOG 0321. Int J Radiat Oncol Biol Phys. 2010;78:751–8. doi:10.1016/j.ijrobp.2009.08.048.
9. Lawton CA, Yan Y, Lee WR, Gillin M, Firat S, Baikadi M, et al. Long-term results of an RTOG Phase II trial (00–19) of external-beam radiation therapy combined with permanent source brachytherapy for intermediate-risk clinically localized adenocarcinoma of the prostate. Int J Radiat Oncol Biol Phys. 2012;82:e795–801. doi:10.1016/j.ijrobp.2011.11.040.
10. Crook JM, Jezioranski J, Grimard L, Esche B, Pond G. Penile brachytherapy: results for 49 patients. Int J Radiat Oncol Biol Phys. 2005;62:460–7. doi:10.1016/j.ijrobp.2004.10.016.
11. Mazeron JJ, Langlois D, Lobo PA, Huart JA, Calitchi E, Lusinchi A, et al. Interstitial radiation therapy for carcinoma of the penis using iridium 192 wires: the Henri Mondor experience (1970–1979). Int J Radiat Oncol Biol Phys. 1984;10:1891–5.
12. Rozan R, Albuisson E, Giraud B, Donnarieix D, Delannes M, Pigneux J, et al. Interstitial brachytherapy for penile carcinoma: a multicentric survey (259 patients). Radiother Oncol. 1995;36:83–93.
13. Crook JM, Haie-Meder C, Demanes DJ, Mazeron JJ, Martinez AA, Rivard MJ. American Brachytherapy Society-Groupe Europeen de Curietherapie-European Society of Therapeutic Radiation Oncology (ABS-GEC-ESTRO) consensus statement for penile brachytherapy. Brachytherapy. 2013;12:191–8. doi:10.1016/j.brachy.2013.01.167.
14. Pollack A, Hanlon AL, Horwitz EM, Feigenberg SJ, Konski AA, Movsas B, et al. Dosimetry and preliminary acute toxicity in the first 100 men treated for prostate cancer on a randomized hypofractionation dose escalation trial. Int J Radiat Oncol Biol Phys. 2006;64:518–26. doi:10.1016/j.ijrobp.2005.07.970.
15. Arcangeli G, Saracino B, Gomellini S, Petrongari MG, Arcangeli S, Sentinelli S, et al. A prospective phase III randomized trial of hypofractionation versus conventional fractionation in patients with high-risk prostate cancer. Int J Radiat Oncol Biol Phys. 2010;78:11–8. doi:10.1016/j.ijrobp.2009.07.1691.
16. Featherstone JM, Aldridge A, Gudgeon AM. Radiotherapy for rectal carcinoma: an unusual cause of foreskin phimosis. Int Urol Nephrol. 2006;38:603–5. doi:10.1007/s11255-005-4758-0.
17. Nair RG, Bensadoun RJ, Oberholzer T, Gopalan V, Young SC, Joubert W. An unusual case of foreskin phimosis after radiotherapy for rectal carcinoma. Cancer Radiother. 2012;16:292–4. doi:10.1016/j.canrad.2012.03.007.
18. Daling JR, Madeleine MM, Johnson LG, Schwartz SM, Shera KA, Wurscher MA, et al. Penile cancer: importance of circumcision, human papillomavirus and smoking in in situ and invasive disease. Int J Cancer. 2005;116:606–16. doi:10.1002/ijc.21009.
19. Dewit L, Ang KK, Van der Schueren E. Acute side effects and late complications after radiotherapy of localized carcinoma of the prostate. Cancer Treat Rev. 1983;10:79–89.
20. Petrovich Z, Lieskovsky G, Langholz B, Luxton G, Jozsef G, Skinner DG. Radiotherapy following radical prostatectomy in patients with adenocarcinoma of the prostate. Int J Radiat Oncol Biol Phys. 1991;21:949–54.
21. Hunter M, Peschel RE. Testicular seminoma. Results of the Yale University experience, 1964–1984. Cancer. 1989;64:1608–11.

10 Gynecologic Cancer

Tracy Sherertz and Jennifer Bohm

Gynecological cancers comprise a heterogeneous group of pelvic malignancies that affect women; these include cervical, uterine, ovarian/fallopian tube, vulvar and vaginal carcinomas. Cervical cancer, in particular, represents a major global health burden, with 528,000 new cases and 266,000 deaths in 2012 [1]. In low- and middle-income countries (LMIC), cervical cancer remains the leading cause of cancer death in women. In high-income countries that utilize widespread screening programs, however, both the incidence and mortality of cervical cancer rates are lower than in LMIC. In the United States, uterine cancer has become the most common cause of gynecological malignancies. Worldwide, there were 320,000 new cases of uterine cancers and 76,000 deaths in 2012 [1]. Ovarian cancer is the seventh most common cancer in women worldwide, with 239,000 new cases diagnosed in 2012 [1], but it carries an exceptionally high mortality rate in advanced stages. The 5-year overall survival for localized ovarian cancer is 92 % compared to only 27 % for advanced disease [2]. Vulvar cancers are much less common, representing only 4 % of gynecological malignancies. Vaginal cancer is even more rare with an expected 4070 cases diagnosed in 2015 in the US, based on estimates from the American Cancer Society [2].

External beam radiotherapy (EBRT) plays an important role in the definitive, adjuvant, and palliative treatment of several gynecological malignancies:

- Definitive treatment for locally advanced or non-operable cervical cancer
- Post-operative adjuvant therapy for high-risk cervical cancer
- Definitive treatment for unresectable uterine cancer
- Post-operative adjuvant therapy for high-risk uterine cancer
- Definitive treatment for vaginal cancer
- Definitive treatment for unresectable vulvar cancer
- Post-operative adjuvant therapy for high-risk vulvar cancer
- Tumor-directed radiotherapy for ovarian, peritoneal, and fallopian tube cancers
- Palliative care for bleeding or painful gynecological tumors in the pelvis

10.1 Treatment-Related Morbidity

Tumors affecting the gynecological organs invariably carry a risk for reproductive, sexual, cosmetic, and emotional consequences due to

T. Sherertz, MD (✉) • J. Bohm, RN, BSN
Department of Radiation Oncology, University of California, San Francisco, Box 1708,
1600 Divisadero, Cancer Centre Room 1029,
San Francisco, CA 94143, USA
e-mail: Tracy.Sherertz@ucsf.edu

B. Fowble et al. (eds.), *Skin Care in Radiation Oncology*, DOI 10.1007/978-3-319-31460-0_10

their unique location. Moreover, due to the proximity to the external genitourinary and lower gastrointestinal tracts, skin toxicity as a result from treatment is one of the most important determinants for patient tolerance and compliance during a course of radiotherapy, especially when the external genitalia is included in the radiation field. Attention to the multitude of side effects from radiotherapy is necessary to maximize its efficacy while minimizing morbidity to the patient. Successfully managing skin toxicity will minimize patient discomfort and treatment interruptions, which is central to high quality care of gynecological tumors.

10.2 Types and Frequency of Skin Reactions

A wide range of skin reactions can occur during a course of pelvic radiotherapy. Acute skin reactions develop because the skin contains a large population of cells that are turning over rapidly. Skin cells are arranged in a hierarchical fashion, with a small number of stem cells that grow into a highly proliferative pool of progenitor cells that in turn become mature, functioning, nonproliferative skin cells [3]. Stem cells and progenitor cells will die first after being exposed to radiation, leaving the mature, non-proliferating skin cells intact until they slough off through normal cell turnover [3]. Skin reactions can occur anywhere in the radiation field, and pelvic radiotherapy fields can cover a variable amount of skin depending on the extent of the target. This can range from a minimal volume of only a few cubic centimeters in small palliative tumor-directed fields, to very large fields that cover the skin of the abdomen, pelvis, inguinal regions, and external genitalia.

Reporting of acute and late toxicity from pelvic radiotherapy has largely been focused on gastrointestinal and hematological toxicity because of the amount of bowel and bone marrow in traditional radiation treatment fields for cervical cancer. Acute radiation dermatitis has not been well-reported, however, despite being a notable occurrence for many patients undergoing EBRT in the pelvis, especially when the inguinal regions and distal genitalia are covered. Several scoring schemes have been used in the past to report toxicity from pelvic radiotherapy with the two more common at present time being the Radiation Therapy Oncology Group (RTOG) and the National NCI/CTC scoring systems [4]. In the RTOG Acute Radiation Morbidity Scoring Criteria for skin toxicity, grade 0 is no change over baseline; grade 1 includes follicular, faint or dull erythema, epilation, dry desquamation, and decreased sweating; grade 2 includes tender or bright erythema, moderate edema, and patchy moist desquamation; grade 3 includes pitting edema, and confluent or moist desquamation other than in skin folds; and grade 4 includes ulceration, hemorrhage, and necrosis [5].

Most published reports about skin toxicity from radiotherapy for gynecological cancers is found in the cervical cancer literature, due to the relatively high incidence of cervical cancer and hence the ability to study in large clinical trials. Table 10.1 [6–12] summarizes the skin toxicity reported in seven major clinical trials where pelvic radiotherapy was used with or without concurrent chemotherapy in the treatment of cervical cancer.

10.3 Typical Course of Reaction

The cell turnover kinetics will determine how quickly the skin in the radiation field demonstrates an effect from radiation. With standard fractionation sizes of 1.8–2.0 Gy per day, the progression of skin reaction is somewhat predictable. In the first 2 weeks of radiotherapy, the skin in the treatment field develops a pink coloration with mild edema and often associated pruritis and discomfort. This may progress to dry desquamation in the second, third, and fourth weeks, characterized by dryness, scaling, and hyperpigmentation of skin. In the fourth through sixth weeks, the reaction can progress to moist desquamation where the skin weeps due to interruption of the epithelial barrier. Final late changes, seen often in the fourth-sixth weeks of radiation, may include pigmentation changes, partial or com-

Table 10.1 Acute skin toxicity reported in cervical cancer trials

	No. of patients reported	Accrual period	Median follow-up (months)	Dose/Fractionation (Gy)	Technique	Concurrent chemo	Toxicity GR 1 (%)	Toxicity GR 2 (%)	Toxicity GR 3 (%)	Toxicity GR 4 (%)	Scoring system
RT alone											
Keys et al. [6]	186	1992–1997	36	45/1.8–2	4-field	None	5.4	3.8	1.6	0.5	NCI/CTC
Morris et al. [7]	193	1990–1997	43	45/1.8	4-field	None	–	–	0	0.5	CGCT (CARMSC)
Peters et al. [8]	112	1991–1996	42	49.3/1.7	4-field	None	1.8	0.9	0	0	SWOG/GOG
Rose et al. [9]	177	1992–1997	35	40.8/1.7 or 50.1/1.7	AP/PA or 4-field	HU	5.6	3.4	1.7	0.6	NCI/CTC
Whitney et al. [10]	188	1986–1990	–	40.8/1.7 or 50.1/1.7 +/– PM boost	AP/PA or 4-field	HU	7.4	3.2	1.6	0	GOG
Roberts et al. [11]	82	1994–1997	–	40/2.0 or 46/2.0	4-field	None	46		1	–	ECOG/RTOG/EORTC [John]
Wong et al. [12]	110	1989–1992	77	40/2.5	–	None	14.5	0	0	0	WHO
RT + Chemo											
Keys et al. [6]	183	1992–1997	36	45/1.8–2	4-field	CDDP	9.8	3.8	0	0	NCI/CTC
Morris et al. [7]	195	1990–1997	43	45/1.8	4-field	CDDP+5FU	–	–	2	0.5	CGCT (CARMSC)
Peters et al. [8]	122	1991–1996	42	49.3/1.7	4-field	CDDP+5FU	1.6	1.6	2.5	0	SWOG/GOG
Rose et al. [9]	176 (RT+Cis) 173 (RT+Cis/5FU/HU)	1992–1997	35	40.8/1.7 or 50.1/1.7	AP/PA or 4-field	CDDP CDDP/5FU/HU	4.0 5.8	3.4 4.0	0.6 1.7	0.6 1.2	NCI/CTC
Whitney et al. [10]	169	1986–1990	–	40.8/1.7 or 50.1/1.7 +/– PN boost	AP/PA or 4-field	CDDP+5FU	14.8	5.3	2.4	0	GOG
Roberts et al. [11]	78	1994–1997	–	40/2.0 or 46/2.0	4-field	MMC	55		4	–	ECOG/RTOG/EORTC [John]
Wong et al. [12]	110	1989–1992	77	40/2.5	–	Epirubicin	18	0	0	0	WHO

AP/PA anterior-posterior/posterior-anterior, *CDDP* Cisplatin, *5FU* 5-Fluorouracil, *HU* Hydroxyurea, *MMC* Mitomycin C, *NCI/CTC* National Cancer Institute Common Toxicity Criteria, *CGCT (CARMSC)* Cooperative Group Common Toxicity Criteria, *WHO* World Health Organization, *GOG* Gynecologic Oncology Group, *ECOG/RTOG/EORTC* Eastern Cooperative Oncology Group/Radiation Therapy Oncology Group/European Organisation for Research and Treatment of Cancer, *SWOG/GOG* Southwest Oncology Group/Gynecologic Oncology Group, – Indicates not reported

plete alopecia, telangiectasia formation, atrophy, ulceration and tissue thickening, and fibrous changes. Once radiation is completed, the skin toxicity gradually resolves over the next 4–5 weeks, although healing can be prolonged in patients with poor wound healing. Multiple patient- and tumor-specific factors affect the onset, severity, and recovery of skin reactions during a course of pelvic radiotherapy, the most significant of which are described below.

10.4 Factors Affecting Skin Toxicity

10.4.1 Appositional Skin in the Radiation Field

Skin in apposition to other skin is at risk for developing more severe skin toxicity when exposed to radiation. Sitton et al. described this observation at treatment sites where skin was in apposition to other skin [13]. In the pelvis, this includes the groin, inner-thighs, perineum, buttocks, and external vagina. Heat and moisture are trapped in these locations, and the skin experiences more friction and less aeration. The proposed mechanism behind the increased dermatitis is that the stratum corneum there is shed more rapidly than the newly forming epithelium [13]. Even areas of the skin experiencing friction from tightly fitting clothing (i.e., skin around waistline and panty-line) are also at risk for this more severe skin reaction. The same is true for bedbound or immobile patients who experience an increase in skin toxicity due to the constant pressure on the skin of their back/buttock.

10.4.2 External Genitalia in the Radiation Field

Not only does skin friction and heat/moisture trapping in these appositional sites worsen the skin toxicity, but the presence of urine and stool over the treated skin also greatly increases the skin irritation and dramatically increases the risk for concomitant skin infection. Radiotherapy for vulvar and vaginal cancer invariably includes the external genitalia in the high-dose treatment fields. For definitive treatment of gross disease, prescribed doses are upwards of 64 Gy, and if EBRT is used in combination with brachytherapy, prescribed doses can reach 65–90 Gy [14]. Due to the high necessary dose, efforts have been focused on using highly conformal techniques such as intensity-modulated radiation therapy (IMRT) to dose-paint, allowing for high doses in the target and lower doses in the normal tissues. Nevertheless, it is common for patients undergoing radiotherapy for vulvar and vaginal cancers to experience severe skin reactions, often necessitating treatment breaks. Table 10.2 [15–18] summarizes the skin toxicity reported in select studies where external radiotherapy was used to treat vulvar or vaginal cancers. Late complications from radiotherapy to the vulvo-vaginal region are important considerations when the vulva and vagina are included in the radiation field. These often include telangiectasia formation, atrophy of the skin, dryness of the mucosa of the vulva and vagina, and narrowing of the vaginal introitus [19]. This plays a central role in the psychosexual consequences following a course of radiotherapy for vulvar or vaginal cancer and can affect long-term quality of life.

In the preoperative series by Beriwal et al, moist desquamation was confined to the vulva and perineum, with no patient experiencing confluent desquamation in the groins. This was suggestive of a possible dosimetric advantage of using intensity-modulated radiation therapy (IMRT) that allows for sparing of the skin dose in the groin regions. With the increased use of IMRT, further investigation may clarify the potential benefit of using IMRT to reduce radiation-related cutaneous toxicity.

10.4.3 Body Habitus

Obese patients, especially those with a pannus or other prominent skin folds, experience increased skin friction in skin folds that worsens their skin reaction from radiation. Not only is there additional friction of the skin, but also deep skin folds

Table 10.2 Skin toxicity in vulvar and vaginal cancer studies

	Disease site	No. of patients reported	Accrual period	Median follow-up (mo)	Fractionation scheme (Gy)	Technique	Concurrent chemotherapy	Toxicity GR 1	Toxicity GR 2	Toxicity GR 3	Toxicity GR 4	Scoring system
Chemo +RT												
Mak et al. [15]	Vulvar (pre-op, post-op and definitive)	44	1988–2008	31.5	Multiple regimens, Median RT dose to vulva = 50.2 Gy	2D or 3D	CDDP or 5FU based	7.7 % (cis) 8.0 % (5FU)	30.8 % (cis) 60 % (5FU)	61.5 % (cis) 32.0 % (5FU)	NR	NCI/CTC
Moore et al. (1998) [16]	Vulvar (pre-op and post-op)	73	1989–1994	50	Split course: 1.7 Gy BID × 4 days, then 1.7 Gy once daily × 6 days 1.5–2.5 week break, then 1.7 Gy BID × 4 days, then 1.7 Gy once daily × 6 days Total = 47.6 Gy	AP/PA	CDDP/5FU	11.3 %	22.5 %	26.8 %	28.2 %	GOG
Beriwal et al. (2008) [17]	Vulvar (pre-op)	18	2002–2007	22	1.6 Gy BID × 10 fx, then 1.8 Gy daily × 7–8fx, then 1.6 Gy BID × 10 fx	IMRT	CDDP/5FU	100 % "acute desquamation in the vulva and/or perineum"		0 %	0 %	RTOG
Moore et al. (2012) [18]	Vulvar (pre-op)	58	2005–2009	24.8	1.8 Gy daily up to 57.6 Gy to gross disease	AP/PA	CDDP	24.1 %	34.5 %	27.6 %	3.4 %	NCI/CTC

NR not reported, *NCI/CTC* National Cancer Institute Common Toxicity Criteria, *RTOG* Radiation Therapy Oncology Group

can create an auto-bolus effect on the skin from incident radiation, effectively increasing the dose deposited in superficial layers of skin. The combination of skin friction, trapping of heat and moisture, and increased dose deposition in skin greatly increase the risk for more severe acute skin reactions. In one review of 61 patients treated with radiotherapy for vulvar carcinoma, multivariate logistic regression analysis confirmed that body mass index was a significant risk factor for the development of dermatitis, $p = 0.034$ [20]. In another review of post-operative radiotherapy for patients with endometrial cancer, increasing body mass index was independently associated with an increased risk for cutaneous radiation-related toxicities [21].

10.4.4 Concurrent Chemotherapy

Several randomized phase III clinical trials have demonstrated the improved local control and overall survival rates when cisplatin chemotherapy is delivered concurrently with radiotherapy for cervical cancer [6, 7, 9, 10, 22]. This was further validated in a meta-analysis [23, 24], and concurrent chemoradiotherapy has remained the standard of care for definitive treatment of cervical cancer. When sensitizing chemotherapy is given concurrently with radiation, however, the combination often increases treatment-related toxicities. While the more prominent and well-reported toxicities are GI and hematological toxicities [20, 21], skin reactions may arise earlier and progress more rapidly when radiotherapy is combined with cisplatin. This has been shown in vulvar cancer where the external genitalia are included in the high dose radiotherapy fields. In Mak et al., grade 3 or greater skin toxicity was seen in 61.5 % of patients receiving cisplatin with radiation compared to 32.0 % when 5FU was combined with radiation [15]. This effect is usually less pronounced outside of the external genitalia, where concurrent chemotherapy may have a minimal, if any, effect on the skin reaction.

10.4.5 Immunocompromised or Actively Smoking Patients

Impaired wound healing is a known risk factor for increased complications from radiotherapy. Patients with any condition that impairs the microvasculature, such as smoking, diabetes, and hypertension, are at an increased risk for more severe skin toxicity due to impaired wound healing. In their retrospective review of definitive radiotherapy for vaginal carcinoma, Frank et al. found a significantly greater risk of complications in current and past smokers compared to never-smokers. At 5 years post-treatment, there was 25 % risk of major complications in current smokers and 18 % risk in patients who claimed to have quit more than 6 months before radiation therapy, versus only 5 % in patients with no smoking history, $p < 0.01$ [14]. While their analysis did not examine skin toxicity independently, this observation is concerning and can be expected to be seen in skin toxicity as well. Multiple case-reports of severe skin toxicities in smokers have been reported. Hoffman et al. described a case of vulvo-vaginal necrosis in a smoker with atherosclerotic disease who required surgical revascularization [25]. Biopsies of the necrotic lesion revealed both acute and chronic inflammation, fibrosis, and focal ulceration all present in the irradiated specimen.

10.4.6 Age

Similar to the immunocompromised patient, elderly patients may tolerate radiation and chemotherapy differently than their younger counterparts. The prognostic role that age plays in cervical cancer has been somewhat controversial, as some studies have shown that younger patients with cervical cancer have a more aggressive biology with a higher mortality rate [26], while other studies have demonstrated that advanced age portends an increased cancer-specific survival [27, 28]. In other series, however, there has been no detectable difference in the outcomes between older and younger patients undergoing treatment [29, 30]. In a recent Brazilian retrospective review of patients over age 65 undergoing definitive chemoradiotherapy for cervical cancer, the authors found that 60% of patients identified completed a full definitive course of chemoradiotherapy [31] with a very low incidence of ≥ grade 3 skin toxicities (CTCAE) [4]. Only one patient treated with cisplatin and radiation experienced a Grade 3 or greater skin toxicity; none of the patients who received carboplatin plus radiation experienced ≥3 skin toxicity [31]. Comorbidities such as diabetes and vasculopathy probably play a more important role in determining skin toxicity than age alone.

10.5 Special Situations

10.5.1 Fungal and Bacterial Infection

Pelvic radiotherapy fields that include the external genitalia and/or groins will cause a skin reaction in these skin folds. Due to heat and moisture trapping, as well as increased skin friction in skin folds, it is very easy for a fungus to overgrow and cause an infection. This can complicate the radiation-related skin reaction by adding to the inflammation, pruritis, and tenderness that patients experience. Moreover, the presence of urine and stool near irritated skin can significantly increase the risk for bacterial infection, especially staph species or enteric organisms. A physician should examine skin in the irradiated field very closely, at least weekly, during a course of radiation therapy in order to diagnose these superimposed infections early so that treatment of the infection can be initiated. Frequent sitz baths and meticulous hygiene are important to help minimize the risk of bacterial infection.

10.6 Photographs and Recommendations

Below are general skin care recommendations (Table 10.3), week-by-week treatment instructions (Table 10.4), and photographs that demonstrate typical skin reactions over time for gynecologic patients undergoing external beam radiation when the external genitalia and/or perianal skin is included in the radiation field. Photographs of special reactions (Table 10.5) and instructions on how to treat these more uncommon cases are also provided. Figure 10.1 shows a suggested treatment algorithm for skin care for patients undergoing radiotherapy for gynecological cancer.

Table 10.3 General principles of skin care for patients with gynecological cancer undergoing external beam radiation

Patient should:
• Cleanse skin of the abdomen and pelvis daily with mild soap and water
• Use sitz baths with diluted 0.5% Hibiclens twice daily for cleansing and comfort (if peri-anal or vaginal involvement)
• Cleanse after each void or bowel movement (i.e., peri bottle with water, or sitz bath)
• Use lotions and creams recommended by provider
• Wear soft absorbent undergarments that provide support and control moisture, and minimize cross contamination (i.e., cotton boxers, underwear, Depends)
• Receive treatment for fungal infections in skin folds and vagina
• When sitting or lying down, use donut seat pillows if perianal region is being treated
• If incontinent of urine or stools, keep area dry with frequent pad and diaper changes and use moisture barrier cream to protect the tissues around the vagina and anus
• Remove zinc containing products, silver ion hydrogels and dressings prior to daily radiation treatment
Patient should not:
• Rub, put pressure on, or scratch radiated area
• Wear tight-fitting clothes or underwear
• Take extremely hot water showers, hot baths, use wash cloths, or use loofahs
• Apply any lotion, cream or ointment in the 3 hours prior to radiation treatment
• Wash off moisturizing lotion, cream, or ointments if applied 3 or more hours before radiation treatment
• Apply drying agents to the skin unless instructed to do so
• Use any tape or adhesives on the radiated skin

Table 10.4 Examples of acute reactions for patients undergoing external beam radiation for gynecological cancer when the external genitalia and/or perianal skin is included in the radiation field

Week	Skin reaction	Reaction type	Treatment and intervention
1–2	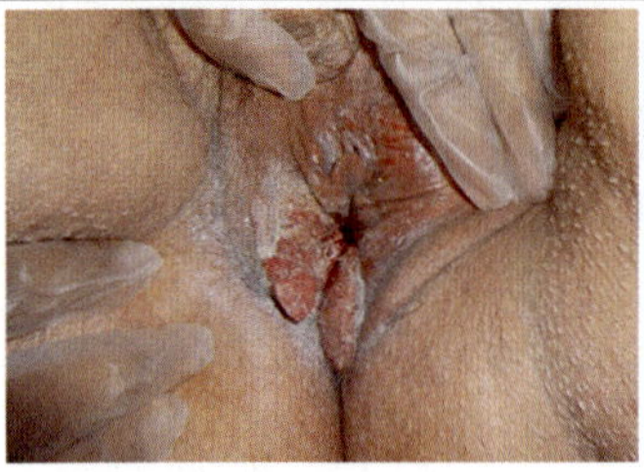 Photo courtesy of Jyoti Mayadev, M.D.	Viable tumor No radiation reaction	• Cleanse daily with mild soap and water or perineal wash • Cleanse after each void or bowel movement • Begin sitz baths with diluted 0.5% Hibiclens for cleansing and comfort at least twice daily and after bowel movements. This should be continued throughout treatment • Apply thin lotion (i.e., Lotion Soft) twice daily to the groins and non-paravaginal/perianal skin
3–4	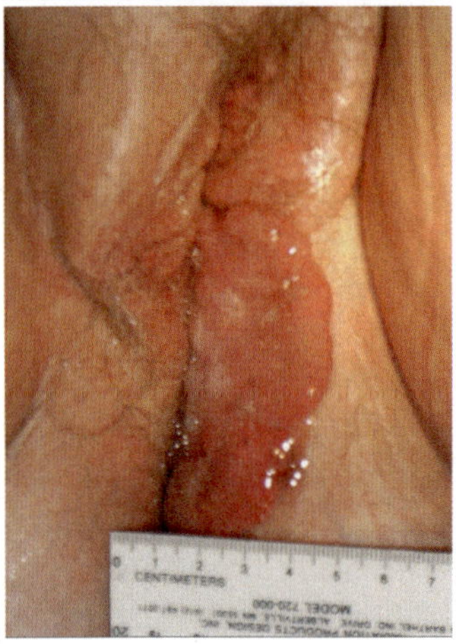 Photo courtesy of Jyoti Mayadev, M.D.	No erythema to mild erythema Anticipate erythema progression with or without moist desquamation Anticipate Discomfort with urination and stools with additional irritation when these come in contact with the skin	• Continue as above • Change moisturizer to a thicker cream such as calendula. Apply twice daily to the groins and non-paravaginal/perianal skin • Aquaphor or A+D ointment may be applied directly to the external mucosa of the genitalia • As irritation progresses, apply a zinc-based moisture barrier cream (or similar: i.e., Carrington, Desitin, zinc oxide) around the external vagina and anus to reduce contact with urine and stools. This may leave a residue but can be cleaned with mineral oil or baza cleanser (medline product or similar) • Continue throughout the course of treatment

(continued)

Table 10.4 (continued)

Week	Skin reaction	Reaction type	Treatment and intervention
4–6		Bright erythema, hyperpigmentation with or without moist desquamation	• Begin Skintegrity wound cleanser spray (or similar). Liberally spray the radiation site daily. Allow the spray to remain on the skin for one to two minutes then rinse with water • Continue sitz baths • May continue calendula cream twice daily to minimally reactive skin in treatment area OR moisturize with the ointments below • Aquaphor or A+D ointment twice a day to the radiation site • Apply moisture barrier cream (or similar, i.e., zinc oxide or Desitin) around the external vagina and anus to reduce contact with urine and stools if needed. This may leave a residue but can be cleaned with mineral oil or baza cleanser • May use lidocaine 5 % cream to anal/perianal areas as needed for discomfort with bowel movements
			• Cover dry desquamated areas with Mepilex Lite to reduce irritation • If moist desquamation develops apply a dressing such as: • Aquacel Ag (or similar silver ion impregnated product) and cover with Mepilex Lite, or Medihoney foam pad or gel (without wax), and cover with Mepilex Lite, or may use Mepilex transfer Ag alone • Continue moisture barrier cream around the external vagina and anus if needed as described above
Week 6–8. Post radiation	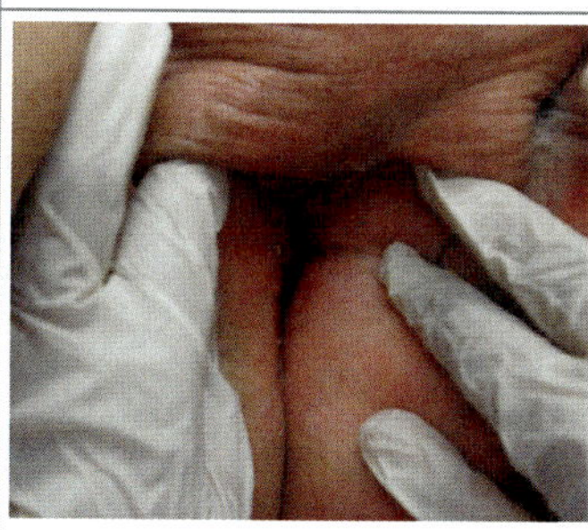 Photo courtesy of Jyoti Mayadev, M.D.	Patchy moist desquamation, dry desquamation with erythema	• Continue cleansing with Skintegrity, leave in place for one to two minutes, and rinse off in shower • Continue sitz baths 1–2 times a day. May discontinue once healed • May transition back to soap and water as skin heals • Continue moisturizing with Aquaphor or A+D ointment twice daily to any area with erythema, hyperpigmentation or dry desquamation • Continue to manage focal areas of moist desquamation as described above • Continue moisture barrier cream as needed (or similar, i.e., zinc oxide or Desitin) around the external vagina and anus to reduce contact with urine and stools if needed • May continue lidocaine 5 % cream to anal/perianal skin for discomfort if needed

Table 10.5 Unique Reaction Types and Suggested Interventions

Special cases and reactions	Reaction type	Treatment and intervention
	Hemorrhoid irritation – Intense perianal itching – Perianal pain, worse with bowel movements – May have spontaneous rectal bleeding or blood with wiping	• Use Preparation H cleansing wipes daily • Increase use of sitz baths • Apply Preparation H ointment to clean/dry area 3–4 times daily • If internal hemorrhoids present, insert Anusol HC or Preparation H suppositories rectally 3–4 times daily • Nutrition consultation for dietary modification • Avoid surgical intervention for at least 6 months following completing of radiotherapy
	Cutaneous candidiasis – Usually presents in skin folds of the groin and pannus – May exhibit odor, bright erythema, and intense pruritus	• Cleanse daily with mild soap and water • Discontinue topical products in the affected area • Treat with clotrimazole 1 % cream TID for 7–10 days, switch to miconazole cream if no improvement in 72 h
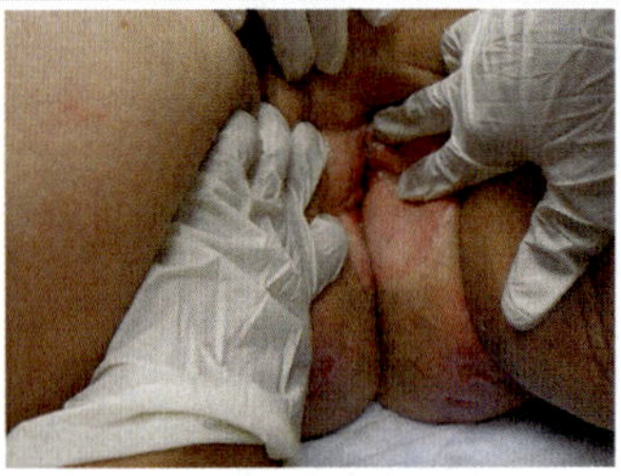 Photo courtesy of Jyoti Mayadev, M.D.	**Bacterial skin infection** – May present during or after completion of radiotherapy – May present with delayed wound-healing, exudate, odor, bright erythema, pruritis, fever/chills	• Cleanse daily with mild soap and water • Discontinue topical products in the affected area • If purulent, obtain culture and treat empirically for MRSA (follow institutional protocol) • If non-purulent, treat empirically for beta-hemolytic strep and MSSA (follow institutional protocol)
	Vaginal yeast infection – Itching and irritation of the vulva and vaginal opening – Pain with urination – Erythematous and swollen vulvar and vaginal tissues – May present with white clumpy (curd-like) or watery discharge	• Fluconazole 150 mg PO × 1 • Repeat 3 and 6 days later if symptoms not improving

Week	Skin Care Overview	Description
1-2	Lotion Soft → Apply 2x/day Sitz baths (if peri-anal or vaginal involvement) → Use 2x/day	Apply thin lotion (i.e. Lotion Soft) twice daily on the non-paravaginal or perianal skin. Use sitz bath with diluted 0.5% Hibiclens for cleansing and comfort at least twice daily. This should be continued throughout treatment.
3	Calendula → Apply 2x/day A+D Ointment OR Aquaphor → Apply 1x/day Mepilex Lite → Apply 1-2x/day Sitz baths (if peri-anal or vaginal involvement) → Use 2x/day	Add calendula (in place of thin lotion) to areas of skin with little to no reaction twice daily. Add A+D Ointment or Aquaphor and apply 1 - 2 times per day to areas with moderate to marked erythema or dry desquamation. May cover with Mepilex Lite or a sheet of interdry in skin folds to reduce skin-on-skin irritation. Apply zinc-based moisture barrier cream (or similar: ie Carrington, Desitin, zinc oxide) can be used around the external vagina and anus to reduce contact with urine and stool if this area is irritated. Use throughout treatment if needed. Must be washed off prior to daily radiation treatments (mineral oil, baza cleanser, or similar)
4-6 (without moist desquamation)	Skintegrity → Apply 1x/day A+D Ointment OR Aquaphor → Apply 2x/day Silvasorb OR Medihoney Gel → Apply 1x/day at night Sitz baths (if peri-anal or vaginal involvement) → Use 2x/day	Continue to apply this combination as erythema progresses. Begin Skintegrity wound cleanser spray (or similar) to the irritated site. Spray liberally and leave in place for 1 - 2 minutes, and rinse off in shower. Continue sitz baths with diluted 0.5% Hibiclens for the perianal and paravaginal tissues. Optional: For comfort and healing: May liberally apply silvasorb hydrogel or medihoney gel to the paravaginal and rectal tissues at night for comfort and rinse away in the morning prior to treatment. For irritated skin in the abdomen or pelvis that is not reached with the sitz baths, apply Skintegrity to the irritated site, leave in place for 1 - 2 minutes, and rinse off in shower.

Fig 10.1 Suggested treatment algorithm for skin care

4-6 (with moist desquamation)	Calendula → Apply 2x/day A+D Ointment OR Aquaphor → Apply 2x/day Skintegrity → Apply 1x/day Sitz baths (if peri-anal or vaginal involvement) → Use 2x/day Dressing Choices → Use 1x/day, replace if it becomes soiled. Aquacel AG (or similar dressing) and cover with Mepilex lite (or similar secondary covering) OR Mepilex Transfer Ag OR Bacitracin with zinc oxide (1:1)	Continue as above. Add a dressing to the desquamated skin, either: Aquacel Ag with or without Mepilex lite (the Aquacel Ag may be tucked into vaginal or groin folds to hold in place). Aquacel may need to be reapplied throughout the day if it becomes soiled with urine or stool OR The Aquacel Ag may be tucked into vaginal or groin folds to hold in place. Aquacel may need to be reapplied throughout the day if it becomes soiled with urine or stool. Mepilex transfer Ag may be applied on the moist desquamation, use care when removing. Mixture of bacitracin/zinc oxide can be slathered on the desquamated area to promote comfort and healing. May cover with Mepilex lite or Depends, etc., as it will be messy. This will need to be cleansed away prior to treatment (mineral oil/baza cleanser, then any residual oil residue should be washed away)
1-3 weeks post-radiation	Calendula → Apply 2x/day A+D Ointment OR Aquaphor → Apply 2x/day Skintegrity → Apply 1x/day Sitz baths (if peri-anal or vaginal involvement) → Use 2x/day	Continue to apply the above combination through at least 1 week post radiation until the skin is no longer peeling. Apply calendula until normal skin color returns.

Fig 10.1 (continued)

References

1. Ferlay J, Soerjomataram I, Ervik M, Eser S, Mathers C, Rebelo M, et al. GLOBOCAN 2012 v1.1, Cancer Incidence and Mortality Worldwide: IARC CancerBase No. 11 International Agency for Research on Cancer; World Health Organization. 2014. http://globocan.iarc.fr/Default.aspx. Accessed 3 August 2015.
2. Siegel R, Ma J, Zou Z, Jemal A. Cancer statistics, 2014. CA Cancer J Clin. 2014;64:9–29. doi:10.3322/caac.21208.
3. McBride WH, Withers R. Biologic basis of radiation therapy. In: Halperin EC, Perez CA, Brady LW, editors. Perez and Brady's principles and practice of radiation oncology. 5th ed. Philadelphia: Lippincott Williams & Wilkins; 2008.
4. Common Terminology Criteria for Adverse Events (CTCAE) Version 4.0. In: Cancer Therapy Evaluation Program. National Cancer Institute, National Institutes of Health, U.S. Department of Health and Human Services. 2010. http://evs.nci.nih.gov/ftp1/CTCAE/CTCAE_4.03_2010-06-14_QuickReference_8.5x11.pdf. Accessed 16 April 2015.
5. RTOG Acute Radiation Morbidity Scoring Criteria. Radiation Therapy Oncology Group. 2015. http://www.rtog.org/ResearchAssociates/AdverseEventReporting/AcuteRadiationMorbidityScoringCriteria.aspx. Accessed 4 May 2015.
6. Keys HM, Bundy BN, Stehman FB, Muderspach LI, Chafe WE, Suggs 3rd CL, et al. Cisplatin, radiation, and adjuvant hysterectomy compared with radiation and adjuvant hysterectomy for bulky stage IB cervical carcinoma. N Engl J Med. 1999;340:1154–61. doi:10.1056/NEJM199904153401503.
7. Morris M, Eifel PJ, Lu J, Grigsby PW, Levenback C, Stevens RE, et al. Pelvic radiation with concurrent chemotherapy compared with pelvic and para-aortic radiation for high-risk cervical cancer. N Engl J Med. 1999;340:1137–43. doi:10.1056/NEJM199904153401501.
8. Peters 3rd WA, Liu PY, Barrett 2nd RJ, Stock RJ, Monk BJ, Berek JS, et al. Concurrent chemotherapy and pelvic radiation therapy compared with pelvic radiation therapy alone as adjuvant therapy after radical surgery in high-risk early-stage cancer of the cervix. J Clin Oncol. 2000;18:1606–13.
9. Rose PG, Bundy BN, Watkins EB, Thigpen JT, Deppe G, Maiman MA, et al. Concurrent cisplatin-based radiotherapy and chemotherapy for locally advanced cervical cancer. N Engl J Med. 1999;340:1144–53. doi:10.1056/NEJM199904153401502.
10. Whitney CW, Sause W, Bundy BN, Malfetano JH, Hannigan EV, Fowler Jr WC, et al. Randomized comparison of fluorouracil plus cisplatin versus hydroxyurea as an adjunct to radiation therapy in stage IIB-IVA carcinoma of the cervix with negative para-aortic lymph nodes: a Gynecologic Oncology Group and Southwest Oncology Group study. J Clin Oncol. 1999;17:1339–48.
11. Roberts KB, Urdaneta N, Vera R, Vera A, Gutierrez E, Aguilar Y, et al. Interim results of a randomized trial of mitomycin C as an adjunct to radical radiotherapy in the treatment of locally advanced squamous-cell carcinoma of the cervix. Int J Cancer. 2000;90:206–23.
12. Wong LC, Ngan HY, Cheung AN, Cheng DK, Ng TY, Choy DT. Chemoradiation and adjuvant chemotherapy in cervical cancer. J Clin Oncol. 1999;17:2055–60.
13. Sitton E. Early and late radiation-induced skin alterations. Part I: Mechanisms of skin changes. Oncol Nurs Forum. 1992;19:801–7.
14. Frank SJ, Jhingran A, Levenback C, Eifel PJ. Definitive radiation therapy for squamous cell carcinoma of the vagina. Int J Radiat Oncol Biol Phys. 2005;62:138–47. doi:10.1016/j.ijrobp.2004.09.032.
15. Mak RH, Halasz LM, Tanaka CK, Ancukiewicz M, Schultz DJ, Russell AH, et al. Outcomes after radiation therapy with concurrent weekly platinum-based chemotherapy or every-3–4-week 5-fluorouracil-containing regimens for squamous cell carcinoma of the vulva. Gynecol Oncol. 2011;120:101–7. doi:10.1016/j.ygyno.2010.09.004.
16. Moore DH, Thomas GM, Montana GS, Saxer A, Gallup DG, Olt G. Preoperative chemoradiation for advanced vulvar cancer: a phase II study of the Gynecologic Oncology Group. Int J Radiat Oncol Biol Phys. 1998;42:79–85.
17. Beriwal S, Coon D, Heron DE, Kelley JL, Edwards RP, Sukumvanich P, et al. Preoperative intensity-modulated radiotherapy and chemotherapy for locally advanced vulvar carcinoma. Gynecol Oncol. 2008;109:291–5. doi:10.1016/j.ygyno.2007.10.026.
18. Moore DH, Ali S, Koh WJ, Michael H, Barnes MN, McCourt CK, et al. A phase II trial of radiation therapy and weekly cisplatin chemotherapy for the treatment of locally-advanced squamous cell carcinoma of the vulva: a gynecologic oncology group study. Gynecol Oncol. 2012;124:529–33. doi:10.1016/j.ygyno.2011.11.003.
19. Montana GS, Kang SK. Carcinoma of the Vulva. In: Halperin EC, Perez CA, Brady LW, editors. Perez and Brady's principles and practice of radiation oncology. 5th ed. Philadelphia: Lippincott Williams & Wilkins; 2008.
20. Kouvaris JR, Kouloulias VE, Plataniotis GA, Balafouta EJ, Vlahos LJ. Dermatitis during radiation for vulvar carcinoma: prevention and treatment with granulocyte-macrophage colony-stimulating factor impregnated gauze. Wound Repair Regen. 2001;9:187–93.
21. Dandapani SV, Zhang Y, Jennelle R, Lin YG. Radiation-Associated Toxicities in Obese Women with Endometrial Cancer: More Than Just BMI? ScientificWorldJournal. 2015;2015:483208. doi:10.1155/2015/483208.
22. Kirwan JM, Symonds P, Green JA, Tierney J, Collingwood M, Williams CJ. A systematic review of acute and late toxicity of concomitant chemoradiation for cervical cancer. Radiother Oncol. 2003;68:217–26.

23. Green J, Kirwan J, Tierney J, Vale C, Symonds P, Fresco L, et al. Concomitant chemotherapy and radiation therapy for cancer of the uterine cervix. Cochrane Database Syst Rev. 2005:CD002225. doi: 10.1002/14651858.CD002225.pub2.
24. Green JA, Kirwan JM, Tierney JF, Symonds P, Fresco L, Collingwood M, et al. Survival and recurrence after concomitant chemotherapy and radiotherapy for cancer of the uterine cervix: a systematic review and meta-analysis. Lancet. 2001;358:781–6. doi:10.1016/S0140-6736(01)05965-7.
25. Hoffman KE, Horowitz NS, Russell AH. Healing of vulvo-vaginal radionecrosis following revascularization. Gynecol Oncol. 2007;106:262–4. doi:10.1016/j.ygyno.2007.03.038.
26. Lybeert ML, Meerwaldt JH, van Putten WL. Age as a prognostic factor in carcinoma of the cervix. Radiother Oncol. 1987;9:147–51.
27. Huang HJ, Chang TC, Hong JH, Tseng CJ, Chou HH, Huang KG, et al. Prognostic value of age and histologic type in neoadjuvant chemotherapy plus radical surgery for bulky (>/=4 cm) stage IB and IIA cervical carcinoma. Int J Gynecol Cancer. 2003; 13:204–11.
28. Wright JD, Gibb RK, Geevarghese S, Powell MA, Herzog TJ, Mutch DG, et al. Cervical carcinoma in the elderly: an analysis of patterns of care and outcome. Cancer. 2005;103:85–91. doi:10.1002/cncr.20751.
29. Spanos Jr WJ, King A, Keeney E, Wagner R, Slater JM. Age as a prognostic factor in carcinoma of the cervix. Gynecol Oncol. 1989;35:66–8.
30. Gao Y, Ma JL, Gao F, Song LP. The evaluation of older patients with cervical cancer. Clin Interv Aging. 2013;8:783–8. doi:10.2147/CIA.S45613.
31. Caires IQ, Souza KT, Negrao MV, de Oliveira JA, Barroso-Sousa R, de Lima RC, et al. Definitive chemoradiotherapy for advanced cervical cancer: should it be different in the elderly? Eur J Obstet Gynecol Reprod Biol. 2015;192:86–9. doi:10.1016/j.ejogrb.2015.05.007.

Central Nervous System

11

Steve E. Braunstein and Florence Yuen

Central nervous system (CNS) neoplasms are a heterogeneous group of brain and spine tumors that include both benign and malignant processes: glioma, meningioma, lymphoma, ependymoma, craniopharyngioma, germinoma, pituitary tumors, nerve sheath tumors, chordomas, chondrosarcomas, and metastatic lesions to brain and spine. Overall, primary CNS tumors are rare, with an estimated US annual incidence of 68,470, of which two thirds are benign and one third are malignant [1]. Both benign and malignant tumors may be associated with high morbidity and mortality. The most common primary brain tumor is meningioma, with a prevalence of approximately 124,000 in the United States, of which the vast majority are non-malignant. The second most common primary brain tumor is glioblastoma, with a prevalence of 54,000 [1]. Brain metastases have a higher incidence than primary brain tumors, with an incidence of 8.3–14.3 per 100,000 [2]. Primary spine tumors are exceptionally rare, with a prevalence of less than 12,000 in the US. [3]. As with brain, metastatic lesions are common to the spine, noted in up to 40 % of cancer patients. However, unlike brain metastases which are intraparenchymal, spine metastases largely involve extradural ossesous vertebral sites rather than intramedullary spinal cord [4].

S.E. Braunstein, MD, PhD (✉)
UCSF Ron Conway Family, Gateway Medical Building, 1825 4th Street, Room M2260, Box 4001, San Francisco, CA 94158, USA

Department of Radiation Oncology, University of California San Francisco, San Francisco, CA, USA
e-mail: Steve.Braunstein@ucsf.edu

F. Yuen, RN, MSN, AOCNP
Department of Radiation Oncology, University of California San Francisco, San Francisco, CA, USA

11.1 Types and Frequency of Skin Reactions

High-dose conventionally fractionated treatments ≥60 Gy involving the brain and skull base are typical for glioblastoma and more rare tumors such as chordoma and malignant meningioma. Routine treatments for diffuse metastatic disease, leptomeningeal dissemination, and poorly differentiated neuro-epithelial tumors commonly employ whole brain and craniospinal axis radiotherapy. These approaches frequently use minimally conformal 2D field setups, often with lower energy to minimize inhomogeneity, but with potential for increased superficial tissue dose. Even highly conformal techniques can still yield appreciable skin dose over treatment course, as target volumes may include cortical brain tissue, meninges, calvarium, and posterior vertebral elements, all of which may lie in proximity to cutaneous tissue. Fortunately, cutaneous craniotomy sites are infrequently included in obligatory treatment volumes, as neuroepithelial tumors rarely recur along surgical tracts. Tanning, erythema, and occasional desquamation

B. Fowble et al. (eds.), *Skin Care in Radiation Oncology*, DOI 10.1007/978-3-319-31460-0_11

may occur during routine fractionated CNS radiotherapy.

11.2 Factors Affecting Skin Reactions

Skin reactions may be more pronounced around skin folds, such as in the peri-auricular region. Thermoplastic masks used for immobilization can produce modest bolus effect, drawing increased skin dose to areas of contact between the mask and skin. The posterior neck and upper spine areas are at higher risk of contact irritation due to clothing contact and pressure. Moreover, as the head, face, and neck are sun-exposed regions of the body, sensitivity is enhanced to even brief UV-exposure with resultant tanning and erythema in treatment-portal distributions, further augmented by early radiation-induced alopecia. In addition, subcutaneous edema and change in facial and cervical soft-tissue anatomy with high-dose and/or protracted steroid-use may increase skin surface area under radiation exposure.

Patients with CNS tumors often require sustained high-dose oral steroid medications to address symptomatic inflammation caused by vasogenic edema or direct-mass effects. Though topical steroids, employed in a variety of dermatologic conditions, are more typically associated with skin-thinning, protracted oral steroid use can result in systemic Cushing's syndrome, and likewise potentiate skin reaction via skin-thinning. Moreover, chronic steroid use can yield impaired immunity and protracted wound healing following radiation-induced desquamation [5, 6]. Furthermore, patients with altered mental status due to their intracranial disease may have difficulty complying with skin care instructions, especially with adherence to wound care protocols after skin breakdown.

Stereotactic radiosurgery employs high-dose treatment of small tissue volumes, routinely used for treatment of limited (1–4) brain metastases. Historically, a frame-fixed technique was first employed. Frame placement entails securing four surgical posts against skull. While considered a noninvasive procedure, superficial wounds are created at these four pin sites, which may result in infection. Though skin reactions have been routinely reported in early stereotactic radiotherapy for thoracic lesions, skin toxicity is not routinely noted for treatment of CNS sites with older reports documenting limited alopecia [7–9]. Newer frameless linear-accelerator-based stereotactic treatments likewise have not been associated with skin toxicity [10–12].

11.3 Interaction with Systemic Therapy

Patients with brain metastases are a special population as they frequently receive systemic therapy as a component of multimodal therapy for advanced disease, with inclusion of novel agents alone or in combination with established chemotherapy, as part of clinical trials. There have been some reports of unexpected significantly increased acute skin toxicity among patients receiving concurrent systemic therapies while undergoing brain metastasis irradiation. Brisk erythema and patchy moist desquamation were reported in patients undergoing limited spine and whole brain radiotherapy for metastatic melanoma with concurrent BRAF-inhibitor therapy [13–15]. EGFR-targeted therapy, employed in treatment of select lung adenocarcinoma brain metastases and in early-phase high-grade glioma studies, is associated with rash but there does not appear to be any increased skin reaction with concurrent radiotherapy [16, 17].

11.4 Photographs and Recommendations

Below are general skin care recommendations (Table 11.1), week by week treatment instructions, and photographs that demonstrate typical skin reactions over time for CNS patients (Table 11.2). Photographs of special reactions and instructions on how to treat these more uncommon cases are also provided (Table 11.3). Figure 11.1 is a general suggested treatment algorithm for skin care for central nervous system patients.

Table 11.1 General principles of skin care for CNS patients

Patient should:
• Cleanse daily with mild soap or baby shampoo and water
• Moisturize the skin
• Protect the radiated site from sun exposure when hair loss occurs by using a soft hat, cap, or scarf
Patient should not:
• Rub, put pressure on, or scratch radiated area
• Take hot water showers, hot baths, use wash cloths
• Apply any lotion, cream, or ointment in the 3 hours prior to radiation treatment
• Wash off lotion, cream, or ointments if applied three or more hours before radiation treatment
• Use drying agents to the skin unless instructed to do so
• Use any tape or adhesives on the radiated skin

Table 11.2 Examples of typical acute skin reactions and recommended interventions for conventionally fractionated high-dose (60 Gy) partial brain radiotherapy for malignant CNS tumors

Week	Skin reaction	Reaction type	Treatment and intervention
1 and 2	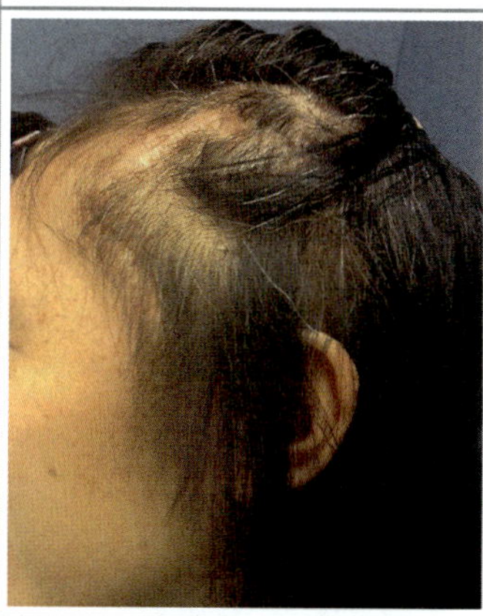	No reaction	• Cleanse daily with mild soap and water or baby shampoo • Apply light moisturizer such as Lotion Soft or Remedy twice daily
3	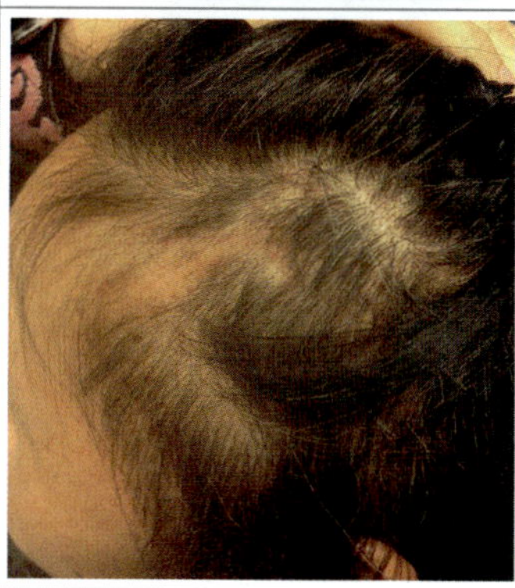	Mild erythema and beginning epilation	• Cleanse daily with mild soap and water or baby shampoo • Continue light moisturizer two times a day • Avoid application three hours prior to receiving radiation

(continued)

Table 11.2 (continued)

Week	Skin reaction	Reaction type	Treatment and intervention
4	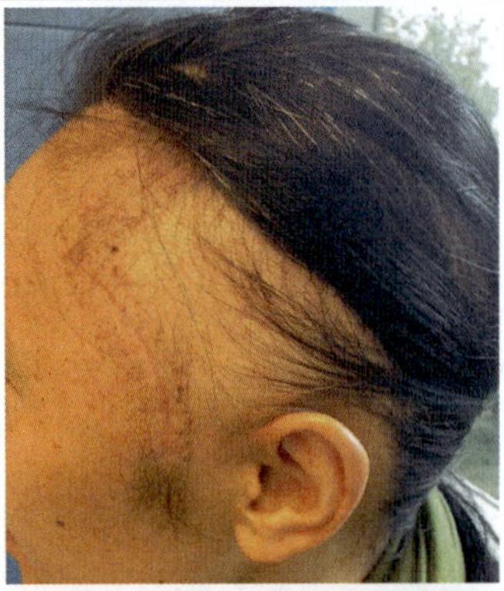	Tanning and epilation	• Cleanse daily with mild soap and water or baby shampoo • Begin calendula cream in place of light moisturizer. Apply a thin coat to the area twice daily
5	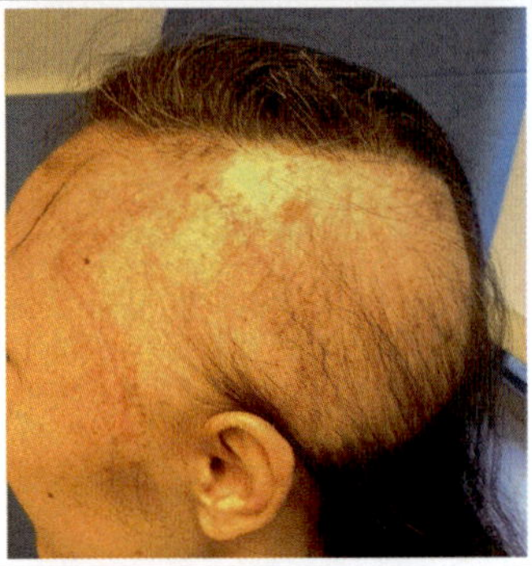	Progressive skin tanning and epilation	• Cleanse daily with mild soap and water or baby shampoo • Continue calendula cream. Apply a thin coat to the area twice daily • Remind the patient to protect the radiated skin from sun exposure by wearing a soft hat, or scarf
6	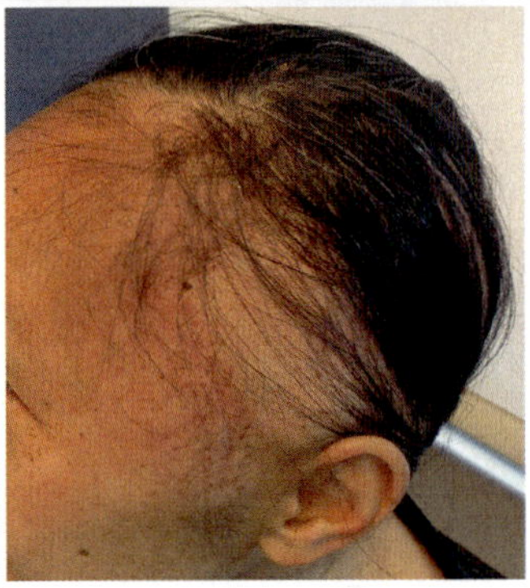	Hyperpigmentation and mild erythema	• Spray Skintegrity daily to radiation site. Allow it to remain on site for one to two minutes, and then rinse it off in the shower. Use in place of soap or shampoo • Continue calendula cream. Apply a thin coat to the area twice daily • Liberally apply A&D or Aquaphor Ointment to radiation site once a day, before bed. The patient should be aware that the A&D can discolor or stain the bedding. Instruct the patient to use on old pillow case. It does not need to be washed off in the morning

(continued)

Table 11.2 (continued)

Week	Skin reaction	Reaction type	Treatment and intervention
7–8	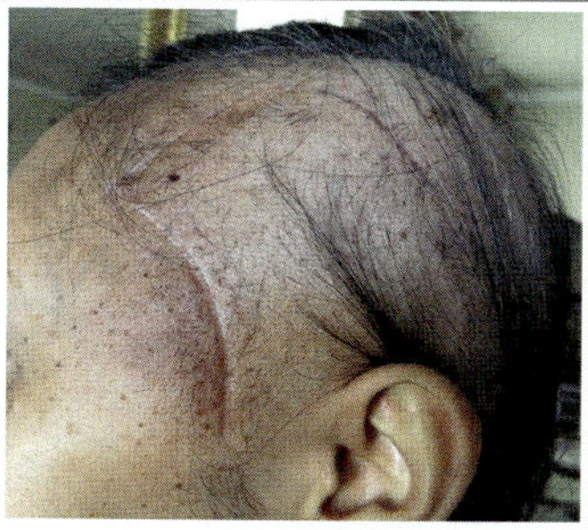 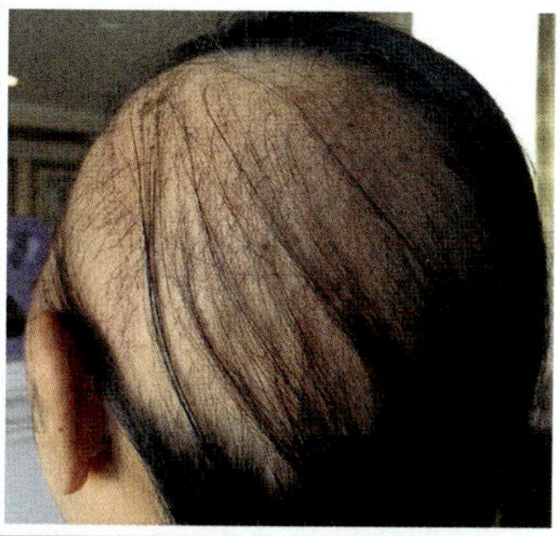	Hyperpigmentation and mild erythema	• Spray Skintegrity daily to radiation site. Allow it to remain on the skin for one to two minutes, and then rinse it off in the shower. Use in place of soap or shampoo • Continue calendula cream. Apply a thin coat to the area twice daily. Continue A&D or Aquaphor ointment to radiation site once a day, before bed
9–10	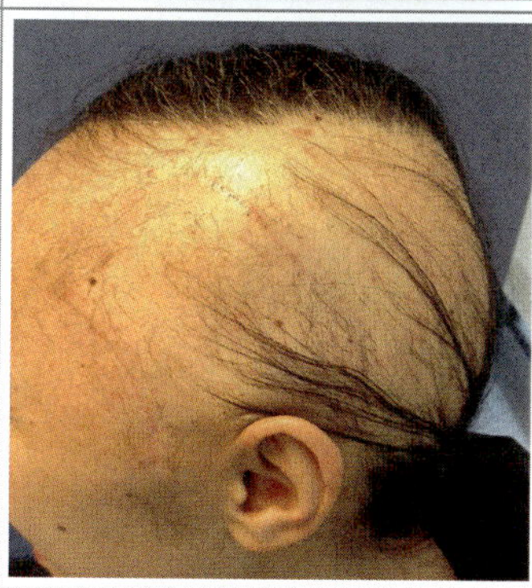	Resolving hyperpigmentation	• Discontinue Skintegrity • Cleanse daily with mild soap and water or baby shampoo • Moisturize daily with an agent of patient's choice

Table 11.3 Special cases and reactions

Special cases and reactions	Reaction type or therapy description	Treatment and intervention
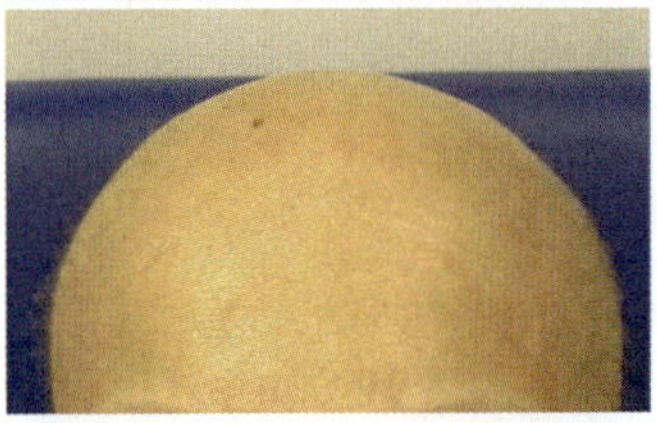 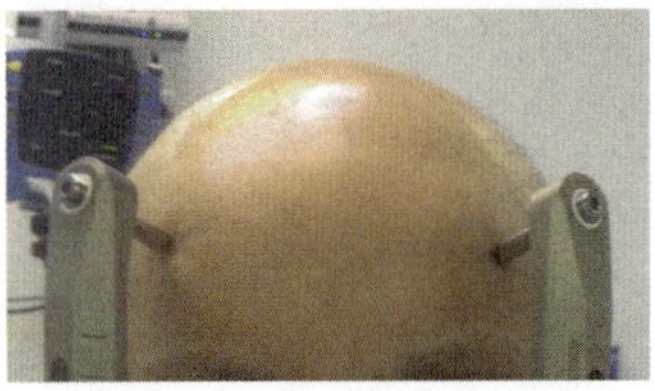 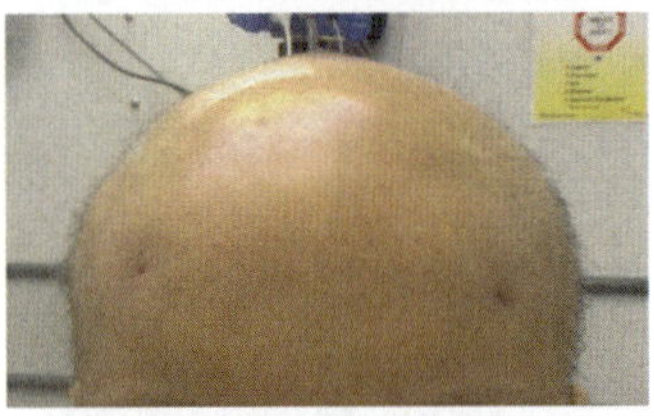	Gamma Knife frame-fixed radiosurgery	• Prior to the frame placement and pin insertion, the site should be prepped per hospital protocol • Following the procedure the pin sites should be kept clean and dry • Cleanse the area with mild soap and water 24 h after frame removal • Periorbital swelling is not uncommon but should be reported to the treatment team as this could be a sign of an infection
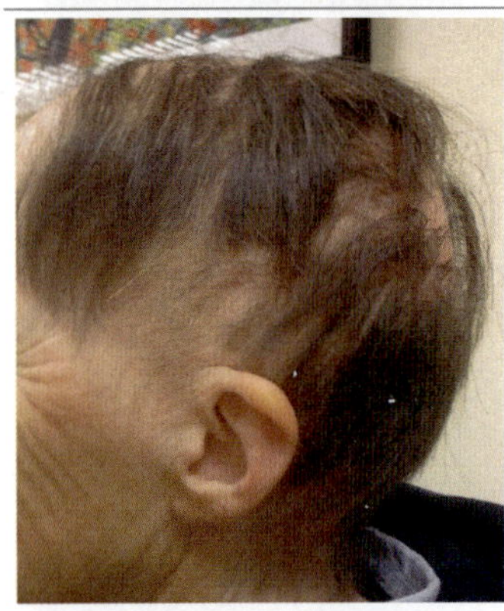 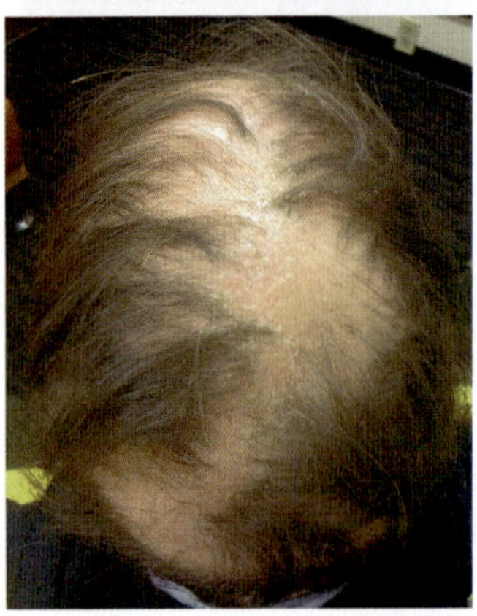	Dry desquamation from whole brain radiotherapy	• Spray Skintegrity daily to radiation site. Allow it to remain on the skin for one to two minutes, and then rinse it off in the shower. May follow with mild baby shampoo if desired • Apply a moisturizing agent such as Lotion Soft or calendula cream to the area twice daily • The patient should protect the area from sun exposure with a soft hat or scarf

(continued)

Table 11.3 (continued)

Special cases and reactions	Reaction type or therapy description	Treatment and intervention
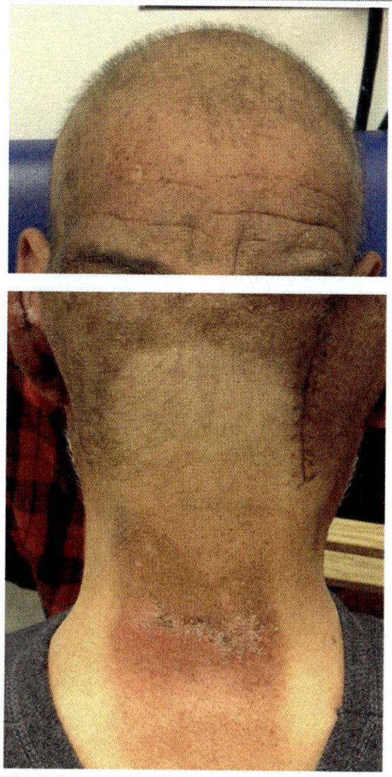	Bolus effect from cranial-spinal mask resulting in dry desquamation	• Spray Skintegrity daily to the hyper-pigmented/desquamated site. Allow it to remain on the skin for one to two minutes, and then rinse it off in the shower. May follow with mild soap or baby shampoo if desired • Apply a moisturizing agent such as calendula cream to the area twice daily • The patient should protect the area from sun exposure with a soft hat or scarf

Week	Apply to Radiated Area	Notes
1-3	Light moisturizer → Apply 2x/day	Optional prior to radiation or chemotherapy related epilation. Apply thin lotion such as Lotion Soft or Remedy that is quickly absorbed, leaves no residue and is not comedogenic.
3+	Switch to calendula → Apply 2x/day	Following epilation, thicker cream can be used to help maintain moisture. Can continue until skin erythema resolves usually two weeks post radiation.
4 - 5+	Calendula + A&D Ointment/Aquaphor + Skintegrity Calendula → Apply 1x/day A&D Ointment/Aquaphor → Apply 1x/day before bed Skintegrity → Spray 1x/day	Begin applying this combination as erythema progresses and moisture loss becomes apparent Spray Skintegrity and wash off after 1 - 2 minutes. Apply A&D until one week post radiation. Apply calendula until normal skin color returns.

Fig. 11.1 Suggested treatment algorithm for skin care

References

1. Ostrom QT, Gittleman H, Liao P, Rouse C, Chen Y, Dowling J, et al. CBTRUS statistical report: primary brain and central nervous system tumors diagnosed in the United States in 2007–2011. Neuro Oncol. 2014;16 Suppl 4:iv1–63. doi:10.1093/neuonc/nou223.
2. Nayak L, Lee EQ, Wen PY. Epidemiology of brain metastases. Curr Oncol Rep. 2012;14:48–54. doi:10.1007/s11912-011-0203-y.
3. Duong LM, McCarthy BJ, McLendon RE, Dolecek TA, Kruchko C, Douglas LL, et al. Descriptive epidemiology of malignant and nonmalignant primary spinal cord, spinal meninges, and cauda equina tumors, United States, 2004–2007. Cancer. 2012;118:4220–7. doi:10.1002/cncr.27390.
4. Klimo Jr P, Kestle JR, Schmidt MH. Treatment of metastatic spinal epidural disease: a review of the literature. Neurosurg Focus. 2003;15:E1.
5. Moghadam-Kia S, Werth VP. Prevention and treatment of systemic glucocorticoid side effects. Int J Dermatol. 2010;49:239–48. doi:10.1111/j.1365-4632.2009.04322.x.
6. Shibli-Rahhal A, Van Beek M, Schlechte JA. Cushing's syndrome. Clin Dermatol. 2006;24:260–5. doi:10.1016/j.clindermatol.2006.04.012.
7. Dunbar SF, Tarbell NJ, Kooy HM, Alexander 3rd E, Black PM, Barnes PD, et al. Stereotactic radiotherapy for pediatric and adult brain tumors: preliminary report. Int J Radiat Oncol Biol Phys. 1994;30:531–9.
8. Solberg TD, Balter JM, Benedict SH, Fraass BA, Kavanagh B, Miyamoto C, et al. Quality and safety considerations in stereotactic radiosurgery and stereotactic body radiation therapy: Executive summary. Pract Radiat Oncol. 2012;2:2–9. doi:10.1016/j.prro.2011.06.014.
9. Staehler M, Haseke N, Nuhn P, Tullmann C, Karl A, Siebels M, et al. Simultaneous anti-angiogenic therapy and single-fraction radiosurgery in clinically relevant metastases from renal cell carcinoma. BJU Int. 2011; 108:673–8. doi:10.1111/j.1464-410X.2010.09895.x.
10. Buatti JM, Bova FJ, Friedman WA, Meeks SL, Marcus Jr RB, Mickle JP, et al. Preliminary experience with frameless stereotactic radiotherapy. Int J Radiat Oncol Biol Phys. 1998;42:591–9.
11. Kelly PJ, Lin YB, Yu AY, Ropper AE, Nguyen PL, Marcus KJ, et al. Linear accelerator-based stereotactic radiosurgery for brainstem metastases: the Dana-Farber/Brigham and Women's Cancer Center experience. J Neurooncol. 2011;104:553–7. doi:10.1007/s11060-010-0514-0.
12. Nath SK, Lawson JD, Simpson DR, Vanderspek L, Wang JZ, Alksne JF, et al. Single-isocenter frameless intensity-modulated stereotactic radiosurgery for simultaneous treatment of multiple brain metastases: clinical experience. Int J Radiat Oncol Biol Phys. 2010;78:91–7. doi:10.1016/j.ijrobp.2009.07.1726.
13. Satzger I, Degen A, Asper H, Kapp A, Hauschild A, Gutzmer R. Serious skin toxicity with the combination of BRAF inhibitors and radiotherapy. J Clin Oncol. 2013;31:e220–2. doi:10.1200/JCO.2012.44.4265.
14. Anker CJ, Ribas A, Grossmann AH, Chen X, Narra KK, Akerley W, et al. Severe liver and skin toxicity after radiation and vemurafenib in metastatic melanoma. J Clin Oncol. 2013;31:e283–7. doi:10.1200/JCO.2012.44.7755.
15. Pulvirenti T, Hong A, Clements A, Forstner D, Suchowersky A, Guminski A, et al. Acute radiation skin toxicity associated with BRAF inhibitors. J Clin Oncol. 2014;34(3):e17–20. doi:10.1200/JCO.2013.49.0565.
16. Raizer JJ, Abrey LE, Lassman AB, Chang SM, Lamborn KR, Kuhn JG, et al. A phase II trial of erlotinib in patients with recurrent malignant gliomas and nonprogressive glioblastoma multiforme postradiation therapy. Neuro Oncol. 2010;12:95–103. doi:10.1093/neuonc/nop015.
17. Sperduto PW, Wang M, Robins HI, Schell MC, Werner-Wasik M, Komaki R, et al. A phase 3 trial of whole brain radiation therapy and stereotactic radiosurgery alone versus WBRT and SRS with temozolomide or erlotinib for non-small cell lung cancer and 1 to 3 brain metastases: Radiation Therapy Oncology Group 0320. Int J Radiat Oncol Biol Phys. 2013; 85:1312–8. doi:10.1016/j.ijrobp.2012.11.042.

12 Pediatrics

Daphne Adele Haas-Kogan, Steve E. Braunstein, Florence Yuen, and Lisa Tsang

Pediatric malignancies are characterized by a highly diverse group of tumors, collectively with involvement across all anatomic compartments and widely varying in severity of prognosis. The estimated number of new pediatric cancer cases in children 0–14 years of age in the United States for 2015 is 10,380 [1]. The most common pediatric malignancies include leukemias and lymphomas with an incidence of 7.1 per 100,000 [2]. Of the non-hematologic malignancies, central nervous system (CNS) tumors have an incidence of 3.1 per 100,000 and include glioma, retinoblastoma, medulloblastoma/PNET, ependymoma, and germ cell tumor [2]. Non-CNS tumors are less common at 2.7 per 100,000 and include neuroblastoma, osteosarcoma, Ewing's sarcoma, Wilm's Tumor, and rhabdomyosarcoma [2].

12.1 Types and Frequency of Skin Reactions

Treatment approaches for the majority of pediatric malignancies are multimodal and include combinations of chemotherapy, surgery, and radiation therapy. While overall survival rates have improved over the past several decades, increasing concern has been drawn to treatment-related toxicity, especially late side-effects that include developmental impairment and secondary malignancies, and thus current focus is largely deescalation of toxic therapies, with the use of radiotherapy declining in pediatric cancer management [3].

While increasingly recognized in several adult malignancies, well-described genetic alterations are distinctive features of pediatric cancers that generally account for the early disease presentation during life. A unique class of pediatric tumors with skin manifestations is the neurocutaneous syndromes that include neurofibromatosis 1/2, tuberous sclerosis, ataxia-telangiectasia, von Hippel–Lindau, and Sturge–Weber syndrome. Notably, treatment is principally directed to the associated malignancies within the CNS compartment, distinct from the cutaneous, generally benign disease.

D.A. Haas-Kogan
Harvard Medical School, Boston, MA, USA

Department of Radiation Oncology, Brigham and Women's Hospital/Dana-Farber Cancer Institute, Boston Children's Hospital, Boston, Boston, MA, USA

S.E. Braunstein, MD, PhD (✉)
UCSF Ron Conway Family, Gateway Medical Building, 1825 4th Street, Room M2260, Box 4001, San Francisco, CA 94158, USA

Department of Radiation Oncology, University of California San Francisco, San Francisco, CA, USA
e-mail: Steve.Braunstein@ucsf.edu

F. Yuen
Department of Radiation Oncology, University of California San Francisco, San Francisco, CA, USA

L. Tsang
Departments of Pediatric Hematology, Oncology, and Bone Marrow Transplant, UCSF Benioff Children's Hospital, San Francisco, CA, USA

B. Fowble et al. (eds.), *Skin Care in Radiation Oncology*, DOI 10.1007/978-3-319-31460-0_12

Inclusion of skin in treatment fields cannot be avoided for many pediatric malignancies. Multimodality interventions including post-operative radiotherapy typify management of several pediatric cancers such as rhabdomyosarcoma, Ewing's sarcoma, and Wilm's tumor. Furthermore, increased surface to body mass ratio and typically more slender physiques position target volumes in proximity to skin. However, technological advancements in radiotherapy have enabled more focal skin-sparing radiotherapy approaches in management of pediatric malignancies. Moreover, dose de-escalation in current protocols may diminish total skin dose. Even with extended field applications, exemplified by craniospinal radiation for disseminated CNS tumors, helical and arc photon-based delivery, as well as particle therapy, may enable increased skin sparing, especially in posterior spinal regions, as compared with historical conventional field setups [4, 5].

Thus, recent reports of acute radiation dermatitis are limited in most modern pediatric radiotherapy protocols. In the recent chemotherapy intensification study AEWS0031 for Ewing's Sarcoma, only 0.4 % of patients experienced high-grade radiation dermatitis with 0.1 % reporting desquamation as part of treatment course [6]. Of note, despite technological advances, skin toxicity cannot be avoided across all anatomic subsites. A recent phase two trial of proton radiotherapy in rhabdomyosarcoma demonstrated 5/35 (14 %) grade 3 acute skin toxicity [7].

12.2 Factors Affecting Skin Reactions

There are significant functional and anatomical differences between adult and pediatric skin [8]. This is particularly important given the role of skin not only in providing a physical barrier, but also in mediating immunological responses. The outermost layer of epidermis, the stratum corneum, protects skin from external environmental exposures. The stratum corneum is present at birth and increases in thickness and hydration capacity as the child grows. Water absorption and water loss are greater in the skin of children than older individuals. Furthermore, skin in children exhibits less protective melanin, thinner stratum corneum and total epidermis, and greater surface area/body mass ratios. Pediatric skin thus exhibits greater vulnerability to insults such as radiation, which in turn translates into more pronounced compromise of barrier integrity and potentially more dramatic effects on skin-related immunological functions such as generation of protective soluble and cellular immune-protective factors. Since chemo-radiation is the norm for the treatment of pediatric malignancies, children are more often neutropenic and hospitalized during their radiation courses, further rendering them particularly susceptible to the risks imposed by radiation therapy.

Importantly, there are special considerations with regard to radiation-related skin effects in the pediatric population. Acute radiation skin injury is related to the loss of basal stem cells from the epidermis. Current pre-clinical evidence supports similar characteristics of the basal stem cell compartment in both young and old populations [9]. Of note, neonates' dermal microstructure is morphologically distinct from adults and may have modestly increased skin fragility [10–12]. However, while most of the pediatric population may not be unique in the essential cutaneous response to ionizing radiation, as body surface area to mass ratio decreases with age, younger patients will often experience greater percentage skin radiation exposure. Pediatric treatment protocols also routinely employ neo-adjuvant and concurrent chemotherapy regimens resulting in immunosuppression and further wound-healing impairment [13–15]. Moreover, given the decreased barrier protection and higher incidence of atopic dermatitis and contact irritant dermatitis in the youngest populations, special care must be afforded to judicially apply topical salves during treatment-related skin care [16]. Finally, there are behavioral and psychosocial considerations with pediatric patients that further complicate adherence with treatment-related wound care [17].

12.3 Photographs and Recommendations

Below are general skin care recommendations (Table 12.1), as well as week by week treatment instructions with photographs that demonstrate skin reactions over time for pediatric patients (Tables 12.2, 12.3, and 12.4). Photographs of special reactions and instructions on how to treat these more uncommon cases are also provided. Figure 12.1 is a general suggested treatment algorithm for skin care for pediatric patients.

Table 12.1 General principles of skin care for pediatric cancer patients

Patient should:
• Cleanse daily with mild soap and water
• Moisturize the skin twice daily while undergoing treatment
• Wear soft garments that minimize friction, irritation and control moisture
Patient should not:
• Rub, put pressure on, or scratch radiated area
• Take hot water showers, hot baths, or use a wash cloth on the radiated skin
• Apply any lotion, cream or ointment in the 3 hours prior to radiation treatment
• Wash off lotion, cream, or ointments if applied 3 or more hours before radiation treatment
• Apply drying agents to the skin unless instructed to do so
• Use any tape or adhesives on the radiated skin

Table 12.2 Acute skin reactions and recommended interventions for pediatric patients undergoing external beam radiation

Week	Skin reaction	Reaction type	Intervention
1–3	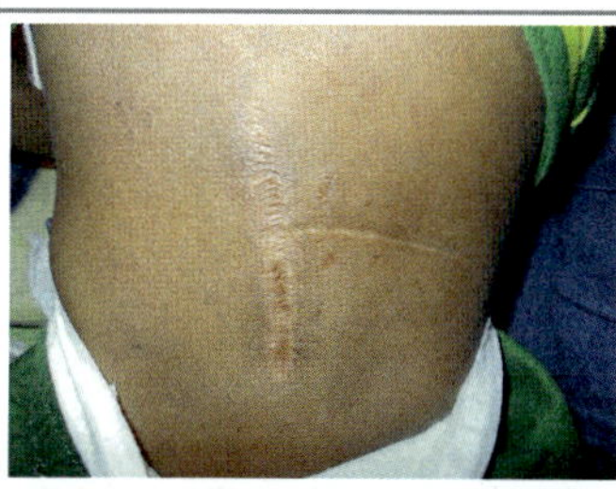	May see no skin reaction or mild hyperpigmentation	• Cleanse daily with mild soap and water • Apply light moisturizer such as Lotion Soft or Remedy twice daily
4	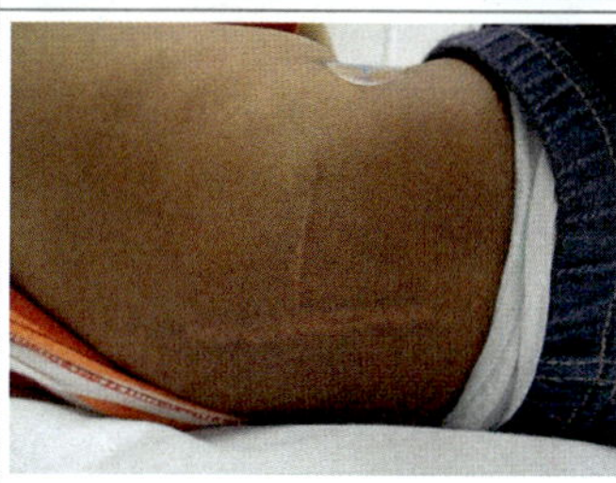	Increasing hyperpigmentation and mild erythema	• Cleanse daily with mild soap and water or spray with Skintegrity cleanser. Allow to remain on the skin for 1–2 min then rinse away • Apply calendula cream twice daily in place of light moisturizer 1–2 times a day • Apply Aquaphor or A&D Ointment in the evening (There is no need to wash this off in the AM)

(continued)

Table 12.2 (continued)

Week	Skin reaction	Reaction type	Intervention
5	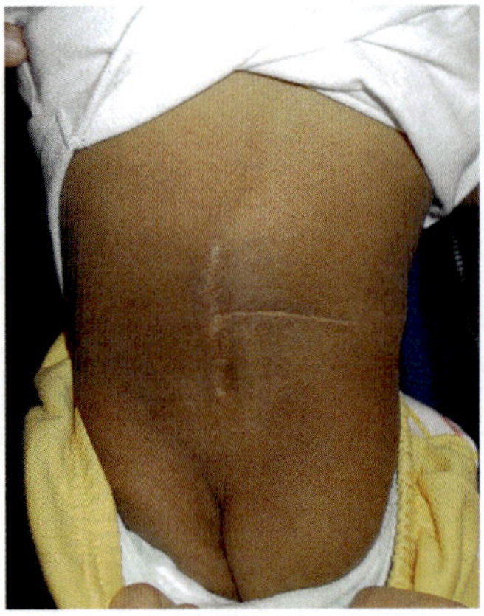	Progressive hyperpigmentation	• Cleanse daily with mild soap and water or spray with Skintegrity cleanser. Allow to remain on the skin for 1–2 min then rinse off • Apply calendula once or twice daily • Apply Aquaphor or A&D Ointment in the evening • Protect the site from friction and irritation (Mepilex Lite if needed and tolerated)

Two-year-old Indian male with a recurrent right flank paraspinous rhabdomyosarcoma

Table 12.3 Acute skin reactions and recommended interventions for pediatric patients undergoing external beam radiation

Week	Skin reaction	Reaction type	Intervention
1	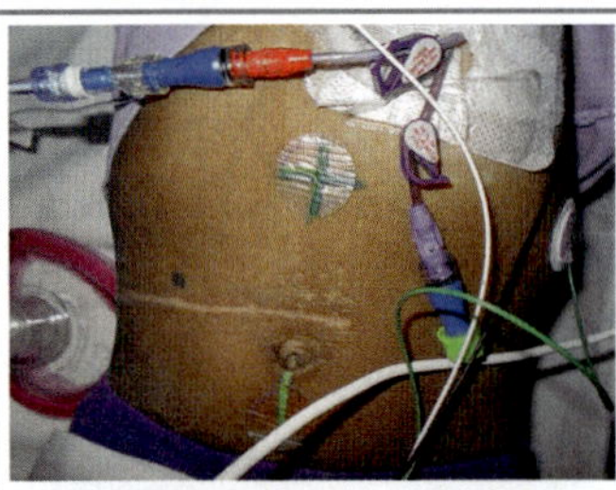	Scattered hyper and hypo skin pigmentation. Post ABMT	• Cleanse daily with mild soap and water • Apply a light moisturizer such as Lotion Soft or Remedy twice daily
2	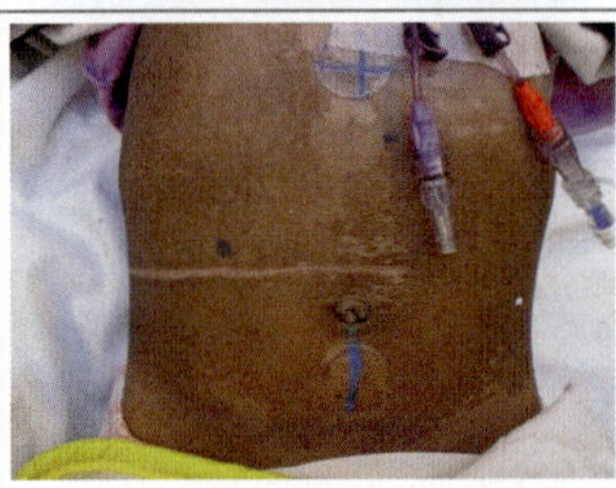	No reaction	• Cleanse daily with mild soap and water • Apply light moisturizer such as Lotion Soft or Remedy twice daily
3–4	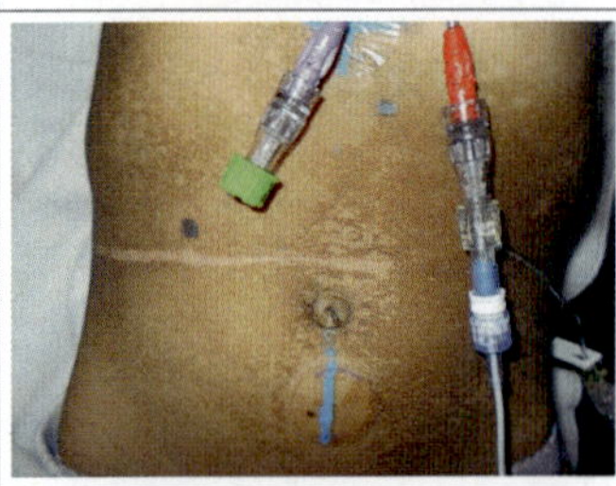	Hyperpigmentation	• Cleanse daily with mild soap and water or spray with Skintegrity cleanser. Allow to remain on the skin for 1–2 min then rinse away • Apply calendula cream twice daily
5–6	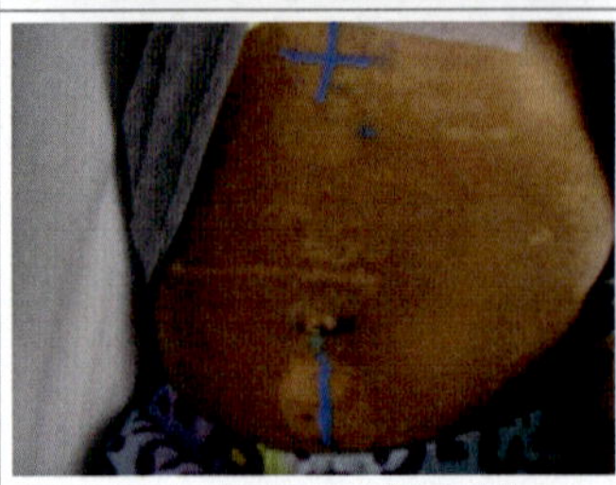	Mild hyperpigmentation	• Cleanse daily with mild soap and water or spray Skintegrity cleanser on skin. Allow to remain on the skin for 1–2 min then rinse away • Apply calendula cream once or twice daily • Apply A&D Ointment or Aquaphor before bed

Four-year-old female stage IV neuroblastoma S/P autologous bone marrow transplant (ABMT) with residual retroperitoneal tumor

Table 12.4 Acute skin reactions and recommended interventions for pediatric patients undergoing external beam radiation

Time post radiation	Skin reaction	Reaction type	Treatment and intervention
Day 1	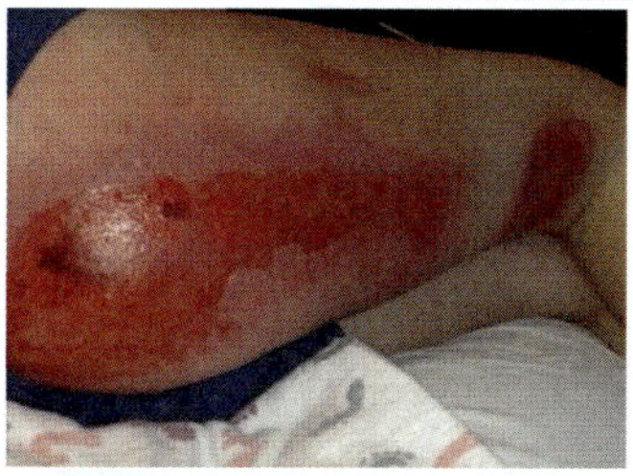	Moderate moist desquamation with marked erythema	• Cleanse daily with mild soap and water • Apply A&D Ointment twice daily
Day 2	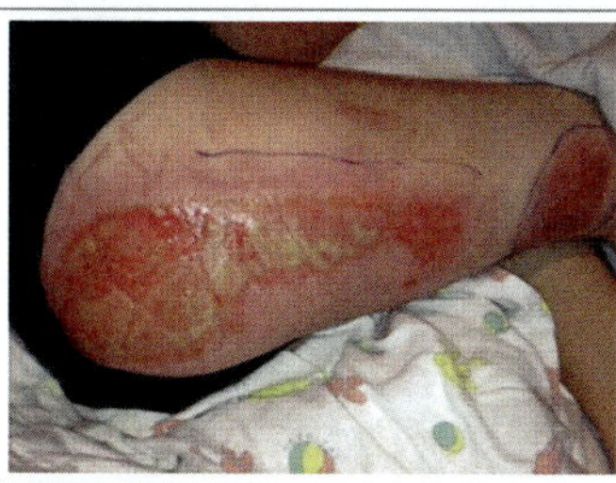	Moist desquamation with purulent exudate *Admitted for fever, neutropenia, and cellulitis	• Cleanse with sterile normal saline • Apply A&D Ointment to intact skin beyond area of moist desquamation • Initiate IV antibiotics

Day 4	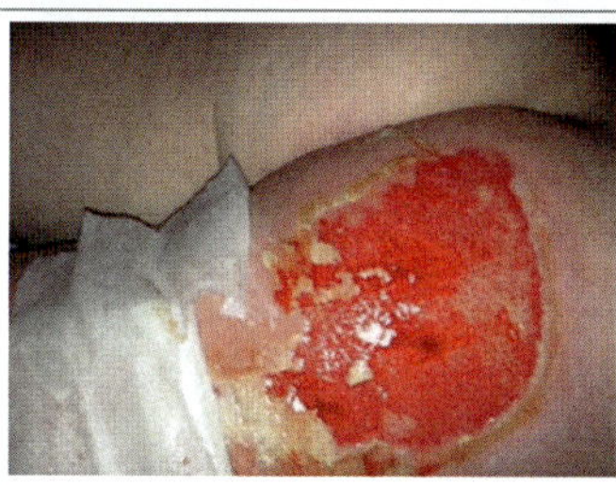	Moist desquamation with bleeding. Exacerbated by the use of vaseline gauze and paper tape	• Initiate/continue IV antibiotics
			• Change skin care regimen
			• Cleanse area with diluted 2 % CHG solution to yield 0.5 % and rinse off
			• Apply Aquacel Ag dressing to areas of moist desquamation
			• Cut dressing to size needed. Aquacel Ag should extend about one-half to one inch over the area of desquamation (shrinks with moisture)
			• Maintain dressing in place for 24 h or change if becomes soiled
			  ◦ The dressing will be moist as it is intended to withdraw moisture and to maintain a moist wound environment
			  ◦ If the dressing is dry and sticking to the wound, moisten with sterile water or saline before removing so as not to disturb the wound
			• Cover this dressing with Mepilex Lite wound dressing
			• Secure with Flexinet or Kerlix. Do not use tape on radiated skin
			• Involve CNS/NP with wound care monitoring

(continued)

Table 12.4 (continued)

Time post radiation	Skin reaction	Reaction type	Treatment and intervention
Day 5 24 h post Aquacel Ag application	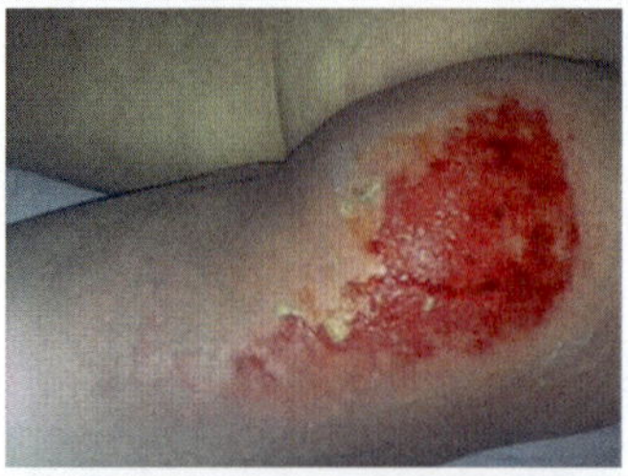	Decreasing erythema. New skin islands forming on desquamated skin Painless debridement of the necrotic tissue was accomplished with the use of the dressing	• Continue skin care and dressing change as above • Apply calendula cream to undressed skin daily with dressing change
Day 7 (1 week post-radiation)	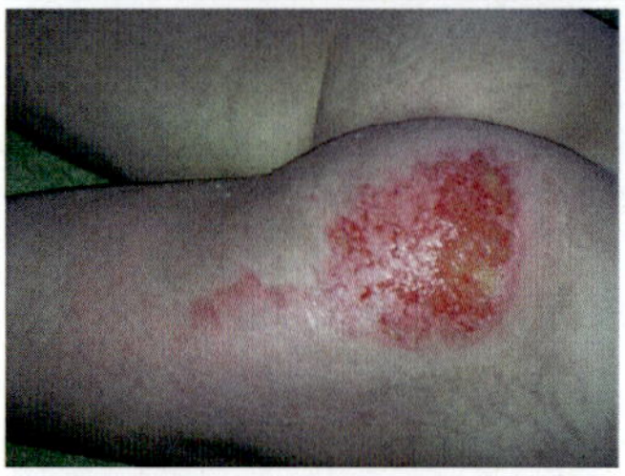	Desquamation improving, marked new tissue granulation (patient discharged home without antibiotics and continued home dressing changes*)	• Continue skin care as above • Avoid agents that will dry the skin or cause discomfort (e.g., Domeboro, aloe vera) *Family was instructed to "float" the dressing off, by wetting it down thoroughly
Day 8	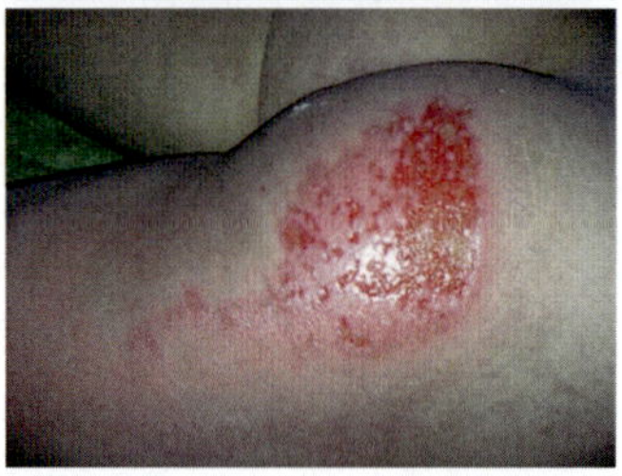		• As above • Instruct the patient and family to continue the process of floating the dressing off to minimize trauma to the new skin • Trim Aquacel Ag to cover only the area of moist desquamation *Patient preferred use of mild soap and water to diluted Hibiclens or Skintegrity spray
Day 9	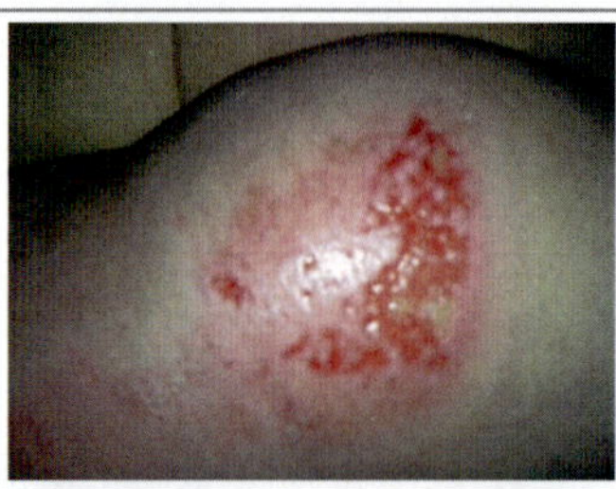		• As above • Ensure the patient and family continue the process of floating the dressing off to minimize trauma to the new skin
Day 10	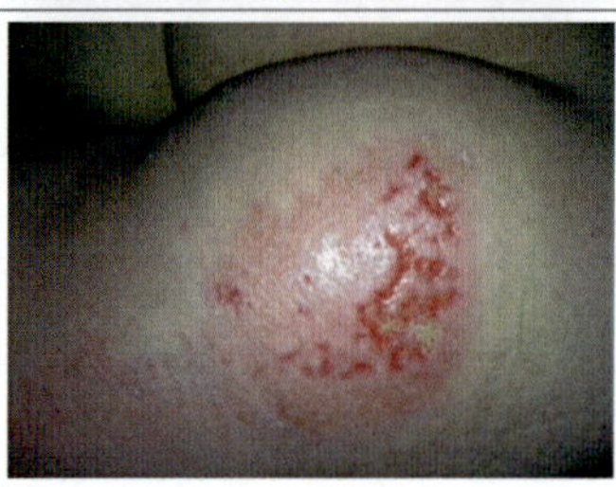		

(continued)

Table 12.4 (continued)

Time post radiation	Skin reaction	Reaction type	Treatment and intervention
Day 11	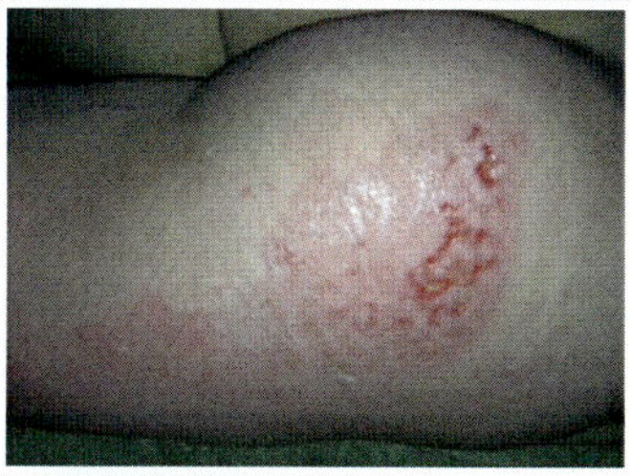		• As above • Trim Aquacel Ag to cover only the area of moist desquamation
Day 12	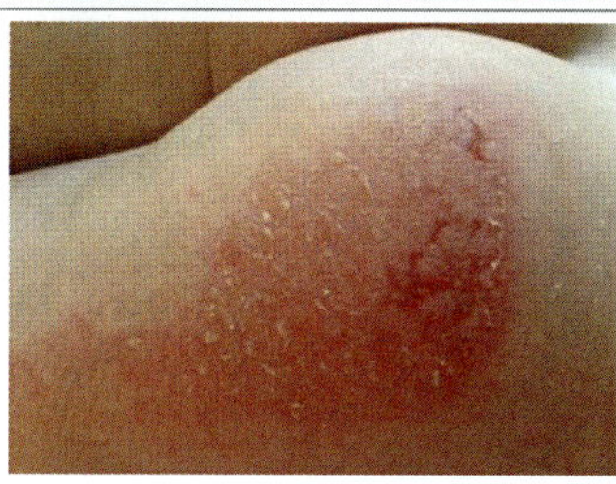	Dry desquamation	• Discontinue Aquacel Ag • Cleanse daily with mild soap and water or use Skintegrity as below • Once daily, spray the desquamated area with Skintegrity. Allow to remain on the skin for 1–2 min then rinse off • Apply calendula cream twice daily • Alternatively, apply calendula cream during the day and A&D or Aquaphor at night • Apply Mepilex Lite to the small area of moist desquamation (for protection)
Day 16 (2 weeks post-radiation)	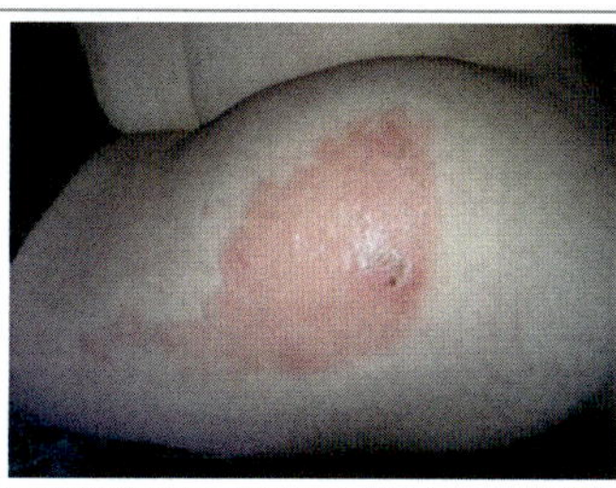	Resolution of desquamation	• Continue to cleanse and moisturize daily with a moisturizing agent of the patient's choice

Twelve-year-old male with Ewing's sarcoma of the right femur. At the completion of radiation he developed moist desquamation complicated by neutropenia, fever, and the development of cellulitis. He was hospitalized and started on Zosyn and Vancomycin

Week	Apply to radiated area	Notes
1-2	Light moisturizer → Apply 2x/day	Apply thin moisturizing lotion such as Lotion Soft or Remedy that is quickly absorbed, leaves no residue and is not comedogenic.
3	Switch to calendula → Apply 2x/day	Thicker cream that can be used to help maintain moisture. Can continue until skin erythema resolves typically 2 weeks post radiation. May continue with calendula if patient does not progress beyond mild to moderate erythema.
4-6 (Without Moist Desquamation)	Calendula or Remedy → Apply 1-2x/day A&D Ointment or Aquaphor → Apply 1x/day at night. Skintegrity if tolerated, or mild soap and water → Skintegrity:, spray 1x/day ; mild soap and water, wash once a day	Apply this combination as erythema progresses and moisture loss becomes apparent. Apply calendula 1-2 times a day. Apply A&D or Aquaphor once at night. Spray Skintegrity and wash off after 1 – 2 minutes. If the child is under anesthesia for treatment, consider performing skin care at the end of treatment, prior to the child awakening.
4-6 (With Moist Desquamation) Moist desquamation should be managed with the pediatric oncology team as patients are at high risk for infection and sepsis. A majority of these patients will be admitted for management of fever, neutropenia and or pain control. If a child is undergoing anesthesia for radiation and requires dressing placement or removal, this can be coordinated to take place while the child is anesthetized.	Skintegrity (or similar wound cleanser): Skintegrity OR Diluted 0.5% Hibiclens Solution Dressing: Aquacel Ag with Mepilex Lite cover dressing or Mepilex Ag Antibiotic (topical antibiotic for early or resolving moist desquamation): Topical mupirocin OR Topical bacitracin *If febrile or neutropenic, admit for IV antibiotics and pain control.	<u>Psycho/social: Child life services, CNS should be involved for care coordination.</u> <u>Cleanser Options as tolerated by the patient</u> Cleanse with 0.5% Hibiclens solution or Skintegrity and wash off after 1 - 2 minutes. Normal saline rinse if the above not tolerated. <u>3 Dressings Options</u> 1. Apply Aquacel Ag and cover with Mepilex lite. 2. Apply Mepilex Ag alone over desquamated area. 3. Apply Mepitel transfer (with or without Ag) to wound and cover with a secondary dressing.
1-3 Weeks Post Radiation	Calendula → Apply 2x/day + A&D Ointment/Aquaphor → Apply 1x/day at night. + Skintegrity or mild soap and water or similar wound cleanser → Daily	Apply calendula twice a day until normal skin color returns. Apply A&D or Aquaphor for 1 - 2 weeks post radiation. Continue Skintegrity until dry desquamation is resolved.

Fig. 12.1 Suggested treatment algorithm for skin care: these are recommended suggestions, but may not be tolerated or accepted by all children. The goal is to keep the skin clean, moisturized, and infection-free

Acknowledgment The editors and authors thank Leanne J. Parsons, RN, MSN for her assistance with obtaining the photos for this chapter.

References

1. Cancer Facts and Figures 2015: American Cancer Society; 2015 [cited 2015 29 April 2015]. Available from: http://www.cancer.org/acs/groups/content/@editorial/documents/document/acspc-044552.pdf.
2. Surveillance, Epidemiology, and End Results Program, Cancer Statistics Review 1975–2012: National Cancer Institute, National Institutes of Health, U.S. Department of Health and Human Services; 2015 [cited 2015 29 April 2015]. Available from: http://seer.cancer.gov/csr/1975_2012/browse_csr.php?sectionSEL=28&pageSEL=sect_28_table.02.html.
3. Jairam V, Roberts KB, Yu JB. Historical trends in the use of radiation therapy for pediatric cancers: 1973–2008. Int J Radiat Oncol Biol Phys. 2013;85:e151–5. doi:10.1016/j.ijrobp.2012.10.007.
4. Min CH, Paganetti H, Winey BA, Adams J, MacDonald SM, Tarbell NJ, et al. Evaluation of permanent alopecia in pediatric medulloblastoma patients treated with proton radiation. Radiat Oncol. 2014;9:220. doi:10.1186/s13014-014-0220-8.
5. St Clair WH, Adams JA, Bues M, Fullerton BC, La Shell S, Kooy HM, et al. Advantage of protons compared to conventional X-ray or IMRT in the treatment of a pediatric patient with medulloblastoma. Int J Radiat Oncol Biol Phys. 2004;58:727–34. doi:10.1016/S0360-3016(03)01574-8.
6. Womer RB, West DC, Krailo MD, Dickman PS, Pawel BR, Grier HE, et al. Randomized controlled trial of interval-compressed chemotherapy for the treatment of localized Ewing sarcoma: a report from the Children's Oncology Group. J Clin Oncol. 2012;30:4148–54. doi:10.1200/JCO.2011.41.5703.
7. Ladra MM, Szymonifka JD, Mahajan A, Friedmann AM, Yong Yeap B, Goebel CP, et al. Preliminary results of a phase II trial of proton radiotherapy for pediatric rhabdomyosarcoma. J Clin Oncol. 2014; 32:3762–70. doi:10.1200/JCO.2014.56.1548.
8. Paller AS, Hawk JL, Honig P, Giam YC, Hoath S, Mack MC, et al. New insights about infant and toddler skin: implications for sun protection. Pediatrics. 2011;128:92–102. doi:10.1542/peds.2010-1079.
9. Liang L, Chinnathambi S, Stern M, Tomanek-Chalkley A, Manuel TD, Bickenbach JR. As epidermal stem cells age they do not substantially change their characteristics. J Investig Dermatol Symp Proc. 2004;9:229–37. doi:10.1111/j.1087-0024.2004.09309.x.
10. Stamatas GN, Nikolovski J, Luedtke MA, Kollias N, Wiegand BC. Infant skin microstructure assessed in vivo differs from adult skin in organization and at the cellular level. Pediatr Dermatol. 2010;27:125–31. doi:10.1111/j.1525-1470.2009.00973.x.
11. Fluhr JW, Darlenski R, Taieb A, Hachem JP, Baudouin C, Msika P, et al. Functional skin adaptation in infancy—almost complete but not fully competent. Exp Dermatol. 2010;19:483–92. doi:10.1111/j.1600-0625.2009.01023.x.
12. Nikolovski J, Stamatas GN, Kollias N, Wiegand BC. Barrier function and water-holding and transport properties of infant stratum corneum are different from adult and continue to develop through the first year of life. J Invest Dermatol. 2008;128:1728–36. doi:10.1038/sj.jid.5701239.
13. Bootun R. Effects of immunosuppressive therapy on wound healing. Int Wound J. 2013;10:98–104. doi:10.1111/j.1742-481X.2012.00950.x.
14. Chan RJ, Webster J, Chung B, Marquart L, Ahmed M, Garantziotis S. Prevention and treatment of acute radiation-induced skin reactions: a systematic review and meta-analysis of randomized controlled trials. BMC Cancer. 2014;14:53. doi:10.1186/1471-2407-14-53.
15. Glover D, Harmer V. Radiotherapy-induced skin reactions: assessment and management. Br J Nurs. 2014;23:S28, S30–5. doi:10.12968/bjon.2014.23.Sup2.S28
16. Stamatas GN, Nikolovski J, Mack MC, Kollias N. Infant skin physiology and development during the first years of life: a review of recent findings based on in vivo studies. Int J Cosmet Sci. 2011;33:17–24. doi:10.1111/j.1468-2494.2010.00611.x.
17. King A, Stellar JJ, Blevins A, Shah KN. Dressings and products in pediatric wound care. Adv Wound Care (New Rochelle). 2014;3:324–34. doi:10.1089/wound.2013.0477.

13 Sarcoma

Anna K. Paulsson, Florence Yuen, and Alex Gottschalk

Soft tissue sarcomas (STS) are a diverse group of rare tumors, which account for less than 1 % of adult malignancies and most commonly occur in the extremities [1, 2]. The American Cancer Society estimates that there will be almost 12,000 new cases and 5000 deaths due to STS in the United States in 2015 [3]. There are over 50 subtypes of STS which include liposarcoma, leiomyosarcoma, malignant fibrous histiocytoma, aggressive fibromatosis, Ewing's sarcoma, chondrosarcoma, clear-cell sarcoma, malignant schwannoma, osteosarcoma, and dermatofibrosarcoma [4]. Subtypes that are more common in the pediatric population include rhabdomyosarcoma, non-rhabdomyosarcoma soft tissue sarcoma, and the Ewing's sarcoma family of tumors [5].

Soft tissue sarcomas often extensively invade the surrounding soft tissues and therefore when treated with wide local excision alone have local recurrence rates of 30–50 % [2]. Previously, radical excision and amputation have been used to improve local control; however, since the 1970s, the addition of radiation to conservative surgery has increased the rate of limb preservation and function without compromising local control [2]. The current paradigm for resection plus local radiation for close or positive margins or high-grade disease has led to five-year local control rates of up to 80–90 % in the extremities [1].

Adjuvant or neo-adjuvant systemic chemotherapy is added for high-risk patients with deep-seated tumors, large tumors, and high-grade disease to decrease the risk of distant failure and improve overall survival [1]. STS have a predilection for early distant metastases. Half of patients die of metastatic disease. While there exists a strong association between local recurrence and the development of metastatic disease with subsequent death, improvements in local control with radiation do not always translate into a survival benefit [2, 6].

Modalities of radiation treatment used to treat STS include intensity-modulated radiation therapy (IMRT), conventional 3D conformal radiation therapy (3DCRT), intraoperative radiation therapy (IORT), and high dose rate brachytherapy (HDR-BT).

13.1 Types and Frequencies of Reactions

Skin reaction tends to be the greatest challenge in the acute management of the STS patient during radiation therapy (RT). As the main goals of RT for STS are limb salvage and minimization of late reactions, little data exist for the severity or frequency of skin reaction in the management of STS.

A.K. Paulsson, MD (✉) • F. Yuen, RN, MSN, AOCNP • A. Gottschalk, MD, PhD
Department of Radiation Oncology, University of California, 1600 Divisadero Street, Suite H1031, San Francisco, CA 94143, USA
e-mail: anna.paulsson@ucsf.edu

B. Fowble et al. (eds.), *Skin Care in Radiation Oncology*, DOI 10.1007/978-3-319-31460-0_13

Inclusion of the skin in RT treatments cannot be avoided, as the surgical scar needs to be included in the RT field for postoperative RT and the biopsy site for preoperative RT. The use of tangential fields, similar to breast cancer, only magnifies the potential for skin reaction. IMRT planning, while not routinely used, may be able to decrease dose to superficial structures, but should be used with caution [7].

Overall between 60 and 90 % of patients develop some degree of acute radiation dermatitis [5, 8, 9]. Radiation dermatitis is frequently graded by the Common Toxicity Criteria of Adverse Events (CTCAE, formerly CTC) published by the NCI [10]. Grade 1 radiation dermatitis is the most common type of adverse skin reaction seen with treatment of STS with an incidence between 32 and 70 % [1, 5, 8]. The incidence of grade 2 radiation dermatitis ranges from 16 to 60 % [1, 5, 8]. The incidence of grades 3 and 4 radiation dermatitis ranges from 0 to 14 % [1, 2, 5, 8]. Of the patients who experienced grade 3 toxicity, in one study, the tumors were located in the foot and in the upper-inner thigh [8].

Postoperatively there may be complications involving wound healing, seroma formation, and deep wound infections. It is difficult, however, to discern what proportion of the postoperative complications are due to surgery or radiation, as the complication rate of surgery alone ranges from 33 to 50 %. Many are likely due to a combination of the multimodality treatment [9]. In two series, one with 50 patients diagnosed with high-risk soft tissue sarcoma treated with neo-adjuvant chemotherapy, surgery with IORT, postoperative EBRT, and adjuvant chemotherapy, the other with 31 patients diagnosed with primary soft tissue sarcoma of the extremity treated with surgery and with preoperative or postoperative IMRT – the wound complication rate ranged from 10 to 25 % and included both noninfectious complications such as wound dehiscence, seroma formation which required drainage, and infectious complications such as abscess formation requiring IV antibiotics and re-operation [1, 8]. The National Cancer Institute of Canada performed a randomized trial of preoperative vs. postoperative radiation therapy for STS [11, 12]. While there were no differences in cancer outcomes, preoperative RT was associated with a high incidence of wound-healing complication (35 % vs. 17 %), while postoperative RT had a higher chance of fibrosis (48 % vs. 31 %). The study did not detect any difference in edema or joint stiffness.

13.2 Factors Affecting Reactions

Clinical variables that affect the development of adverse radiation reactions include tumor location, neutropenia and absolute neutrophil count (ANC), chemotherapy delivery prior to or during radiation, race or ethnicity, treatment volume, and radiation treatment breaks of more than a day [5]. In a series of 82 pediatric or young-adult patients diagnosed with primary musculoskeletal tumor of the head and neck and trunk or extremity, analysis of the impact of these factors demonstrated that tumor location, ANC, use of concurrent chemotherapy (cyclophosphamide, doxorubicin, dactinomycin), treatment breaks, gross tumor volume, and beam energy did not significantly impact toxicity [5]. Tumor types included in this study were rhabdomyosarcoma, non-rhabdomyosarcoma soft tissue sarcoma, Ewing's sarcoma, and other musculoskeletal tumors, and patients were treated with either 3D conformal radiation treatment or IMRT to a dose ranging from 4140 to 7020 cGy.

Krasin et al. [5] noted that ethnicity was significantly correlated with skin toxicity such that those of Caucasian descent had a higher incidence of grade 1 and 2 toxicity when compared to African Americans. The confounding factor in this analysis, however, is that erythema was part of the National Cancer Institute's Common Toxicity Criteria for grade 1 and 2 reactions, which is less apparent in those with darker skin. This bias could be substantiated by the fact that there was no difference between the rate of grade 3 and 4 toxicity with regard to race.

Factors that significantly impact on acute radiation skin reactions included total radiation dose, the volume of skin receiving more than 4000 cGy, and the presence of a bolus [5]. Bolus is a material with properties akin to human tissue, which is placed on the skin and decreases the skin-sparing properties of megavoltage photon beams, therefore increasing the superficial skin dose and expected toxicity.

There are a variety of modalities available with which to deliver radiation treatment for STS, and the types and frequencies of radiation reactions differ among the different modalities. The use of tangential fields, similar to breast cancer, only magnifies the potential for skin reaction. For patients where conventional radiation would have included the entire circumference of the extremity to provide adequate tumor coverage or who would have needed amputation to achieve a gross total resection, IMRT is an option which can be utilized to avoid circumferential treatment of the limb and underlying bone [8]. Doses used with IMRT are similar to those used with 3DCRT with adequate skin flash and scar coverage to ensure comparable build up doses [8].

13.2.1 Interactions with Systemic Therapy

Many systemic chemotherapy agents, including doxorubicin and dactinomycin, are believed to have some inherent radiosensitizing activity [5]. When systemic therapy is not given during radiation treatment and held immediately after the completion of radiation treatment, the degree of radiation dermatitis is not significantly impacted by systemic treatment [1, 5]. When chemotherapy was given concurrently with radiation, however, the incidence of complications was significantly higher among patients receiving chemotherapy, with one study reporting complication rates of 43 % with chemotherapy compared to 8.3 % without concurrent treatment [2].

Sorafenib is a molecular inhibitor of several tyrosine kinases and functions as an anti-angiogenesis agent. It is one of the systemic agents that can be used to treat STS. In a small phase I study using sorafenib in the neo-adjuvant setting, the distinct adverse skin effects observed included a grade 2 macular-papular rash not tolerating drug reintroduction, hand-foot syndrome, or palmar-plantar erythrodysesthesia [13]. Thirty-eight percent of patients in this study had grade 3 postsurgical wound complications [13].

Systemic therapy does increase the risk for radiation recall dermatitis, which is a poorly understood acute inflammatory skin reaction seen in previously irradiated areas after complete resolution of the acute radiation reaction [1]. In a study where the systemic agents used included ifosfamide, doxorubicin, and etoposide, doxorubicin had an increased risk for radiation recall dermatitis when compared to the other agents [1]. In this study, 12 % of the patients receiving postoperative chemotherapy developed recall dermatitis between 12 and 41 days after radiation during the first or second cycle of adjuvant chemotherapy [1]. The reaction resolved in all patients without the need to dose-reduce chemotherapy and there were no recurrences of recall dermatitis [1]. Furthermore, the severity of the recall dermatitis was not associated with the severity of the acute skin reaction during external beam radiation treatment [1].

13.3 Late Effects

Late effects most commonly include progressive lymphedema, hyperpigmentation, fibrosis, and joint stiffness. Generally, the radiation treatment volume has been predictive of the incidence of late effects [2]. Hyperpigmentation is the most common late effect with an incidence of up to 60 % [1]. Severe fibrosis (which can occur in up to 29 % of patients), edema, and joint stiffness as a result of radiation therapy are associated with increased field size. IORT has the advantage of potentially decreasing the external beam field size and can reduce late radiation toxicity and improve functional outcomes [1].

The incidence of lymphedema ranges from 5 to 33 % [1, 2] at 1–2 years posttreatment. Alektiar et al. reported that the majority (19 %) of patients who developed lymphedema presented with an interlimb discrepancy of 5–10 %, while 13 % had a 10–30 % interlimb discrepancy, and no patients had a >30 % interlimb discrepancy. Lymphedema may be reversible. Roeder et al. observed that while 33 % of patients had lymphedema at 1 year posttreatment, the number decreased to 15 % at 2 years after the completion of treatment. Attempts to minimize the risk of lymphedema include sparing at least one-third of the extremity circumference [1, 2] and the use of IMRT [8]. IORT has the potential to decrease late toxicity as it enables the application of higher total doses to a smaller target volume to spare more normal tissue [14].

The different modalities of radiation treatment confer different risks of late toxicity. Patients who receive EBRT have approximately double the risk of chronic pain or neuritis and fibrosis and almost sevenfold risk of chronic edema [9]. Although more focal IORT can potentially decrease the size of the treatment field receiving a higher dose of radiation, it is generally associated with a higher risk of limb edema, as well as fistula formation within the scar, thus must be applied to appropriate clinical scenarios [14].

13.4 Photographs and Recommendations

Below are general skin care recommendations (Table 13.1), as well as week-by-week treatment instructions and photographs that demonstrate typical skin reactions over time for sarcoma patients (Table 13.2). Photographs of special reactions are also provided (Table 13.3). Figure 13.1 is a suggested general treatment algorithm for skin care for sarcoma patients.

Table 13.1 General principles of skin care for sarcoma patients

Patient should:
• Cleanse daily with mild soap and water
• Moisturize the skin
• Protect the radiated site from sun exposure
Patient should not:
• Rub, put pressure on, or scratch radiated area
• Take hot water showers, hot baths; use washcloths
• Apply any lotion, cream, or ointment in the 3 hours prior to radiation treatment
• Wash off lotion, cream, or ointments if applied 3 or more hours before radiation treatment
• Use drying agents to the skin unless instructed to do so
• Use any tape of adhesives on the radiated skin

Table 13.2 Examples of typical acute skin reactions and recommended interventions for patients with extremity sarcomas undergoing external beam radiation

Week	Skin reaction	Reaction type	Treatment and intervention
1–2	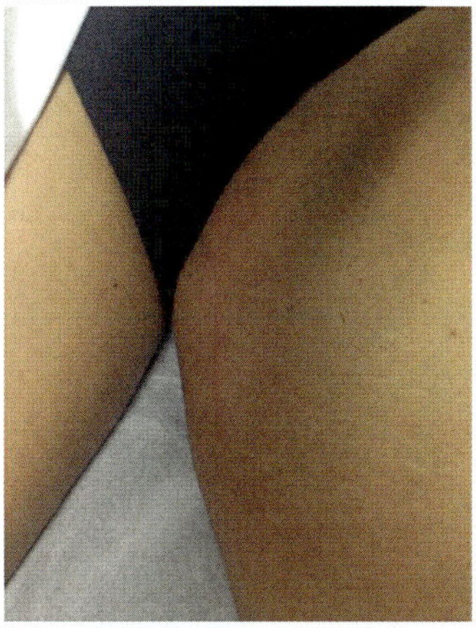	No reaction	• Cleanse daily with mild soap and water • Apply a light moisturizer such as Lotion Soft twice a day
3	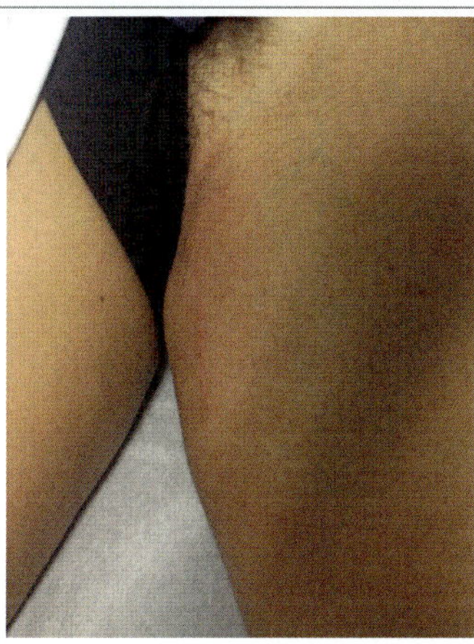	Darker skin with tanning and early erythema	• Continue to cleanse daily with mild soap and water • Begin calendula cream in place of light moisturizer. Apply a thin coat to the area twice daily
4	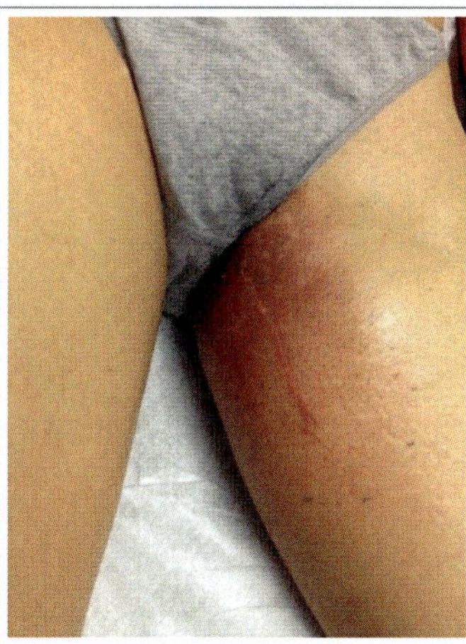	Erythema and hyperpigmentation	• Begin Skintegrity and spray daily to radiation site. Allow it to remain on the site for 1–2 min, and then rinse it off in the shower. Use in place of soap • Continue calendula cream. Apply a thin coat to the area twice daily • Liberally apply A&D or Aquaphor Ointment to radiation site once a day, before bed. The patient should be aware that the A&D can discolor or stain clothing. It does not need to be washed off in the morning

(continued)

Table 13.2 (continued)

Week	Skin reaction	Reaction type	Treatment and intervention
5–6	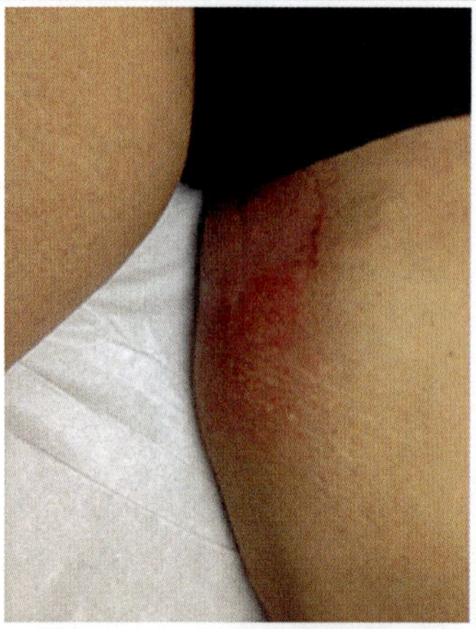	Hyperpigmentation and dry desquamation	• Continue Skintegrity spray once a day • Continue calendula twice a day • Continue A&D Ointment once a day before bed • Manually debride peeling skin if needed • Apply Mepliex Lite to protect the skin and allow healing to the site • Ensure the dressing is removed prior to daily radiation • Avoid agents that will dry the skin (Domeboro, aloe vera) as they will cause discomfort to the patient
1 week postradiation	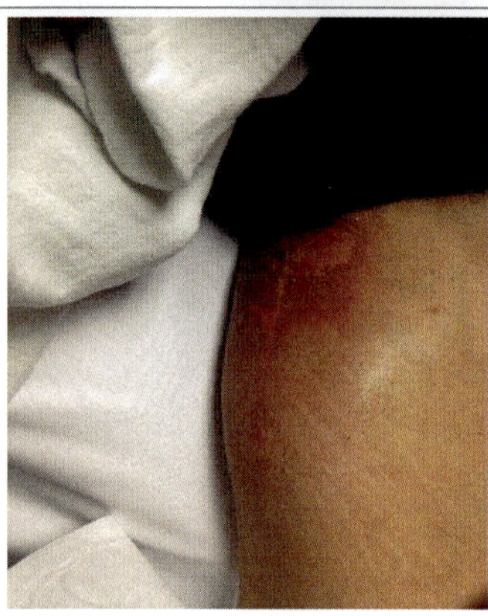	Resolution of desquamation and resolving of hyperpigmentation	• Cleanse daily with mild soap and water • Moisturize daily with an agent of patient's choice until the discoloration resolves • May continue or discontinue Skintegrity once discoloration resolves

Table 13.3 Examples of typical acute skin reactions and recommended interventions for patients with extremity sarcomas undergoing external beam radiation

Special cases	Reaction type	Treatment and intervention
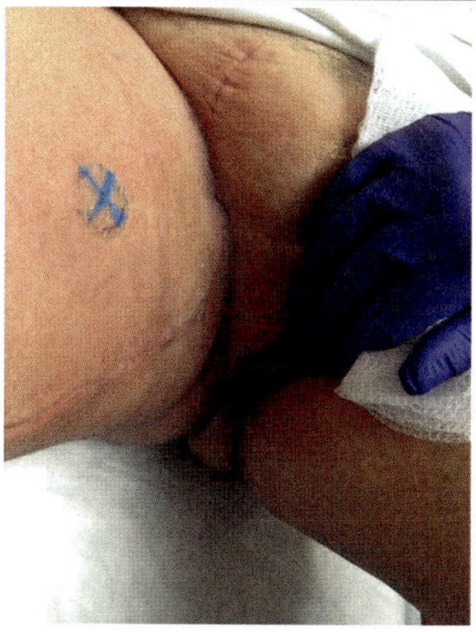 Status: Week 5, IMRT. 69-year-old Caucasian female with undifferentiated pleomorphic sarcoma of the right femur	Moist desquamation in the groin fold.	• Spray Skintegrity daily to the entire radiation site. Allow it to remain on the site for 1–2 min, and then rinse it off in the shower. Use in place of soap • Continue calendula cream on the intact skin. Apply a thin coat to the area twice daily • Liberally apply A&D or Aquaphor Ointment to radiation site once a day, before bed • Apply Aquacel Ag, cut to fit into to the skin fold. Allow ¼ inch extra over the desquamated site. Many times the Aquacel Ag will stay in place in the groin or gluteal folds without a secondary dressing. Secure with Mepilex Lite and snug fitting boxers. Change dressing daily. If the Aquacel Ag is sticking to the skin, wet it down so that it falls off easily and does not disrupt the new skin formation • Remove all dressings prior to daily radiation treatments
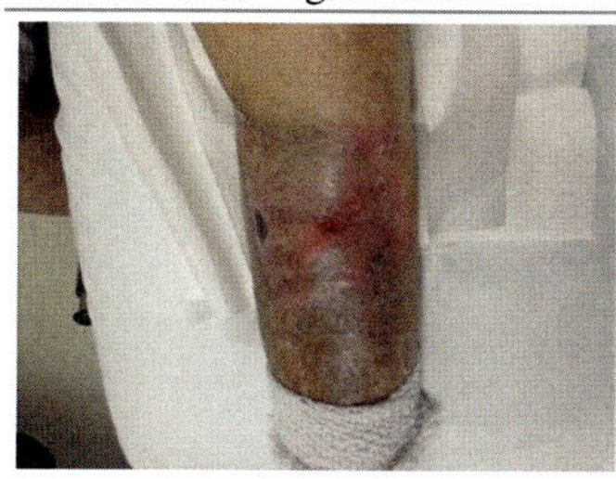 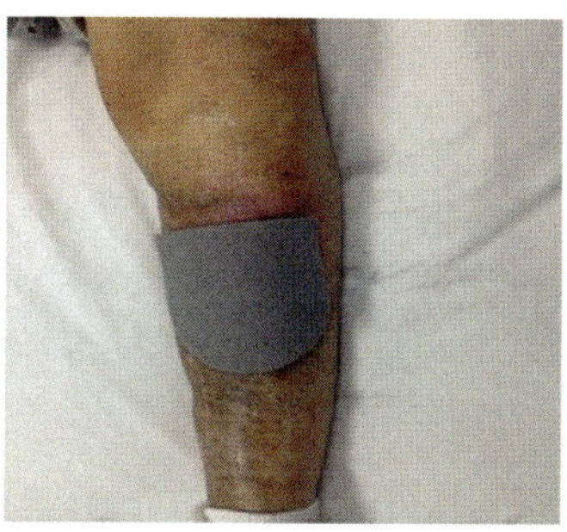 Status: Week 2, external beam radiation. 84-year-old Asian male with recurrent left lower extremity pleomorphic undifferentiated sarcoma. Post 15 Gy of intraoperative radiation therapy	Cellulitis	• Cleanse daily with mild soap and water or Skintegrity spray • Apply a light moisturizer such as Lotion Soft twice a day, to the intact skin • Apply a self-adherent silver ion dressing (Mepilex Ag) over the wound. May be left in place for 24–72 h, but site should be assessed daily • Culture wound • Initiate oral antibiotics in consultation with referring service. Septra DS, doxycycline, clindamycin • Follow-up in 24–48 hours • Remove dressing prior to radiation treatment

(continued)

Table 13.3 (continued)

Special cases	Reaction type	Treatment and intervention
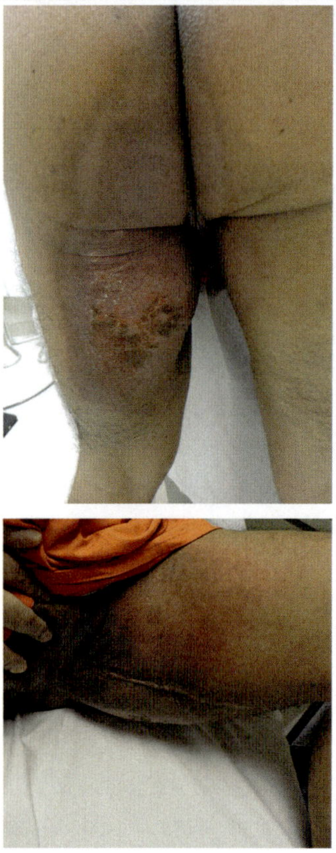 Status: Week 6, External Beam Radiation. 50-year-old Hispanic male with recurrent liposarcoma of the left thigh	Erythema and dry desquamation	• Manually debride peeling skin if needed • Skintegrity. Spray liberally over the radiated area and allow it to remain on the skin for 1–2 min then rinse or shower • Apply calendula to the radiation site twice a day • Apply A&D Ointment to the radiation site before bedtime

(continued)

Table 13.3 (continued)

Special cases	Reaction type	Treatment and intervention
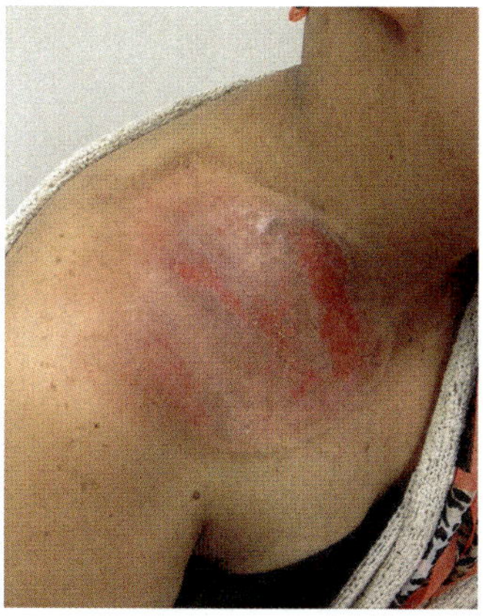	Mixture of moist and dry desquamation Resolving desquamation	• Manually debride peeling skin if needed • Spray Skintegrity over the radiation site area and allow it to stay on the skin for 1–2 min then rinse or shower • Apply calendula to the radiation site twice a day • Apply A&D Ointment to the radiation site before bedtime • May apply Mepilex Lite cut to fit, following application of moisturizing agents for comfort • Cleanse daily with mild soap and water or Skintegrity spray
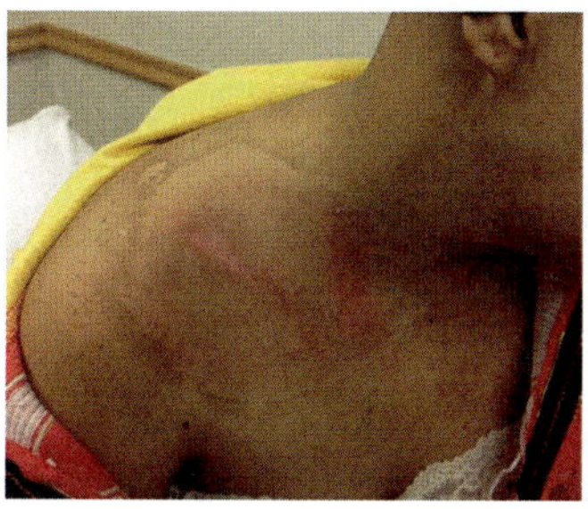 Status: Week 6, External Beam Radiation. 22-year-old Hispanic female with Ewing's sarcoma of the right shoulder		• Apply a moisturizer such as calendula twice a day to the intact skin • May provide a protective barrier for the new skin such as Mepilex Lite or a hydrogel pad

Week	Apply to Radiated Area	Notes
1-3	Light Moisturizer → Apply 2x/day	Apply a light moisturizer that is quickly absorbed, leaves no residue and is not comedogenic..
3+	Switch to Calendula → Apply 2x/day	Thicker cream that can be used to help maintain moisture. Can continue until skin erythema resolves, typically 2 weeks post radiation.
4+	Calendula + A&D Ointment/Aquaphor + Skintegrity Calendula → Apply 1x/day A&D Ointment/Aquaphor → Apply 1x/day before bed Skintegrity → Spray 1x/day	Begin applying this combination as erythema progresses and moisture loss becomes apparent. Spray Skintegrity and wash off after 1 - 2 minutes. Apply A&D or Aquaphor until 1 week post radiation. Apply calendula until normal skin color returns.

Fig. 13.1 Suggested treatment algorithm for skin care

References

1. Roeder F, Lehner B, Schmitt T, Kasper B, Egerer G, Sedlaczek O, et al. Excellent local control with IOERT and postoperative EBRT in high grade extremity sarcoma: results from a subgroup analysis of a prospective trial. BMC Cancer. 2014;14:350. doi:10.1186/1471-2407-14-350.
2. Lee J, Park YJ, Yang DS, Yoon WS, Lee JA, Rim CH, et al. Treatment outcome of conservative surgery plus postoperative radiotherapy for extremity soft tissue sarcoma. Radiat Oncol J. 2012;30:62–9. doi:10.3857/roj.2012.30.2.62.
3. American Cancer Society. Cancer Facts and Figures 2015. 2015. http://www.cancer.org/acs/groups/content/@editorial/documents/document/acspc-044552.pdf. Accessed 29 April 2015.
4. Montero A, Polo A, Hernanz de Lucas R, Sanchez del Campo I, Perez Aguilar D, Fernandez Lizarbe E, et al. Intraoperative radiotherapy (IORT) combined with external beam radiotherapy (EBRT) for the treatment of musculoskeletal tumors. Radiother Oncol. 2011; 99:S9. doi: 10.1016/S0167–8140(11)70137–2.
5. Krasin MJ, Hoth KA, Hua C, Gray JM, Wu S, Xiong X. Incidence and correlates of radiation dermatitis in children and adolescents receiving radiation therapy for the treatment of paediatric sarcomas. Clin Oncol (R Coll Radiol). 2009;21:781–5. doi:10.1016/j.clon.2009.09.022.
6. Yang JC, Chang AE, Baker AR, Sindelar WF, Danforth DN, Topalian SL, et al. Randomized prospective study of the benefit of adjuvant radiation therapy in the treatment of soft tissue sarcomas of the extremity. J Clin Oncol. 1998;16:197–203.
7. Griffin AM, Euler CI, Sharpe MB, Ferguson PC, Wunder JS, Bell RS, et al. Radiation planning comparison for superficial tissue avoidance in radiotherapy for soft tissue sarcoma of the lower extremity. Int J Radiat Oncol Biol Phys. 2007;67:847–56. doi:10.1016/j.ijrobp.2006.09.048.
8. Alektiar KM, Hong L, Brennan MF, Della-Biancia C, Singer S. Intensity modulated radiation therapy for primary soft tissue sarcoma of the extremity: preliminary results. Int J Radiat Oncol Biol Phys. 2007;68:458–64. doi:10.1016/j.ijrobp.2006.12.054.
9. Emory CL, Montgomery CO, Potter BK, Keisch ME, Conway SA. Early complications of high-dose-rate brachytherapy in soft tissue sarcoma: a comparison with traditional external-beam radiotherapy. Clin Orthop Relat Res. 2012;470:751–8. doi:10.1007/s11999-011-2106-5.
10. Common Terminology Criteria for Adverse Events (CTCAE) Version 4.0. In: Cancer Therapy Evaluation Program. National Cancer Institute, National Institutes of Health, U.S. Department of Health and Human Services. 2010. http://evs.nci.nih.gov/ftp1/CTCAE/CTCAE_4.03_2010–06–14_QuickReference_8.5x11.pdf. Accessed 16 April 2015.
11. O'Sullivan B, Davis AM, Turcotte R, Bell R, Catton C, Chabot P, et al. Preoperative versus postoperative radiotherapy in soft-tissue sarcoma of the limbs: a randomised trial. Lancet. 2002;359:2235–41. doi:10.1016/S0140-6736(02)09292-9.
12. Davis AM, O'Sullivan B, Turcotte R, Bell R, Catton C, Chabot P, et al. Late radiation morbidity following randomization to preoperative versus postoperative radiotherapy in extremity soft tissue sarcoma. Radiother Oncol. 2005;75:48–53.
13. Canter RJ, Borys D, Olusanya A, Li CS, Lee LY, Boutin RD, et al. Phase I trial of neoadjuvant conformal radiotherapy plus sorafenib for patients with locally advanced soft tissue sarcoma of the extremity. Ann Surg Oncol. 2014;21:1616–23. doi:10.1245/s10434-014-3543-7.
14. Niewald M, Fleckenstein J, Licht N, Bleuzen C, Ruebe C. Intraoperative radiotherapy (IORT) combined with external beam radiotherapy (EBRT) for soft-tissue sarcomas—a retrospective evaluation of the Homburg experience in the years 1995–2007. Radiat Oncol. 2009;4:32. doi:10.1186/1748-717X-4-32.

14 Skin Cancer

Sue S. Yom and Sarah Arron

Skin cancers are typically divided into the two very broad categories of melanomas and non-melanomatous skin cancers (NMSCs). Within both of these categories are a number of subtypes based on the site of origin or histologic features. NMSC encompasses the three major subcategories of basal cell carcinoma (BCC), cutaneous squamous cell carcinoma (cSCC), and Merkel cell carcinoma (MCC).

In 2015, there were 73,870 new cases of melanoma diagnosed in the USA, and melanoma accounted for 9940 deaths [1]. In developed countries, the incidence of melanoma has risen faster than any other cancer types since the 1950s, and it is estimated that the incidence rate of melanoma has been increasing approximately 3–7 % per year worldwide for Caucasians [2]. The annual costs of melanoma care in the USA may be as high as $932.5 million among newly diagnosed cases across all age groups [3, 4].

In contrast to the fairly clearly defined incidence of melanoma, the exact number of NMSC diagnoses is a matter of debate. While traditionally cited estimates are in the range of about 1 million cases per annum in the USA [5], updated projections are that there may be as many as 3.5 million cases [6]. NMSC are thought to comprise between 33 and 50 % of all cancers diagnosed in the USA [7]. Costs for NMSC management in the USA are thought to amount to $2 billion a year [8].

Efforts to estimate NMSC incidence in a more accurate fashion have focused on the USA, Australia, and Europe. A systematic review indicated that Australia has the highest incidence of skin cancers in the world, where incidence has risen the most for BCC and in the population over 60 years of age. In an attempt to counteract these trends, Australia has funded nationwide awareness programs encouraging sun protection since the 1980s, and new legislation has just been passed in several Australian states to ban commercial tanning beds. The Southwestern United States is one area of the world where rates of BCC are considered comparable to those in Australia [9], and the area specifically known as the "sunbelt" region sees the highest annual incidences of all types of skin cancers in the USA.

Skin cancers can occur in any area of the body, although the most common occurrences are on sun-exposed areas such as the face, scalp and ears, dorsal hands and arms, and back [10, 11]. Ninety percent of NMSC and 86 % of melanoma are attributed to UV radiation exposure [12, 13].

S.S. Yom, MD, PhD (✉)
Department of Radiation Oncology,
University of California, San Francisco, Box 1708,
1600 Divisadero Street, Suite H1031, San Francisco,
CA 94143, USA
e-mail: yoms@radonc.ucsf.edu

S. Arron, MD, PhD
Department of Dermatology, University of California,
San Francisco, Box 0316, 1701 Divisadero Street,
San Francisco, CA 94115, USA

B. Fowble et al. (eds.), *Skin Care in Radiation Oncology*, DOI 10.1007/978-3-319-31460-0_14

Patients who have received an organ transplant have a higher incidence of all skin cancers as compared to the general population, up to 65-fold higher incidence for cSCC, 10-fold for BCC, and 3.4-fold for melanoma. Because of their complex immunosuppressive regimens, which are the predisposing factor for skin cancer development, these patients present a special challenge in their requirement for closely coordinated multidisciplinary management. Approximately 140,000 organ transplant recipients are alive in the USA [14].

14.1 Skin Cancer Treatment

Among melanomas, 91 % are of cutaneous origin, 5 % are ocular, 1 % are mucosally based, and 2 % are from an unknown primary site [15]. For cutaneous melanoma, while prognosis of early stage disease is highly dependent on increasing tumor thickness and ulceration, in advanced stages, survival is related to the number and disease burden of involved lymph nodes, the presence of satellite or in-transit metastasis, and the presence of visceral disease [16].

Among the NMSC, BCC contains a number of histologically defined subtypes. The most common nodular and cystic types are relatively indolent, but micronodular, superficial, morpheaform, and infiltrative subtypes are more aggressive [17]. cSCC is characterized by its level of differentiation, defined as well, moderately or poorly differentiated. Early stage NMSC is quite curable, with rates of cure on the order of 95–99 % after surgical removal and for small tumors less than 2 cm in size, 90–93 % after definitive radiotherapy [18–20]. However, tumors with perineural invasion or those with lymph node metastasis or close or positive margins obtain local-regional control rates of only 50–88 % at 5 years [21, 22].

Merkel cell carcinoma (MCC) is considered a distinct type of non-melanomatous skin cancer; it arises from the pluripotent basal cells of the epithelium and is considered highly aggressive due to its ability to invade rapidly through local tissues and metastasize early [23]. MCC patients who present with local disease have 64 % survival at 5 years, those with regional nodal disease 39 %, and those with distant metastatic disease 18 % [24]. Less than half of MCC patients present with localized disease [25].

In general, for early stage melanoma and NMSC, surgery alone is usually appropriate, but postoperative radiation may be required if negative prognostic features are discovered at the time of operation. For Merkel cell carcinoma, because rates of recurrence after surgery alone are high, postoperative radiation is routinely delivered. For patients who are not surgical candidates or who prefer definitive radiation, radiotherapy alone can be used with high rates of success in NMSC and Merkel cell carcinoma and present a viable alternative to surgery in cosmetically sensitive areas. However, for melanoma, as radiotherapy is much less successful, upfront surgery is highly preferred.

Radiation is frequently used for advanced-stage skin cancer cases as a postoperative treatment. In the case of cSCC, it is sometimes delivered with a concurrent systemic therapy, which can greatly increase the cutaneous, mucosal, and hematologic toxicity burden.

Radiation may be used as palliation for skin cancers that are incurable, recurrent, or metastatic, especially for symptoms of bleeding, dysphagia, and pain.

14.2 Types and Frequency of Skin Reactions

Treatment of skin cancers with radiation is somewhat unique in that the skin surface itself must be part of the target. For most patients receiving radiation therapy, skin reaction is an off-target ancillary reaction, but in the treatment of skin cancers, a skin reaction is anticipated and desired. Recurrence of skin cancers may be enabled along small lymphatic and perineural channels located within the skin around the primary tumor location, and an additional margin must therefore be treated around the clinically involved area to prevent peripheral recurrence. This margin can range from a few millimeters in the case of early stage NMSC to several centimeters for MCC. In any case, a clinically visible skin reaction at the surface is desired as an indication of adequate treatment. The level of expected reaction can be reasonably estimated in advance by an experienced clinician depending on the technique, dose, and location of the radiotherapy treatment.

Very little data exists on acute or late toxicity resulting from radiotherapy for skin cancers. For superficial treatments such as orthovoltage or electron treatments, which are typically intended for stages I–II NMSC, the area of skin to be treated is very small. These treatments typically result in grade 1 skin reactions for the most part. On the rare occasion that an extremely aggressive superficial treatment is needed, such as that carried out in the nonsurgical treatment of lentigo maligna, the visibly impressive grades 3–4 skin reactions that are elicited still tend to be of a relatively minimal clinical impact on the patient's overall health.

In general, the reactions due to skin cancer irradiation tend to be moderate in nature, because the actual area of targeted skin in the vast majority of cases is usually not extremely large. A recent review of the published medical literature on radiotherapy treatment of BCC identified 13 studies, including one prospective cohort study and two randomized studies comparing radiotherapy with either surgery or cryotherapy. Of these, only four studies described cosmetic outcome; overall 90 % or more of patients achieved a good or excellent aesthetic outcome [26]. The best results were seen in a study that delivered 57 Gy over 19 fractions; in this study, 38 % of patients had excellent outcome and 56 % had good outcome [27]. On the other hand, patients in another study were given a much more hypofractionated regimen of 30.6 Gy in three fractions over 14 days, with 48 % having only a good outcome and 50 % having a fair outcome and half of patients having a visible permanent scar and 3 % having complications such as ulceration or blocked nasolacrimal duct [28]. Long-term complications identified in the literature review included alopecia, pigmentation change, telangiectasia, fibrosis/scar, atrophy/contraction, epiphora, and, rarely, soft tissue necrosis, bone necrosis, cataracts, dry eye, conjunctival scarring, and eyelid deformity [26]. The rates of severe late complications are generally very low (<5 %), but may be highest for skin cancer treatments on the pinna, where cartilage necrosis rates have ranged between 0 and 13 % [29].

Electron beam radiation therapy has been studied for superficial NMSC and has not been found to be inferior to superficial X-ray therapy in either outcome or cosmesis [30]. A Dutch pilot study using blinded photographs to compare cosmetic results of two fractionation regimens of either 54 Gy in 18 fractions or 44 Gy in 10 fractions found essentially no differences in the ratings of ten independent observers; the 54 Gy schedule results were 38 % good, 49 % fair, and 13 % poor, and the 44 Gy schedules were 33 % good, 50 % fair, and 17 % poor [31].

Larger-scale treatments, such as those given in the advanced-stage postoperative setting, usually encompass the primary skin tumor area as well as a large area of draining regional lymphatics. For deep or extensive basal cell carcinomas or inoperable squamous cell carcinomas, where surgery is deemed not feasible or overly morbid, similarly large-scale radiation therapy fields are required. The skin reaction will vary depending on the anatomic regions that are included in the treatment area. For example, anticipated reactions in the face or neck region will necessarily differ from those seen during a treatment delivered to the trunk or extremity or axilla or groin. Many advanced-stage skin cancers occur in the head and neck region. These are typically addressed with initial surgery, and the postoperative therapy is conducted according to principles that are very similar to other forms of postoperative head and neck irradiation.

Very few prospective data have been collected in advanced-stage skin cancer. Two studies were conducted combining an inhibitor of the epidermal growth factor receptor (EGFR) with surgery and postoperative radiotherapy. In a small phase I study, 150 mg of daily erlotinib was given for

14 days prior to surgery and then given concurrently with radiation therapy for 6 weeks. Of the 15 patients on this study, 11 (73 %) had grades 2–3 dermatitis attributed to erlotinib, and 10 (67 %) had grades 2–3 skin reaction attributed to radiation dermatitis. Of the 15 patients, 47 % had a grade 2 skin reaction and 53 % had a grade 3 skin reaction. Three (20 %) patients required a dose reduction of erlotinib and antibiotics due to intolerable rash [32]. In a phase II study, 250 mg gefitinib was given by mouth daily for 60 days prior to surgery and postoperative radiotherapy, and patients received 12 months maintenance of gefitinib. Patients who had stable disease after the first 15 days were dose escalated to 500 mg gefitinib daily. Of 22 evaluable patients, grade 1 acneiform rash was seen in 10 (45 %) patients over the entire course of the study, and grade 2 toxicity was seen in 7 (32 %) patients. There was no grade 3 toxicity, and gefitinib given during the radiotherapy did not increase the in-field toxicity [33].

The Trans Tasman Radiation Oncology Group (TROG) conducted two studies exploring postoperative regional radiotherapy after surgery for melanoma. Radiation was specified to the neck, axilla, or groin to a dose of 48 Gy in 20 fractions, with 50 Gy in 21 fractions allowed for positive margins. Lymphedema was the most common toxicity, with rates as high as 46 % of grades 1–2 and 19 % grades 3–4 in the groin. Grades 1–2 skin changes were reported in 55 % of patients receiving radiotherapy to the head and neck region but no grades 3–4 toxicities were recorded. In the axilla, grades 1–2 skin changes were recorded in 37 % of patients and 1 % had grades 3–4. In the groin, grades 1–2 skin toxicity occurred in 50 % of patients and grades 3–4 occurred in 2 % [34]. The follow-up randomized TROG phase III study of adjuvant radiotherapy versus no radiotherapy reported slightly higher recorded rates of grades 3–4 dermatitis in the radiotherapy arm. At 2 weeks after completion of radiotherapy, the head and neck group had 3 % acute grades 3–4 dermatitis, the axilla group had 10 %, and the groin group had 6 % [35].

14.3 Impact of Technical Choices on the Skin

There are many means of delivering superficial radiation therapy to the skin. These include superficial X-ray therapy, electron therapy, and brachytherapy. In any case, the important aspects that determine the extent of skin reaction are the total dose and fractionation scheme that are chosen, as well as whether dosimetric or physical shielding is used to protect adjacent nontargeted skin.

In general, fractionation schemes of 3 Gy per fraction or less will result in mild to moderate effects, mostly consisting of skin erythema and superficial dry desquamation. Larger fraction sizes, such as 4–6 Gy per fraction or higher, are more likely to produce confluent wet desquamation within the field at an earlier dose level and can rarely result in soft tissue or cartilage necrosis. In sensitive areas, even with conventional fractionation schedules (1.8–2.0 Gy/fraction given once daily), toward the end of the treatment course, there can be confined moist desquamation within the field or within creases lying near skin folds or irregular surfaces.

Electrons will usually yield the same degree of skin reaction as superficial X-ray therapy or brachytherapy. However, with either electron or photon therapy, bolus is sometimes used on the surface of the skin to raise the dose to the superficial surface or to increase the delivered dose to surgical scars that are considered at risk for recurrence. The area that is covered with bolus will show a very pronounced reaction. It is an excellent and recommended practice when targeting a superficial skin area to measure the actual received radiation dose with thermoluminescent dosimetry to confirm the calculations.

Megavoltage photon therapy has skin-sparing effects, making it most appropriate for deep-seated treatment areas. For skin cancers that have spread to cranial nerves or lymph node basins, megavoltage photon therapy is used to achieve coverage of these regions. In these situations when three-dimensional or intensity-modulated radiation therapy is used, wax or commercial bolus of density similar to human tissue is frequently used to bring the primary tumor bed at the skin surface to an adequate dose.

14.4 Other Factors Affecting Acute Skin Toxicity

14.4.1 Prior UV Damage

Patients who have extensive history of UV skin damage are prone to greater skin reactions during therapeutic radiotherapy [36].

14.4.2 Prior Surgery and/or Reconstruction

Radiation therapy delivered to a recently operated surgical bed predisposes to nonhealing and wound complications. While reconstructed musculocutaneous flaps tend to have less reaction than the surrounding native skin, thin skin grafts are very fragile.

14.4.3 Concurrent Systemic Therapy

The use of systemic radiosensitizers in combination with radiation therapy has no clearly established role in skin cancers. However, based on studies from the head and neck cancer literature, many treating physicians will extrapolate that operative findings of positive margins or extracapsular extension are reasonable indications for the addition of concurrent systemic therapy during the postoperative radiation therapy course.

14.5 Management of Skin Reaction

The field of dermatology is experienced at handling postoperative skin reactions, but expertise in managing radiation-related skin reactions is just now emerging, and the evidence base remains very limited. The management of skin reactions from skin cancer treatment is not different from treatment of any other subsite. Readers are encouraged to refer to the chapters about the specific anatomic area that is involved, e.g., head and neck, gastrointestinal tract, etc.

The first important step is education. The patient and any involved caregivers should be instructed on the expected side effects to the skin, with special attention to sensitive areas such the inframammary, axillary, or inguinal areas where large skin folds naturally occur and there is frequent occurrence of rubbing or friction. Self-care measures should be encouraged, such as gentle rinsing with mild soap and water, patting the area dry, applying frequent moisturization, and reporting any itching or erythema to the treating physician. Lotion moisturizer (Eucerin, Lubriderm, Lotion Soft) is encouraged.

The physician and patient should both engage in assessment of the progress of the reaction. Grading of dermatologic side effects may be based on clinician-observed ratings or incorporate patient-reported outcomes. Assessment should take place at least weekly. The most commonly used grading is the CTCAE skin toxicity scale, but patients' experiences are not incorporated into it as it is based on clinician observership.

Erythema and discomfort often begin at around 20–30 Gy with capillary dilatation and increased blood flow. Patients should avoid localized irritation to the skin area under treatment, such as nonelectric razors, metal-containing deodorant, perfumes or powders, or rubbing or pressure from clothing. Treatment areas exposed to chlorinated water from swimming should be rinsed afterward with fresh water and moisturized. Use of tape in the radiated area of the skin should be avoided in favor of light removable netting. As the treatment course progresses to 40–50 Gy, the skin can become hyperpigmented, dry, and xerotic as the glandular cells produce less. An emollient such as Aquaphor or vitamin A&D ointment can help to reduce discomfort due to the dryness of the skin. If there is mild to moderate dry peel or slough, a medical honey dressing (MediHoney HCS) can assist with gentle autolytic debridement.

Wet desquamation may start to appear at around 50–60 Gy and can progress rapidly to superficial tissue hemorrhage, ulceration, and necrosis. It is important to note that for an appropriate treatment of a superficial skin cancer, an adequate dosage should be expected to produce a moderate moist reaction. Therefore, the patient should be prepared for this reaction and trained on care of the skin. The treating team should be prepared to manage this reaction to minimize discomfort and facilitate healing.

Depending on the extent of the wet desquamation, our practice is to utilize soft silicone (Mepilex) or sheet hydrogel (CoolMagic) dressings for their soothing properties and protection of the skin. Small amounts of silver-containing amorphous hydrogel (Silvasorb) can be useful to address the risk of bacterial overgrowth in small cracked areas of wet desquamation. For larger areas of wet desquamation or tissue ulceration, patients are treated with daily wound cleansing and application of silver-impregnated hydrofiber or alginate dressings, with netting to secure the dressing in place.

14.6 Photographs and Recommendations

Below are general skin care recommendations (Table 14.1), week-by-week treatment instructions, and photographs that demonstrate typical skin reactions over time for skin cancer patients (Table 14.2). Photographs of special reactions and instructions on how to treat these more uncommon cases are also provided (Table 14.3). Figure 14.1 is a general suggested treatment algorithm for skin care for patients receiving radiotherapy for cutaneous primary cancers.

Table 14.1 General principles of skin care for skin cancer patients

Patient should:
• Cleanse daily with mild soap and water or baby shampoo if lesion is on the scalp
• Use lotions and creams recommended by your provider
• Wash off lotion, cream, or ointments if applied within 3 hours before radiation treatment
• Wear soft garments that control moisture and minimize friction
• After cleansing or washing, pat dry gently
Patient should not:
• Rub, put pressure on, or scratch radiated area
• Take hot water showers or hot baths; use rough washcloth or rub dry on the radiated skin
• Apply any lotion, cream, or ointment in the 3 hours prior to radiation treatment
• Apply drying agents to the skin unless instructed to do so
• Use any tape or adhesives on the radiated skin

Table 14.2 Examples of typical acute skin reactions and recommended intervention for a skin cancer patient undergoing postoperative radiation therapy to the scalp

<table>
<tr><th>Week</th><th>Skin reaction</th><th>Intervention</th></tr>
<tr><td>1</td><td>57-year-old Caucasian female on immunosuppressive therapy for pancreas and kidney transplants with multiple skin cancers, treated with Mohs micrographic surgery for squamous cell carcinoma of the scalp vertex with residual disease, planned to undergo radiation therapy to 70 Gy using 1 cm wax bolus
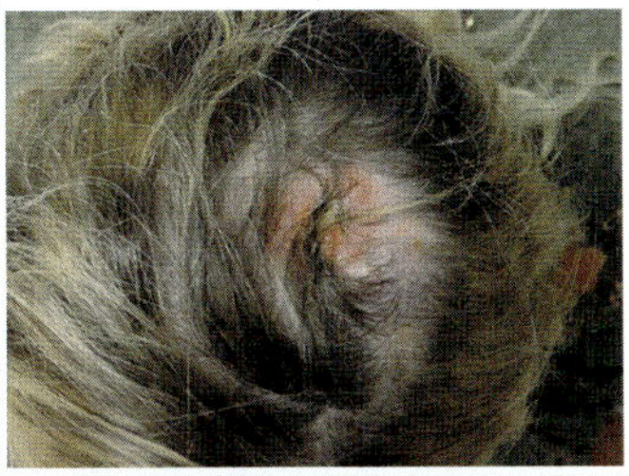</td><td>• Cleanse daily with baby shampoo or mild soap and water
• Apply a light moisturizing lotion, such as Lotion Soft, twice a day
• Protect the radiated site from sun exposure and friction. Continue this throughout treatment</td></tr>
<tr><td>2</td><td>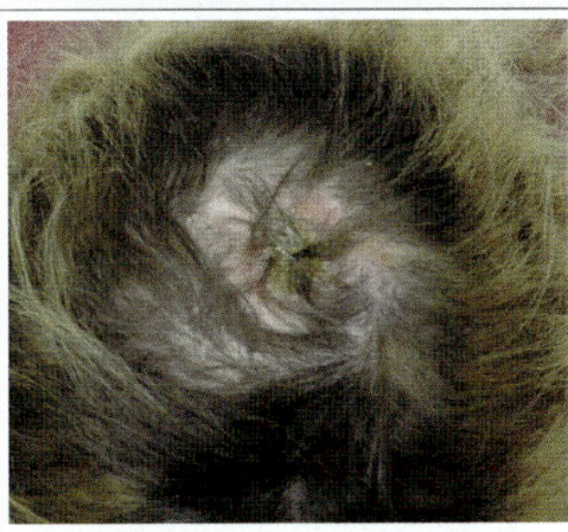</td><td>• Continue to cleanse daily with baby shampoo or mild soap and water
• Continue light moisturizing lotion, such as Lotion Soft, twice a day</td></tr>
<tr><td>3</td><td>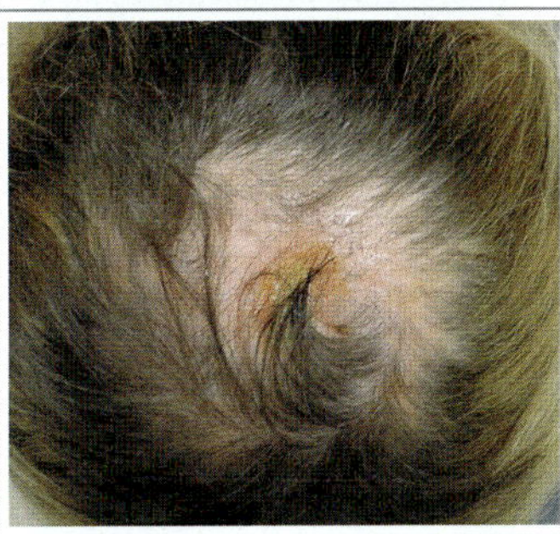</td><td>• Cleanse the ulcer and surrounding skin with mild soap and water or Skintegrity wound cleanser spray (or similar). Spray Skintegrity over the entire site. Allow it to remain on the skin for 1–2 min then rinse away
• Apply a light moisturizer to the surrounding intact skin
• Apply Aquaphor to the ulceration twice daily
• Cover the ulcer with Mepilex Lite, Mepilex Transfer Ag, or similar nonstick dressing</td></tr>
<tr><td>4</td><td>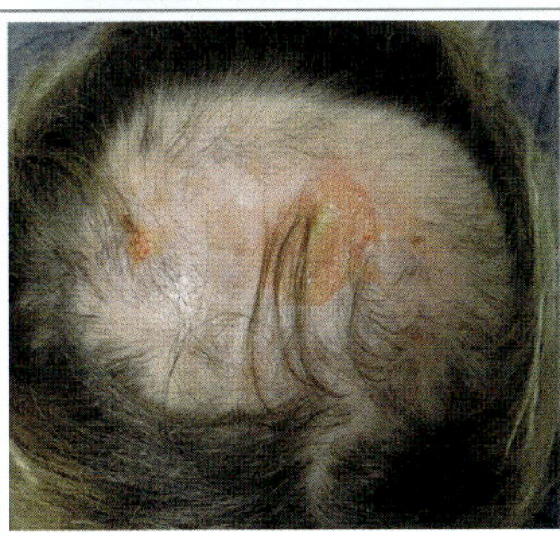</td><td>• Continue to cleanse the skin and ulcer as above
• Apply a dressing to the ulceration, such as Aquacel Ag (or similar), and cover with Mepilex Lite. Ensure the primary dressing lifts off easily. If it sticks to the wound, wet it thoroughly with normal saline or water then gently remove
• Alternatively Mepilex Transfer Ag or Mepilex Ag may be used alone
• Apply Aquaphor to the remaining undressed skin twice daily
• Continue this regimen until radiation is complete and the moist desquamation has healed</td></tr>
</table>

Table 14.3 Special cases and reactions

	Description	Reaction type	Treatment and intervention
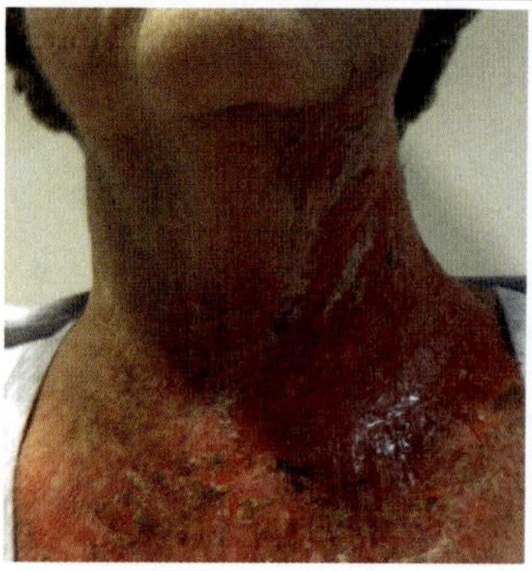	63-year-old female with history of repeated kidney transplants on immuno-suppression, who received deliberately desquamating electron therapy to a large field on the side of the neck for an aggressive multiply recurrent desmoplastic skin cancer Supportive care measures included cleaning, disinfecting, and moisturizing the wound bed	Mixed moist desquamation with light to moderate exudate and erythema with dry desquamation along the periphery	• Cleanse the area with Skintegrity wound cleanser spray (or similar). Spray Skintegrity over the entire site. Allow it to remain on the skin for 1–2 min then gently rinse away • Apply a moisturizer such as Aquaphor to the surrounding intact skin • Apply a silver ion dressing to the moist desquamtion, such as Aquacel Ag (or similar), and cover with Mepilex Lite or roller gauze. Ensure the primary dressing extends over the edge of the moist wound and that it lifts off easily. If it sticks to the wound, wet it thoroughly with normal saline or water and gently remove • Alternatively Mepilex Transfer Ag or Mepilex Ag may be used alone and secured with Flexinet or roller gauze • Ensure the dressings are removed prior to daily radiation treatments • Continue this regimen daily until radiation is complete and the moist desquamation has healed. At the completion of radiation, dressings may be changed or left in place per manufacturer's recommendations or changed every 24–72 hours as clinically indicated

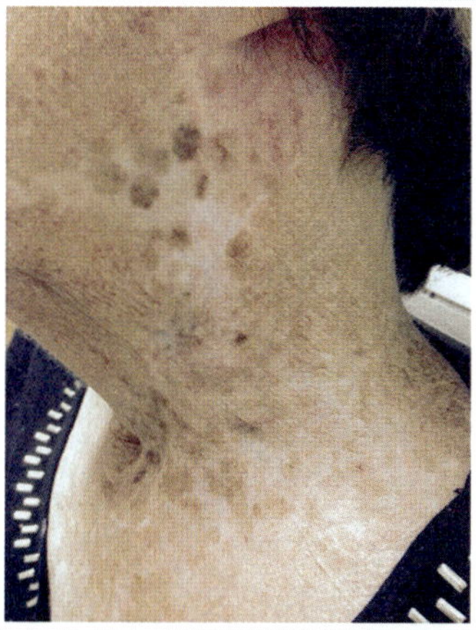		4-year follow-up photo shows hyperpigmentary changes on a background of hypopigmentation	
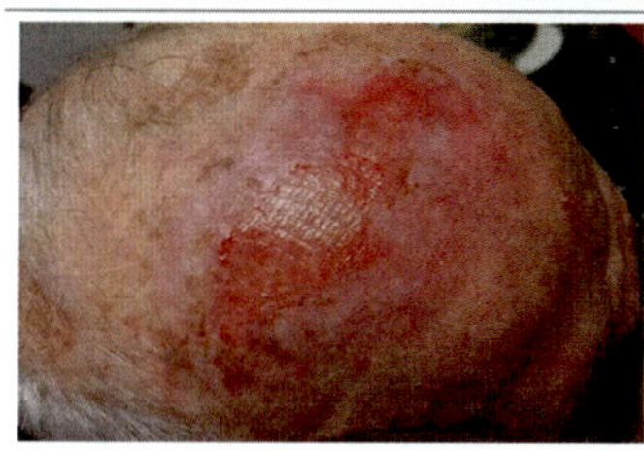	91-year-old male who received 100 KV superficial X-ray therapy for mixed squamous and basal cell carcinoma of the scalp, to 3600 cGy in 6 fractions twice a week, at fraction 6 of treatment		• Cleanse the site with mild soap and water or Skintegrity wound cleanser spray (or similar). Spray Skintegrity over the entire site. Allow it to remain on the skin for 1–2 min then rinse away • Apply Aquaphor to the site twice daily • If needed, cover the area with Mepilex Lite, Mepilex Transfer Ag or similar nonstick dressing

Week	Apply to Radiated Area	Notes
1-3	Lotion Soft OR Remedy ↓ Apply 2x/day	Thin lotion that is quickly absorbed, leaves no residue and does not clog pores.
3+	Calendula OR Aquaphor ↓ Apply 2x/day	Liberally apply over radiated site twice a day. Continue to utilize the emollients for 2-3 weeks post radiation.
4+ (without moist desquamation)	Skintegrity ↓ Apply 1x/day Calendula OR Aquaphor ↓ Apply 2x/day Mepilex Lite ↓ Apply 1x/day before bed if needed	Continue as above. Add Skintegrity, which is used to cleanse and disinfect the area. Spray Skintegrity onto radiated site and surrounding skin, leave in place for 1 - 2 minutes, and then rinse. Mepilex Lite reduces friction and trauma to the area.
4+ (with moist desquamation)	Skintegrity ↓ Apply 1x/day Calendula OR Aquaphor ↓ Apply 2x/day Silver Ion Dressing ↓ Apply 1x/day	Continue as above. Silver ion dressings such as Aquacel Ag, Mepitel Transfer, and Mepilex Ag can promote healing and maintain moisture balance.

Fig. 14.1 Suggested treatment algorithm for skin care

References

1. Siegel RL, Miller KD, Jemal A. Cancer statistics, 2015. CA Cancer J Clin. 2015;65:5–29. doi:10.3322/caac.21254.
2. Parkin DM, Bray F, Ferlay J, Pisani P. Estimating the world cancer burden: Globocan 2000. Int J Cancer. 2001;94:153–6.
3. Tsao H, Rogers GS, Sober AJ. An estimate of the annual direct cost of treating cutaneous melanoma. J Am Acad Dermatol. 1998;38:669–80.
4. Guy Jr GP, Ekwueme DU, Tangka FK, Richardson LC. Melanoma treatment costs: a systematic review of the literature, 1990-2011. Am J Prev Med. 2012; 43:537–45. doi:10.1016/j.amepre.2012.07.031.
5. Higashi MK, Veenstra DL, Langley PC. Health economic evaluation of non-melanoma skin cancer and actinic keratosis. Pharmacoeconomics. 2004;22:83–94.
6. Rogers HW, Weinstock MA, Harris AR, Hinckley MR, Feldman SR, Fleischer AB, et al. Incidence estimate of nonmelanoma skin cancer in the United States, 2006. Arch Dermatol. 2010;146:283–7. doi:10.1001/archdermatol.2010.19.

7. Acarturk TO, Edington H. Nonmelanoma skin cancer. Clin Plast Surg. 2005;32:237–48. doi:10.1016/j.cps.2004.11.009.
8. Donaldson MR, Coldiron BM. No end in sight: the skin cancer epidemic continues. Semin Cutan Med Surg. 2011;30:3–5. doi:10.1016/j.sder.2011.01.002.
9. Harris RB, Griffith K, Moon TE. Trends in the incidence of nonmelanoma skin cancers in southeastern Arizona, 1985-1996. J Am Acad Dermatol. 2001;45:528–36. doi:10.1067/mjd.2001.114742.
10. Elwood JM, Gallagher RP. Body site distribution of cutaneous malignant melanoma in relationship to patterns of sun exposure. Int J Cancer. 1998;78:276–80. doi:10.1002/(SICI)1097-0215(19981029)78:3<276::AID-IJC2>3.0.CO;2-S.
11. Youl PH, Janda M, Aitken JF, Del Mar CB, Whiteman DC, Baade PD. Body-site distribution of skin cancer, pre-malignant and common benign pigmented lesions excised in general practice. Br J Dermatol. 2011;165:35–43. doi:10.1111/j.1365-2133.2011.10337.x.
12. Chen AC, Halliday GM, Damian DL. Non-melanoma skin cancer: carcinogenesis and chemoprevention. Pathology. 2013;45:331–41. doi:10.1097/PAT.0b013e32835f515c.
13. Parkin DM, Mesher D, Sasieni P. Cancers attributable to solar (ultraviolet) radiation exposure in the UK in 2010. Br J Cancer. 2011;105 Suppl 2:S66–9. doi:10.1038/bjc.2011.486.
14. Berg D, Otley CC. Skin cancer in organ transplant recipients: Epidemiology, pathogenesis, and management. J Am Acad Dermatol. 2002;47:1–17. quiz 8-20.
15. Day TA, Hornig JD, Sharma AK, Brescia F, Gillespie MB, Lathers D. Melanoma of the head and neck. Curr Treat Options Oncol. 2005;6:19–30.
16. Balch CM, Soong SJ, Atkins MB, Buzaid AC, Cascinelli N, Coit DG, et al. An evidence-based staging system for cutaneous melanoma. CA Cancer J Clin. 2004;54:131–49. quiz 82-4.
17. Sexton M, Jones DB, Maloney ME. Histologic pattern analysis of basal cell carcinoma. Study of a series of 1039 consecutive neoplasms. J Am Acad Dermatol. 1990;23:1118–26.
18. Mosterd K, Krekels GA, Nieman FH, Ostertag JU, Essers BA, Dirksen CD, et al. Surgical excision versus Mohs' micrographic surgery for primary and recurrent basal-cell carcinoma of the face: a prospective randomised controlled trial with 5-years' follow-up. Lancet Oncol. 2008;9:1149–56. doi:10.1016/S1470-2045(08)70260-2.
19. Voss N, Kim-Sing C. Radiotherapy in the treatment of dermatologic malignancies. Dermatol Clin. 1998;16:313–20.
20. Silverman MK, Kopf AW, Gladstein AH, Bart RS, Grin CM, Levenstein MJ. Recurrence rates of treated basal cell carcinomas. Part 4: X-ray therapy. J Dermatol Surg Oncol. 1992;18:549–54.
21. Han A, Ratner D. What is the role of adjuvant radiotherapy in the treatment of cutaneous squamous cell carcinoma with perineural invasion? Cancer. 2007;109:1053–9. doi:10.1002/cncr.22509.
22. Langendijk JA, Slotman BJ, van der Waal I, Doornaert P, Berkof J, Leemans CR. Risk-group definition by recursive partitioning analysis of patients with squamous cell head and neck carcinoma treated with surgery and postoperative radiotherapy. Cancer. 2005;104:1408–17. doi:10.1002/cncr.21340.
23. Hughes MP, Hardee ME, Cornelius LA, Hutchins LF, Becker JC, Gao L. Merkel cell carcinoma: epidemiology, target, and therapy. Curr Dermatol Rep. 2014;3:46–53. doi:10.1007/s13671-014-0068-z.
24. Lemos BD, Storer BE, Iyer JG, Phillips JL, Bichakjian CK, Fang LC, et al. Pathologic nodal evaluation improves prognostic accuracy in Merkel cell carcinoma: analysis of 5823 cases as the basis of the first consensus staging system. J Am Acad Dermatol. 2010;63:751–61. doi:10.1016/j.jaad.2010.02.056.
25. Agelli M, Clegg LX. Epidemiology of primary Merkel cell carcinoma in the United States. J Am Acad Dermatol. 2003;49:832–41. doi:10.1067/S0190.
26. Cho M, Gordon L, Rembielak A, Woo TC. Utility of radiotherapy for treatment of basal cell carcinoma: a review. Br J Dermatol. 2014;171:968–73. doi:10.1111/bjd.13253.
27. Olschewski T, Bajor K, Lang B, Lang E, Seegenschmiedt MH. [Radiotherapy of basal cell carcinoma of the face and head: Importance of low dose per fraction on long-term outcome]. J Dtsch Dermatol Ges. 2006;4:124–30. doi:10.1111/j.1610-0387.2006.05880.x.
28. Abbatucci JS, Boulier N, Laforge T, Lozier JC. Radiation therapy of skin carcinomas: results of a hypofractionated irradiation schedule in 675 cases followed more than 2 years. Radiother Oncol. 1989;14:113–9.
29. Silva JJ, Tsang RW, Panzarella T, Levin W, Wells W. Results of radiotherapy for epithelial skin cancer of the pinna: the Princess Margaret Hospital experience, 1982-1993. Int J Radiat Oncol Biol Phys. 2000;47:451–9.
30. Griep C, Davelaar J, Scholten AN, Chin A, Leer JW. Electron beam therapy is not inferior to superficial x-ray therapy in the treatment of skin carcinoma. Int J Radiat Oncol Biol Phys. 1995;32:1347–50. doi:10.1016/0360-3016(94)00603-I.
31. van Hezewijk M, Creutzberg CL, Putter H, Chin A, Schneider I, Hoogeveen M, et al. Efficacy of a hypofractionated schedule in electron beam radiotherapy for epithelial skin cancer: Analysis of 434 cases. Radiother Oncol. 2010;95:245–9. doi:10.1016/j.radonc.2010.02.024.
32. Heath CH, Deep NL, Nabell L, Carroll WR, Desmond R, Clemons L, et al. Phase 1 study of erlotinib plus radiation therapy in patients with advanced cutaneous squamous cell carcinoma. Int J Radiat Oncol Biol

Phys. 2013;85:1275–81. doi:10.1016/j.ijrobp.2012.09.030.

33. Lewis CM, Glisson BS, Feng L, Wan F, Tang X, Wistuba II, et al. A phase II study of gefitinib for aggressive cutaneous squamous cell carcinoma of the head and neck. Clin Cancer Res. 2012;18:1435–46. doi:10.1158/1078-0432.CCR-11-1951.
34. Burmeister BH, Mark Smithers B, Burmeister E, Baumann K, Davis S, Krawitz H, et al. A prospective phase II study of adjuvant postoperative radiation therapy following nodal surgery in malignant melanoma-Trans Tasman Radiation Oncology Group (TROG) Study 96.06. Radiother Oncol. 2006;81:136–42. doi:10.1016/j.radonc.2006.10.001.
35. Burmeister BH, Henderson MA, Ainslie J, Fisher R, Di Iulio J, Smithers BM, et al. Adjuvant radiotherapy versus observation alone for patients at risk of lymph-node field relapse after therapeutic lymphadenectomy for melanoma: a randomised trial. Lancet Oncol. 2012;13:589–97. doi:10.1016/S1470-2045(12)70138-9.
36. Porock D, Kristjanson L, Nikoletti S, Cameron F, Pedler P. Predicting the severity of radiation skin reactions in women with breast cancer. Oncol Nurs Forum. 1998;25:1019–29.

Locally Advanced Cancers

15

Florence Yuen and Diane Sandman

Locally advanced fungating and ulcerative tumors present a challenge in management both for the patient and the provider. It is estimated that approximately 5–10 % of cancer wounds may be fungating [1–4].

Fungating tumors are the result of the proliferation of uncontrolled malignant cells which eventually protrude through and erode the skin and tissue [3–5]. These tumors may be the result of a rapidly progressive cancer, recurrent cancer, or ignored disease. They may initially present as small, raised erythematous, discrete, or confluent nodules, with or without tenderness, which progress to a cauliflower-like mass, deep ulceration, or a combination of any of these features [5]. Fungating tumors can occur anywhere on the body. The most common sites include the head, neck, and breast [6].

Radiation therapy in the form of external beam treatment with or without hyperthermia may be used for control of the tumor, ulceration, drainage, and reduction of pain [7]. Linthorst et al. [8] reported a complete clinical response rate of 70 % in 248 women with locally recurrent breast cancer treated with re-irradiation and hyperthermia. The median duration of local control was 15 months. However, at 5 years, local control was 39 %. Therefore, 60 % of these patients continued to have gross disease with its associated morbidity. The goal of palliative radiotherapy is to provide temporary local control, which assists in reducing untoward symptoms and promoting quality of life [5, 7]. Radiation dermatitis is a potential complication of palliative radiation therapy and can pose an additional management challenge to the patient with a chronic fungating wound.

Wounds heal well in a well vascularized, moist environment, free from infection and necrotic tissue [9, 10] This is not the case with a fungating malignant wound. A malignant wound is often a mixture of friable, vascular, poorly oxygenated, necrotic tissue. The moist necrotic tissue produces an environment that allows bacteria to thrive with an associated odor. The wound exudate which is produced may be copious and can severely macerate the surrounding normal dermal tissue [3, 5]. Chronic non-healing malignant wounds have a profound impact on the patient's quality of life and activities of daily living [3, 5, 6]. Some patients don't seek treatment due to the embarrassment caused by the wound [4]. Treatment of these wounds should be individualized and should take into consideration some of the following points: pain (due to the cancer itself or caused by dressing management), management of drainage, odor,

F. Yuen, MSN, AOCNP (✉)
Department of Radiation Oncology, University of California, San Francisco,
Box 1708, 1600 Divisadero, Cancer Center Room 1031, San Francisco, CA 94143, USA

Department of Nursing, University of California San Francisco Medical Center, San Francisco, CA, USA
e-mail: Florence.Yuen@ucsf.edu

D. Sandman, RN, CWOCN, MSN, FNP
Department of Nursing, University of California San Francisco Medical Center, San Francisco, CA, USA

B. Fowble et al. (eds.), *Skin Care in Radiation Oncology*, DOI 10.1007/978-3-319-31460-0_15

bleeding, infection, prevention of healthy skin maceration, the patient/caregiver's ability to dress the wound, and cost-effectiveness of dressing supplies [3, 5, 6, 11]. The goal of wound healing and closure is usually not realistic or expected in this setting. Instead, goals should focus on improving the patient's quality of life by effectively managing wound bioburden, exudate, bleeding, odor, and promotion of comfort [3, 6, 11, 12].

Presently, there are no evidence-based standards or guidelines for the management of these wounds. Significant differences in practice occur within organizations and across the nation as a result of historical practices and limited evidence to guide practice.

General principles in the care of malignant chronic wounds include cleansing of the area, the use of dressings to facilitate a balance between a moist and dry environment, decreasing wound bioburden, minimizing infection, minimizing scab formation (which can trap bacteria), controlling pain, and promoting quality of life [3, 6, 10–12].

Certain products should be avoided, so as not to irritate the wound more. These include neosporin and polysporin which may cause an allergic reaction and skin sensitivity, Betadine which inhibits healing by damaging fibroblasts [5], occlusive dressings and over-the-counter products such as Ben-Gay, Gold Bond, milk of magnesia, and menthol camphor. Alginate dressings are effective for absorbing exudates but should be selectively chosen as they have the potential to break apart leaving debris in the wound that may form a granuloma. Silvadene, although previously very popular, may result in an allergic reaction, especially in patients with a known allergy to sulfa, as well as cause the patient discomfort with the dressing changes [13].

Many of our patients who present for palliative radiation therapy will have the dressing removed and replaced in the department when receiving active radiation treatment. The following are suggestions for the management of fungating and ulcerative wounds in patients who are undergoing radiation therapy.

15.1 Cleansing

Cleansing of the wound is important as it decreases the wound's bacterial bioburden and assists with odor control. Wounds can be cleansed directly with normal saline, tap water, or a mild wound cleanser [3, 5]. In order to prevent the spread of bacteria and cross contamination, the use of washcloths, hand, or bath towels on the wound should be avoided; instead opt for disposable items such as 4×4 gauze pads or soft paper towels. Using products such as hydrogen peroxide or alcohol is not recommended as they may be irritating to the wound, can cause maceration of the tissues, and can delay or prevent wound healing [3]. Iodine, with the exception of cadexomer iodine (Iodosorb gel), has been noted to be cytotoxic to cells [3, 5]. If the patient is able, encourage the patient to shower daily or every other day. Mild soap (such as Dove or Neutrogena) can be used in the shower, but not directly on the wound as it can be irritating. Instead, the patient can wash around the wound and allow the soapy water to run over it.

15.2 Drainage

Fungating, ulcerative tumors can obstruct lymphatic flow. The drainage produced by these tumors varies from light to copious. It has also been noted that the pH of the fungating tumor wound exudate can be irritating to the surrounding normal tissue and result in tissue maceration. There are multiple dressings and products available for the management of small, moderate, and heavy drainage. These include less expensive over-the-counter items such as baby diapers, menstrual pads ("Kotex") or plastic backed liners (Chux), and abdominal (ABD) pads. For wounds that have a small amount of drainage, Mepilex Lite or various medical grade honey products can be used. Calcium alginate (seaweed) dressings will absorb small amounts of exudate and then turn to a gel. For moderate to heavy drainage, Mepilex transfer or another absorbent nonstick dressing can be used as the primary dressing with secondary dressings of an abdominal (ABD) pads and/or Chux. Abdominal or mesh binders are useful for wounds on the chest, thorax, abdomen, or limbs, to keep the dressings in place and thereby avoid the use of tape. Cavilon No Sting skin barrier can be applied to the peri-wound area to protect the skin from maceration. This does not need to be washed off if the patient is undergoing concurrent radiation. Coban or silicone tapes are an alternative to tape and roller gauze (Kerlix) to secure dressings and prevent additional skin denudement, pain, and infection.

15.3 Odor

Severe and profound odor may be present in patients with fungating, exudative wounds. Wound odor is the result of bacteria that are present in the necrotic tissue [3, 11]. Many of these wounds contain both aerobic and anaerobic bacteria. The anaerobic bacteria emit by-products that produce an intensely nauseating foul odor [11]. Wound cleansing and debridement of necrotic debris to decrease bacterial count is helpful in the management of odor. Topical metronidazole (tablets, gel, or cream) has been found to be effective in decreasing wound odor [3, 5, 11].

Metronidazole tablets (250 mg) can be finely crushed and sprinkled over the wound (put in salt shaker) prior to placing the dressing. This is an inexpensive and effective method for controlling odor, as well as managing bacterial burden. This can be used for long-term management of the wound [3, 5, 11]. Charcoal-embedded dressings, as either a primary or secondary dressing, are excellent for odor control; however they may be cost prohibitive [3].

For the home environment, charcoal briquettes or cat litter under the bed, essential oils, and aromatherapy products have been used to absorb odors [3, 12].

15.4 Bleeding

The malignant wound can be very friable. Bleeding may occur easily with manipulation of the wound and dressing [3]. Consideration should be given to using a nonadherent primary dressing to prevent bleeding and minimize traumatizing the wound. Care should be taken with dressing removal to avoid and minimize bleeding. If the primary dressing adheres to the tumor, it should be moistened with normal saline for ease of removal. For significant areas of bleeding, pressure should be applied using gauze moistened with water or normal saline for a full 5 min. The application of a paste made from mixing a sucralfate tablet (1 g) with a teaspoon of water may assist with the control of oozing [3, 14]. Other interventions include Gelfoam or Surgicel applied to the site of bleeding. The use of silver nitrate sticks is effective for managing small areas of bleeding [3].

15.5 Infection

In patients with chronic wounds, decreasing bioburden or lowering bacterial counts to subinfection levels assists in controlling both local and systemic mediators of inflammation, which can assist in promoting healing [10, 15]. This is an essential component of caring for chronic, fungating malignant wounds as well. Chronic wounds have been noted to become colonized with bacteria that can promote both infection and odor. β[beta]-hemolytic streptococci and bacteria concentrations in excess of 10^5 units per gram of tissue have been noted to impair healing [10]. Commonly identified wound bacteria include *Staphylococcus aureus*, methicillin-resistant *Staphylococcus aureus* (20–50 % of cases), and *Pseudomonas aeruginosa* [10, 16]. Systemic antibiotics should be reserved for systemic infections, evidenced by erythema, increased pain, leukocytosis, or fever. They tend to have limited value with stable chronic or fungating wounds due to limited blood supply to the necrotic areas [3, 10]. For localized, clinically infected areas, topically applied antimicrobials, in addition to debridement and cleansing, may be effective [3, 17, 18]. The use of antimicrobial dressings, such as Xeroform gauze, silver ion, and medical grade (Leptospermum) honey, may assist with managing bioburden, thereby decreasing infection.

Debridement and cleansing assist in lowering the bacterial burden in chronic wounds [17, 18]. Infection can develop under a scab or eschar. Wounds that have scabs or eschars in places other than the heels, toes, nose, and ears should be debrided of dry adherent dead tissue. There are four forms of debridement: sharp (scalpel, scissors), autolytic (using the body's own enzymes), enzymatic (topical collagenase), and mechanical (wet to dry gauze, tweezers, mist therapy, pulse lavage, hydro surgical, low frequency ultrasound). Our practice is to use very mild forms of debridement, such as tweezers, dry gauze, and hydrocolloidal or medical grade honey for the debridement of necrotic tissue. Occasionally we will utilize sharp debridement for hyperkeratotic, nonvascular tissue. Vascular or friable sites are not debrided due to the risk of bleeding.

15.6 Pain

There may be various types of pain associated with a fungating tumor mass, due to the spread of disease and the tumor itself. Many of these patients will already be on systemic opioids for management of their pain. If the patient is experiencing pain at the wound site, it is important to premedicate the patient prior to treatment and dressing change. Topical lidocaine may be applied for 10–15 min immediately upon removing the dressing and prior to debridement [3]. Off-label use of topically applied opioids has been used to reduce severe pain. The opioid product is thought to exert its action by binding with peripheral opioid receptors [19]. The final product needs to be compounded and may include a combination of opioids (cocaine, morphine), cream, or ointment base (Silvadene, Intrasite Gel, Aquaphor, etc.) and numbing (lidocaine) agents [3, 19–21].

15.7 Dressing the Wound and Securing Dressings

Many times the patient will present to the radiation oncology setting with a dressing and cleansing regimen already in place. This may or may not suffice for the patient who is undergoing active radiation therapy. It is not uncommon for a fungating, ulcerative tumor undergoing radiation to get worse before it begins to improve. Many of these tumors will have increased tissue edema, increased erythema, tissue necrosis, exudates in addition to the development of "radiation dermatitis" to the surrounding skin. The choice for specific primary and secondary dressings should take into consideration the wound location and extent; the amount of exudate, odor, and pain; the type(s) of tissue in the wound base; the status of the surrounding skin; and the availability and expertise of the primary wound care provider. There are numerous dressings currently available for wound management.

Xeroform is a bacteriostatic, primary dressing containing bismuth on petroleum mesh [3]. It is generally covered with a secondary absorbable dressing (abdominal pad, menstrual pads, etc.) It is inexpensive and is commonly used by many patients on presentation to the department.

As the patient progresses through radiation, we will often change to a dressing that will facilitate decreasing bioburden, manage moisture and exudates, and promote healing of moist desquamation. Antimicrobial silicone (such as Mepilex Ag, Mepilex Ag transfer, Mepitel Ag), silver ion hydrofiber (i.e, Aquacel Ag), silver ion alginate, and foam dressings have been found to be effective in our practice. They are also well accepted by our patients and are easy to use, promoting patient compliance. We have also utilized gels containing medical grade (Leptospermum) honey and honey-impregnated calcium alginate for the debridement of hyperkeratotic and necrotic tissue as well as dry fissures. We have found these dressings and gels to be most beneficial in our practice for the acute management of the wound and radiation site while the patient is actively undergoing radiation and recovery.

Standard tape should not be used on the radiated or fragile skin. Some dressings have self-adhesive edges and do not need additional securing (care must be used to ensure the adhesive edge does not traumatize the skin). Dressings may be secured with roller gauze (Kerlix), Coban, Mepilex, Mepitel, or silicone tape. Additional products to secure dressings include abdominal binders, netting, disposable underwear, mesh underwear, Montgomery dressings, or hydrofiber dressing straps.

15.8 Cost Containment of Chronic Wound Management

If a patient is being seen by home health, palliative care, or hospice nurses, they will provide the supplies the patient needs. If the patient is being cared for by a family member, loved one, private nurse, or caregiver, the supplies may come from a medical supply company or be bought by the family depending on insurance coverage. Simple efforts to minimize cost include the use of a homemade solution of normal saline. Two level teaspoons of table salt (non-iodized) added to four cups of tap water and boiled for 15 min will create a 0.9 % solution of sodium chloride that can be stored in a sterile jar for 48 h. Other measures include thoughtful dressing selection to keep the wound clean, contain exudate, odor and promote comfort.

15.9 Photographs and Recommendations

Below are general skin care recommendations (Table 15.1) and photographs that demonstrate typical skin reactions over time for locally advanced cancers (Table 15.2). Photographs of special reactions and instructions on how to treat these cases are also provided (Table 15.3). No general suggested treatment algorithm for skin care management for locally advanced cancer patients undergoing radiotherapy is provided because of the highly unique nature of these skin reactions and the treatment regimens.

Table 15.1 General principles of skin care for chronic wounds

Patient should:
• Continue daily dressing changes while on treatment
• Remove all dressings prior to radiation treatment
• Cleanse daily with mild soap and water or wound cleanser such as Skintegrity
• Moisturize intact undressed skin in the radiation field
• Wear soft garments that control moisture and minimize friction
• After cleansing or washing, pat dry gently
Patient should not:
• Rub, put pressure on, or scratch radiated area
• Take hot water showers, hot baths; use rough washcloth or rub dry on the radiated skin
• Apply any lotion, cream or ointment in the 3 hours prior to radiation treatment
• Apply drying agents to the skin unless instructed to do so
• Use any tape or adhesives on the radiated

Table 15.2 Patient with chronic wound undergoing radiation therapy

Week	Skin Reaction	Reaction Type	Intervention
1	65-year-old- Caucasian female with neglected breast cancer 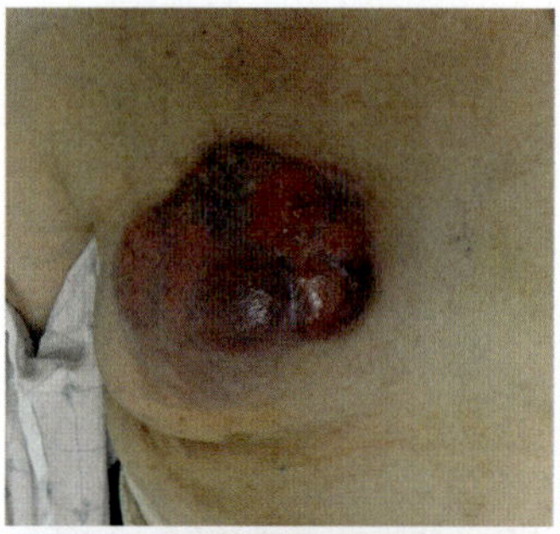 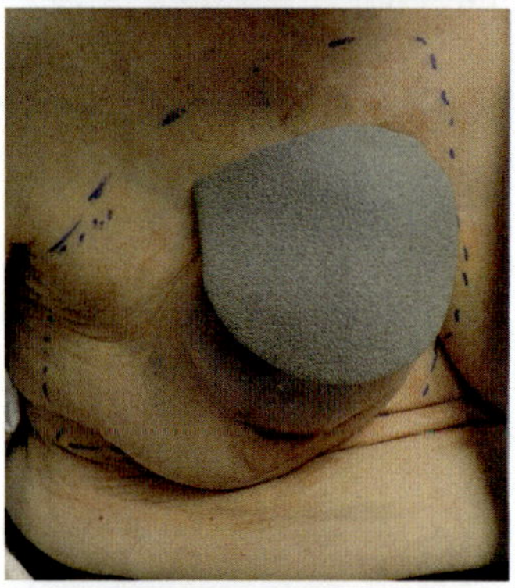 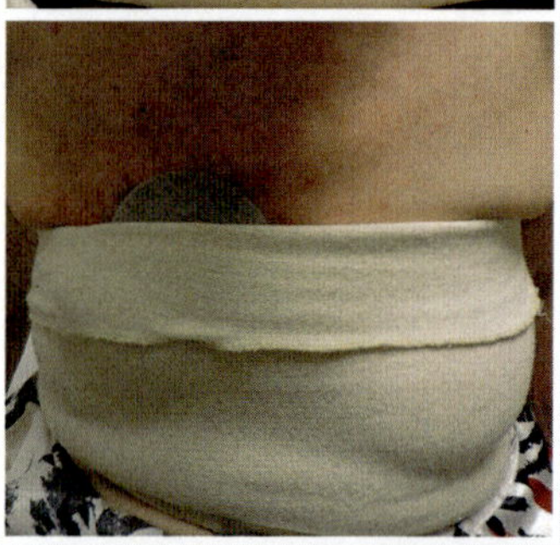	Fungating breast cancer with areas of necrosis at start of palliative radiation	• Spray Skintegrity once a day to the skin (entire radiation site) before shower and rinse off after 1–2 min • Apply a light moisturizer such as Lotion Soft twice a day to intact skin in the radiation field • Apply Mepilex Ag or similar nonstick dressing over fungating wound. The goal of this intervention is to absorb exudate, maintain moisture, and prevent infection throughout radiation treatment • Remove the dressing prior to each treatment • Repeat procedure daily • May use an abdominal binder to hold the dressing in place
2	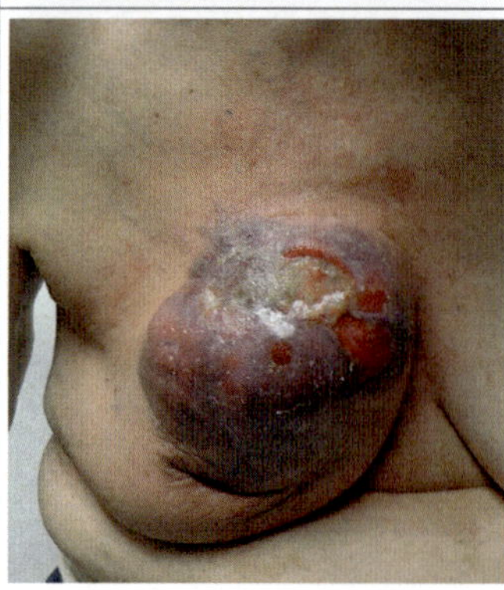	Edema and maceration of the right breast and treatment area	• Spray Skintegrity once a day to the skin before shower and rinse off after 1–2 min • Apply Lotion Soft twice a day to intact skin • Debride any necrotic tissue and fibrotic biofilms • Debridement can be done manually or with the use of hydrocolloidal dressings and enzymatic cleansers • May apply silver nitrate to bleeding areas • Continue to apply Mepliex Ag or similar nonstick, absorbable dressing after each treatment. May use an abdominal binder to hold the dressing in place

(continued)

Table 15.2 (continued)

Week	Skin Reaction	Reaction Type	Intervention
3	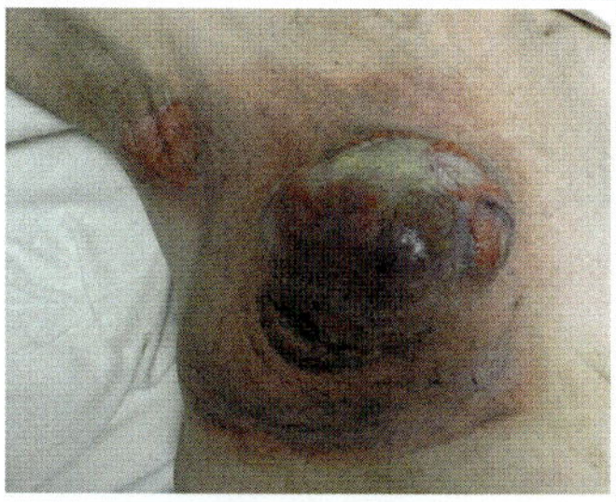 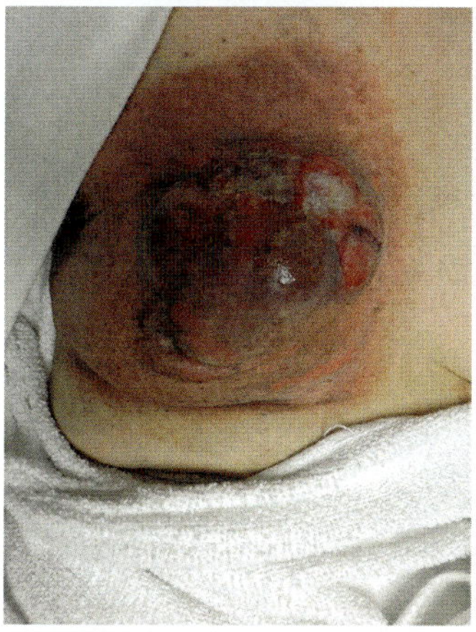 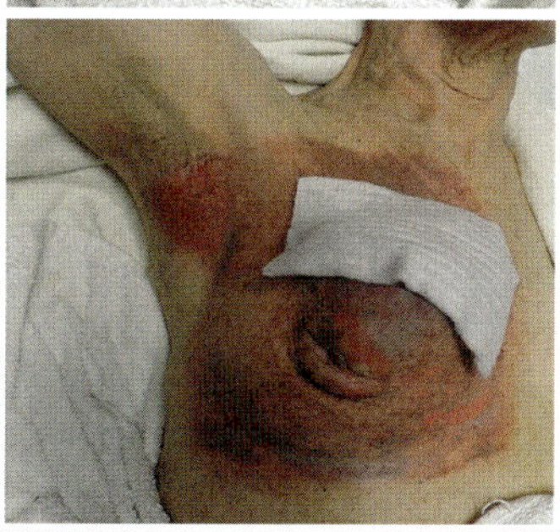	Mixture of moist and dry desquamation along with build-up of white hyperkeratotic/biofilm tissue over the fungating mass	• Spray Skintegrity once a day to the skin before shower and rinse off after 1–2 min • Debride necrotic areas and biofilm (yellow/white area) • Apply calendula (in place of light moisturizer) once or twice a day to the remaining undressed skin • Switch to a dressing that will assist in decreasing bioburden, debridement and absorption of excess exudate. Aquacel Ag was used here and covered with a secondary dressing (abdominal pad) • May secure again with an abdominal binder • A hydrocolloidal dressing containing Manuka honey or an alginate is also an appropriate option in place of the Aquacel Ag
1 week postradiation	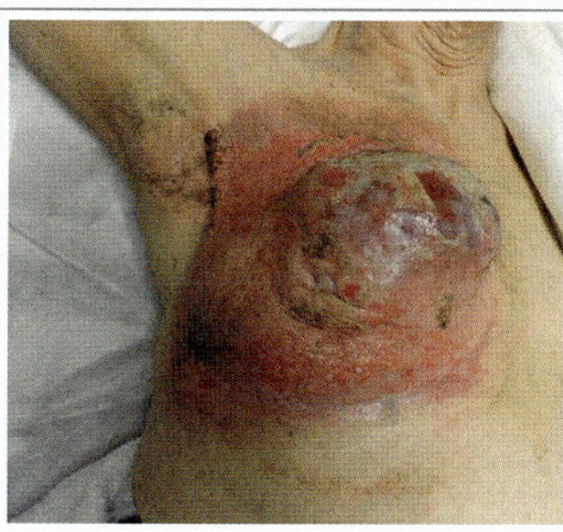	Mixture of moist and dry desquamation along with white biofilm/hyperkeratotic tissue and new skin islands beneath fungating mass	• Spray Skintegrity once a day to the skin (entire radiation site) before shower and rinse off after 1–2 min • Debride necrotic areas and biofilm • Apply calendula once or twice a day to the remaining undressed skin • Continue use of a dressing that will assist in debriding the wound and absorbing excess exudate • Patient preferred to resume Mepilex Ag for its ease of use
2 weeks postradiation	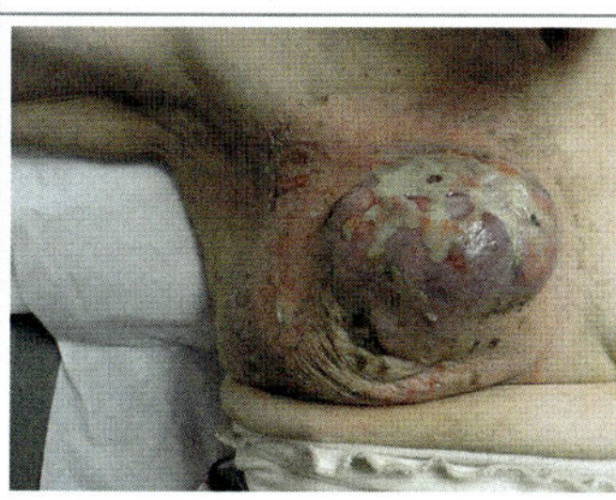	Dry desquamation along the periphery with white biofilm/hyperkeratotic tissue and new skin islands on fungating mass	• Spray Skintegrity once a day to the skin (entire radiated site) before shower and rinse off after 1–2 min • Manually debride necrotic areas and biofilm. (tweezers, dry gauze) • Apply calendula once or twice a day to the skin around the dressing • Continue with daily dressing procedure as described above

(continued)

Table 15.2 (continued)

Week	Skin Reaction	Reaction Type	Intervention
3 weeks postradiation	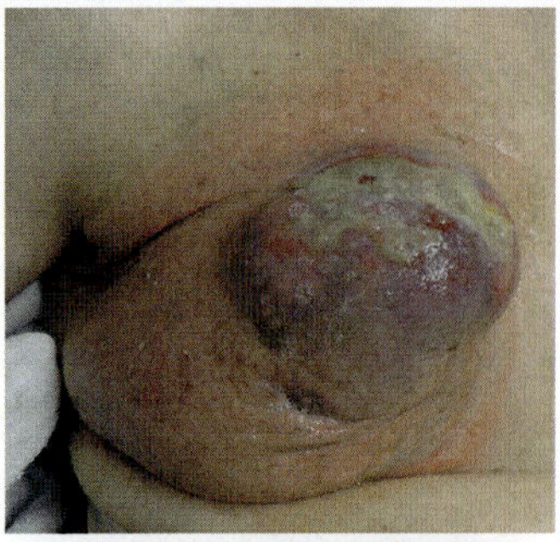 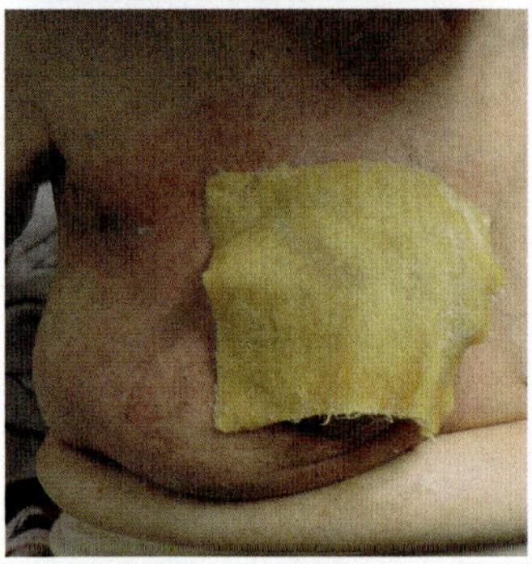	Resolving dry desquamation. Mass decreasing in size with continued moist hyperkeratotic tissue	• Spray Skintegrity once a day to skin before shower and rinse off after 1–2 min • Debride necrotic areas and biofilm (white area) • Apply calendula once or twice a day to the skin around the dressing • Apply calcium alginate dressing impregnated with Leptospermum honey to assist with wound debridement. An ABD pad and trimmed plastic back liner (Chux) was used as a secondary dressing. This was effective in absorbing the moisture from the honey dressing • The patient continued the use of the abdominal binder to keep the dressing in place
4 weeks postradiation	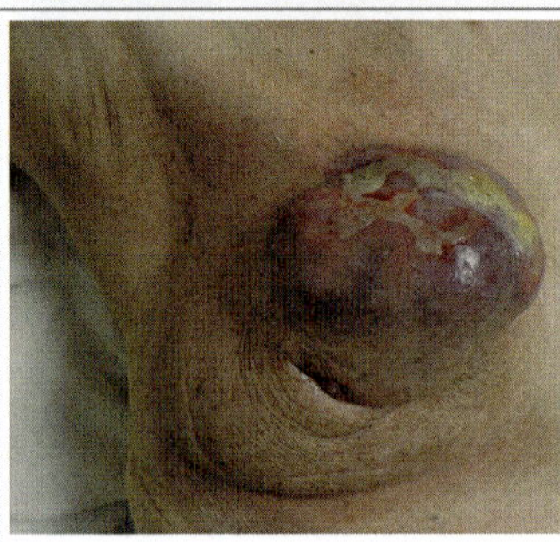	Residual tumor with decreasing hyperkeratotic tissue	• Spray Skintegrity once a day to the skin before shower and rinse off after 1–2 min • Debride necrotic areas and biofilm (white area) • Apply calendula once or twice a day to the remaining undressed skin • Apply calcium alginate dressing with Leptospermum honey to assist with wound debridement. (Patient used this twice a week rather than daily) • May also switch back to normal dressing procedure
5 weeks postradiation	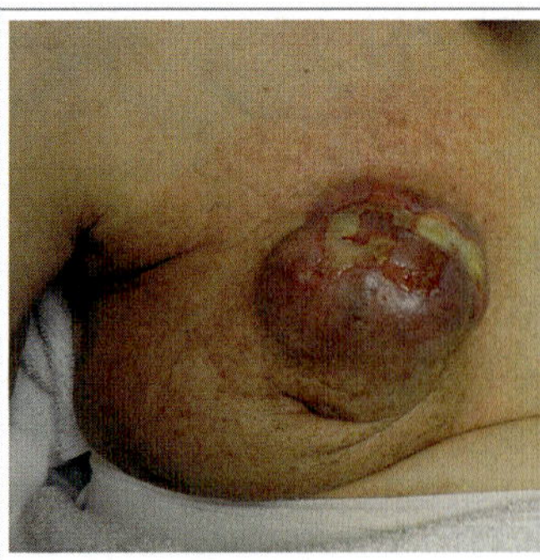	Residual hyperpigmentation of the radiation field with a decreasing mass and continued hyperkeratotic area	• Spray Skintegrity once a day to skin before shower and rinse off after 1–2 min • Debride necrotic areas and biofilm (white/yellow area) • Apply calendula once or twice a day to the remaining undressed skin • Patient applied calcium alginate dressing with Leptospermum honey once a week to assist with wound debridement • Resume Mepilex Ag

(continued)

Table 15.2 (continued)

Week	Skin Reaction	Reaction Type	Intervention
12 weeks postradiation	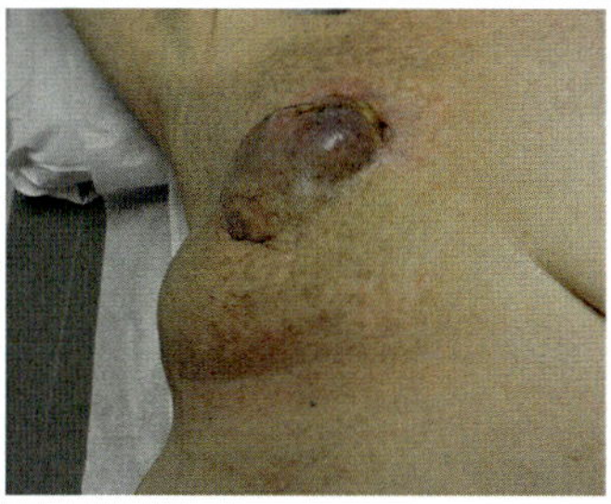	Mass is now resectable	• May resume pre- radiation dressing change procedure or continue with the above

The dressings are tailored to the patient's phase of therapy and wound care needs and goals

Table 15.3 Special cases and reactions

Special cases and reactions	Reaction Type	Treatment and intervention
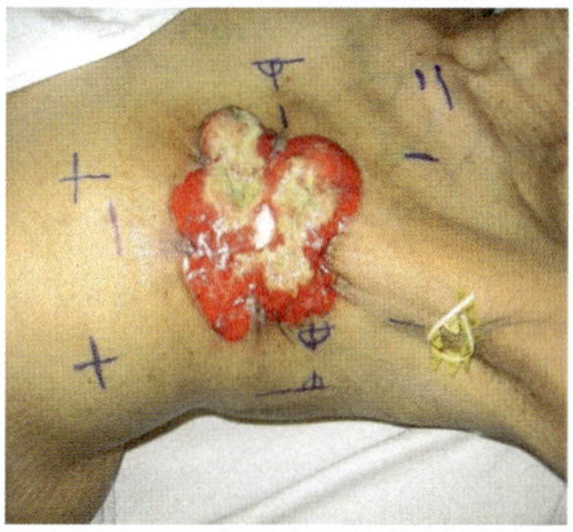	74-year-old Asian female Planning for neglected fungating breast cancer Patient changing dressing twice daily on presentation with complaints of wound odor	• Cleanse daily in shower with mild soap and water. Allow the soapy water to run over wound and then rinse • Pat dry • Silver nitrate applied as needed to wound edges for control of bleeding • Sprinkle the wound with crushed Flagyl daily • Cover the wound with Telfa, followed by abdominal pad and a Chux trimmed to fit to absorb drainage • Secure in place with large Flexinet wrap around the chest
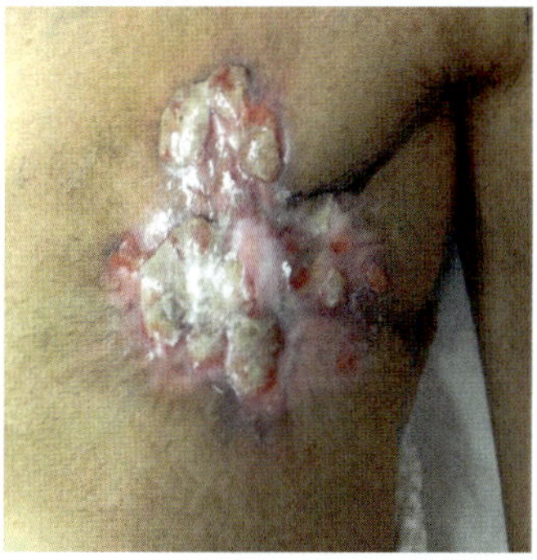	S/P radiation of fungating mass with a daily dressing change	• Skintegrity spray. Spray generously on the wound. Rinse off in the shower after 1–2 min • Apply Aquacel Ag dressing to the wound • Cover with ABD pad (secondary dressing) • Apply calendula cream to the skin around the open wound daily with the dressing change • Cover with Chux (to absorb any potential exudate) • Secure the entire dressing using a large Flexinet around the chest
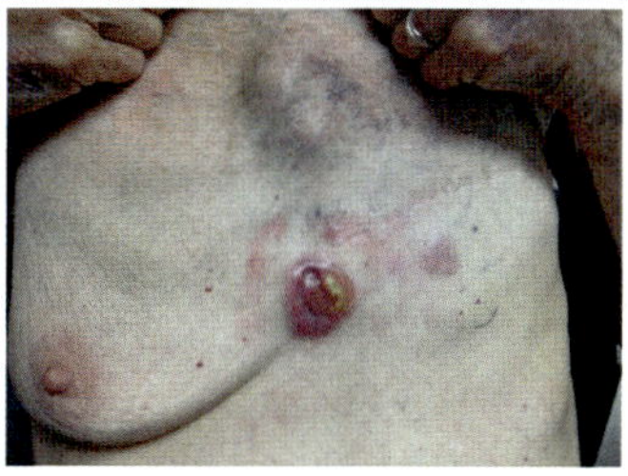	69-year-old Caucasian female. Postmastectomy. Recurrent breast cancer undergoing hyperthermia	• Cleanse daily with mild soap and water • Hydrocolloidal dressing (Manuka honey, silver ion) to the affected area. Left in place for 24–48 hours. Removed in the shower prior to treatments • Reapplied following treatment • Calendula cream applied one to two times a day to undressed skin surrounding the tumor

(continued)

Table 15.3 (continued)

Special cases and reactions	Reaction Type	Treatment and intervention
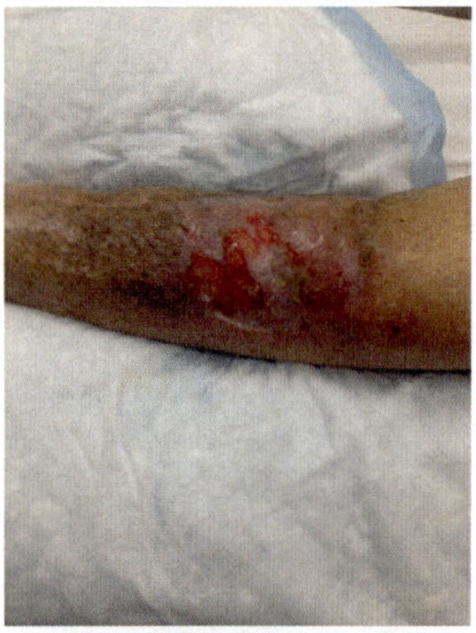 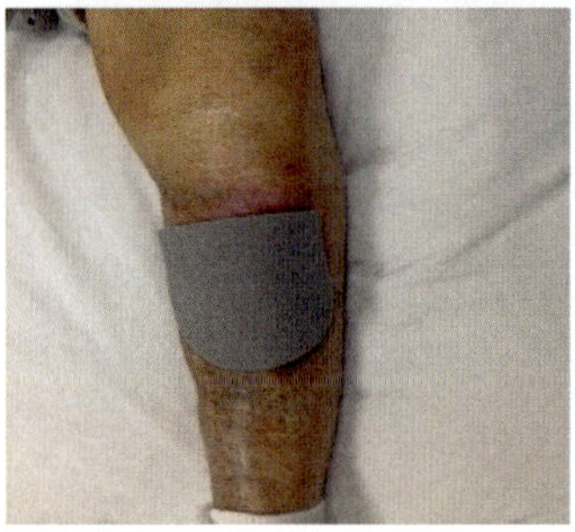	84-year-old Asian male with recurrent left lower extremity pleomorphic undifferentiated sarcoma. Last day of radiation therapy	• Spray the wound and radiation site with Skintegrity daily. Allow it to remain on the skin for 1–2 min and blot dry with clean gauze (the patient was unable to shower daily) • Apply Mepilex Ag to the wound • The dressing was left in place for 24–72 h and was removed prior to the patient receiving radiation treatments • Secure the Mepilex Ag with mesh. No tape was applied to the skin as the patient was undergoing daily treatments

References

1. Alexander S. Malignant fungating wounds: epidemiology, aetiology, presentation and assessment. J Wound Care. 2009;18:273–4, 6–8, 80. doi:http://dx.doi.org/10.12968/jowc.2009.18.7.43110
2. Probst S, Vellone D. The effective management of wounds with high levels of exudate. Br J Nurs. 2013; 22:S34. doi:http://dx.doi.org/10.12968/bjon.2013.22.Sup4.S34
3. Seaman S. Management of malignant fungating wounds in advanced cancer. Semin Oncol Nurs. 2006;22:185–93. doi:10.1016/j.soncn.2006.04.006.
4. Adderley UJ, Holt IGS. Topical agents and dressings for fungating wounds. Cochrane Database Syst Rev. 2014;2:CD003948. doi:10.1002/14651858.Cd003948.Pub3.
5. Alvarez OM, Kalinski C, Nusbaum J, Hernandez L, Pappous E, Kyriannis C, et al. Incorporating wound healing strategies to improve palliation (symptom management) in patients with chronic wounds. J Palliat Med. 2007;10:1161–89. doi:10.1089/jpm.2007.9909.
6. Selby T. Managing exudate in malignant fungating wounds and solving problems for patients. Nurs Times. 2009;105:14–7.
7. van Oorschot B, Rades D, Schulze W, Beckmann G, Feyer P. Palliative radiotherapy—new approaches. Semin Oncol. 2011;38:443–9. doi:10.1053/j.seminoncol.2011.03.015.
8. Linthorst M, Baaijens M, Wiggenraad R, Creutzberg C, Ghidey W, van Rhoon GC, et al. Local control rate after the combination of re-irradiation and hyperthermia for irresectable recurrent breast cancer: Results in 248 patients. Radiother Oncol. 2015;117(2):217–22. doi:10.1016/j.radonc.2015.04.019.
9. Armstrong DG, Meyr DPM. UpToDate: Basic principles of wound management Wolters Kluwer. 2015. http://www.uptodate.com/contents/basic-principles-of-wound-management. Accessed 27 May 2015.
10. Werdin F, Tennenhaus M, Schaller HE, Rennekampff HO. Evidence-based management strategies for treatment of chronic wounds. Eplasty. 2009;9, e19.
11. O'Brien C. Malignant wounds managing odour. Can Fam Phys. 2012;58:272–4.
12. Symptom Management Guidelines: Care of Malignant Wounds. BC Cancer Agency. 2015. http://www.bccancer.bc.ca/nursing-site/Documents/9.%20

Malignant%20Wounds.pdf. Accessed 11 September 2015.
13. Black JS, Drake DB. A prospective randomized trial comparing silver sulfadiazine cream with a water-soluble polyantimicrobial gel in partial-thickness burn wounds. Plast Surg Nurs. 2015;35:46–9. doi:10.1097/PSN.0000000000000081.
14. Masuelli L, Tumino G, Turriziani M, Modesti A, Bei R. Topical use of sucralfate in epithelial wound healing: clinical evidences and molecular mechanisms of action. Recent Pat Inflamm Allergy Drug Discov. 2010;4:25–36.
15. Mustoe T. Understanding chronic wounds: a unifying hypothesis on their pathogenesis and implications for therapy. Am J Surg. 2004;187:65S–70. doi:10.1016/S0002-9610(03)00306-4.
16. Gjodsbol K, Christensen JJ, Karlsmark T, Jorgensen B, Klein BM, Krogfelt KA. Multiple bacterial species reside in chronic wounds: a longitudinal study. Int Wound J. 2006;3:225–31. doi:10.1111/j.1742-481X.2006.00159.x.
17. Sibbald RG, Williamson D, Orsted HL, Campbell K, Keast D, Krasner D, et al. Preparing the wound bed—debridement, bacterial balance, and moisture balance. Ostomy Wound Manage. 2000;46:14–22, 4–8, 30–5; quiz 6–7.
18. Diehr S, Hamp A, Jamieson B, Mendoza M. Clinical inquiries. Do topical antibiotics improve wound healing? J Fam Pract. 2007;56:140–4.
19. Sawynok J. Topical and peripherally acting analgesics. Pharmacol Rev. 2003;55:1–20. doi:10.1124/pr.55.1.1.
20. Krajnik M, Zylicz Z. Topical morphine for cutaneous cancer pain. Palliat Med. 1997;11:325.
21. Guidelines for the use of topical morphine for painful skin ulcers in palliative care. Northamptonshire Healthcare. 2014. http://www.neneccg.nhs.uk/resources/uploads/files/use%20of%20topical%20Morphine.pdf. Accessed 11 September 2015.

Appendix: Skin Care Products Commonly Used in Radiation Oncology

B. Fowble et al. (eds.), *Skin Care in Radiation Oncology*, DOI 10.1007/978-3-319-31460-0

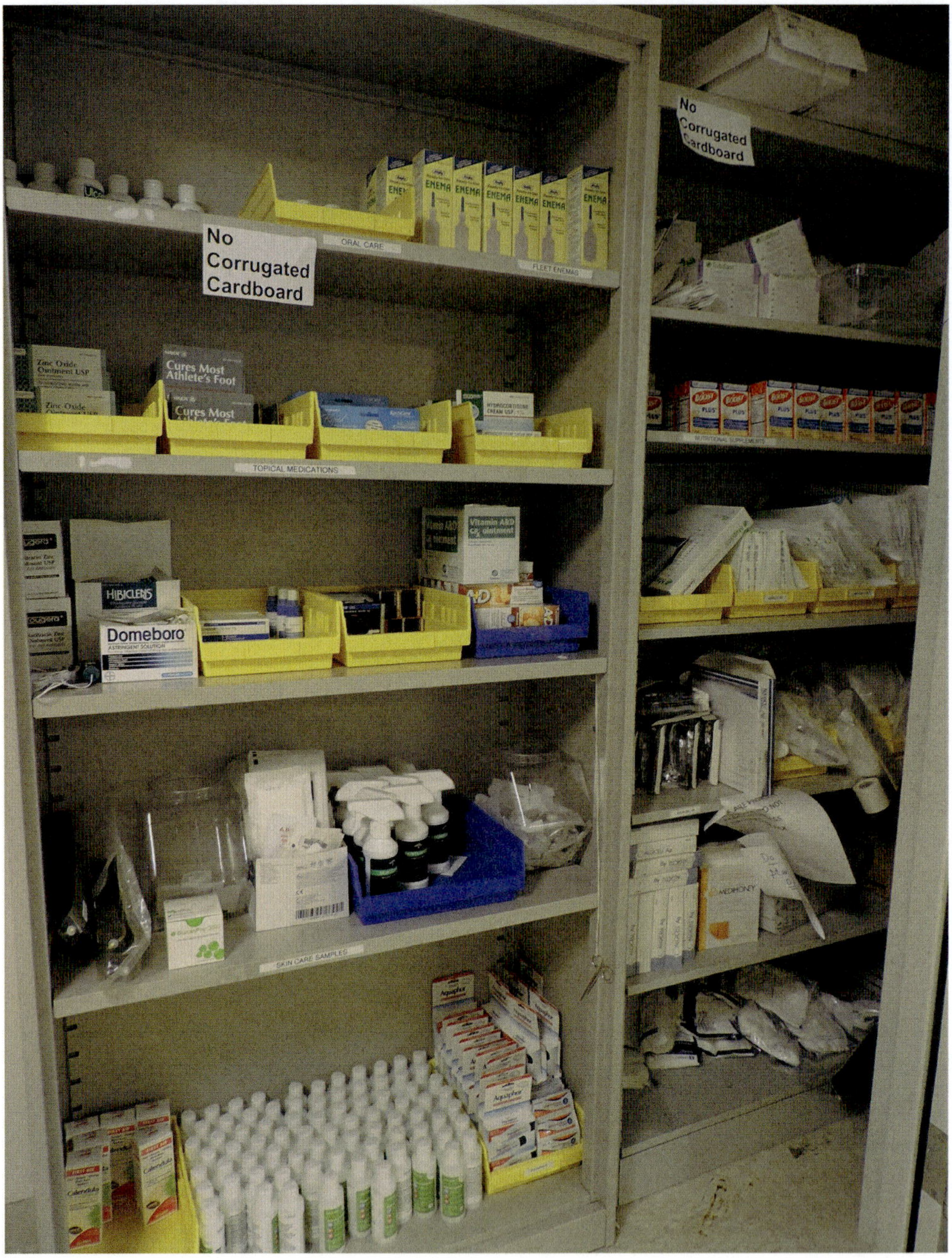

Closet for storage of skin care products

1. *Moisturizers*

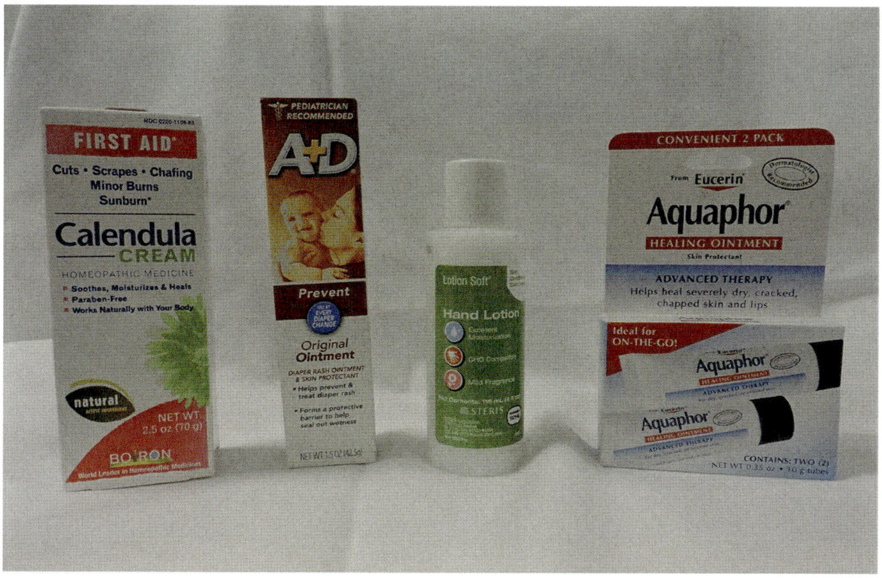

Calendula, A+D Ointment, Lotion Soft, Aquaphor

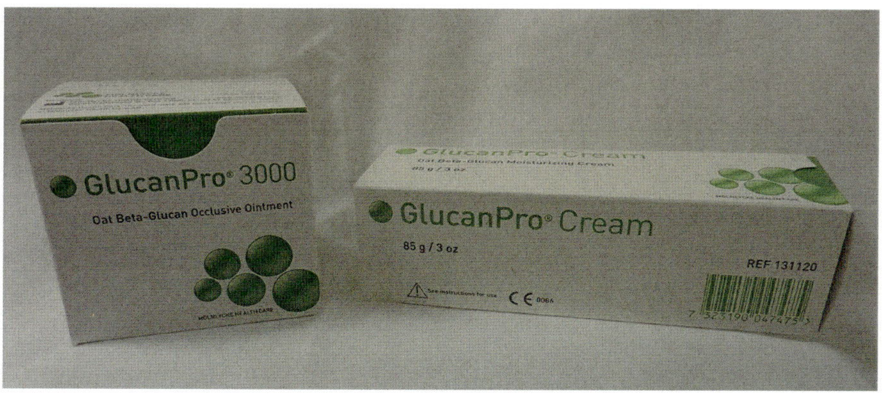

GlucanPro 3000 and GlucanPro Cream

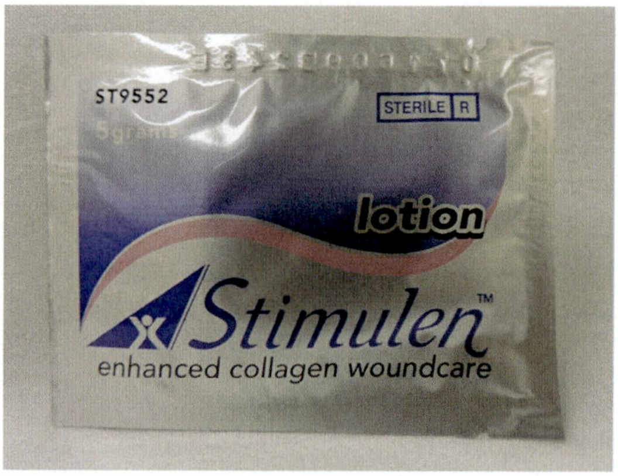

Stimulen lotion

2. *Topical Steroids*

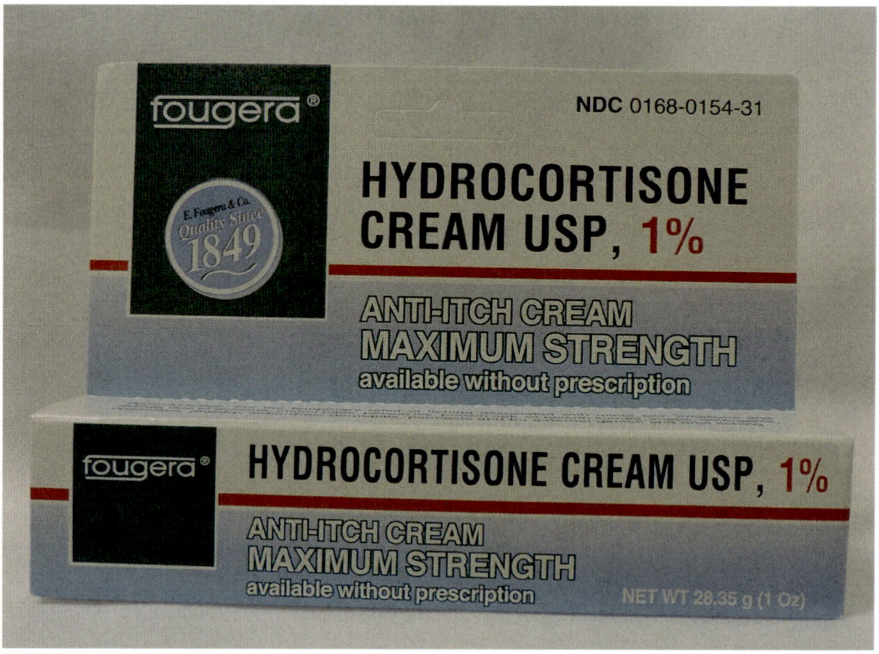

Hydrocortisone cream

3. *Cleansers*

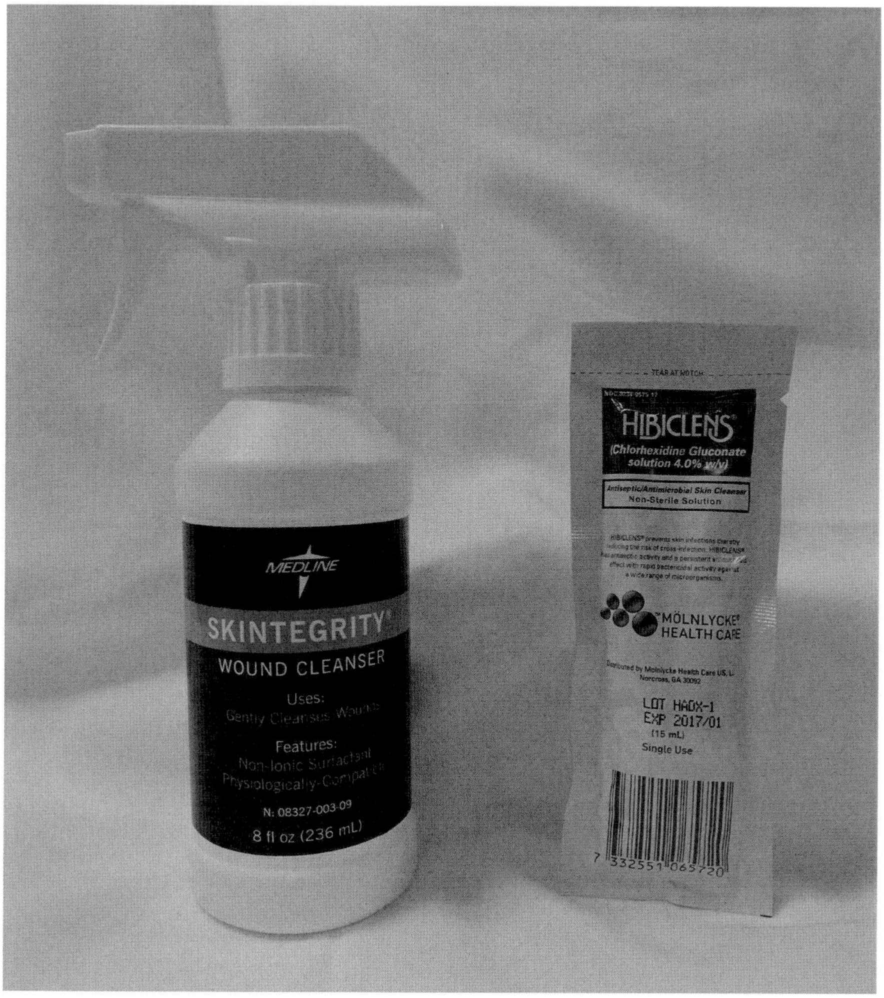

Skintegrity and Hibiclens

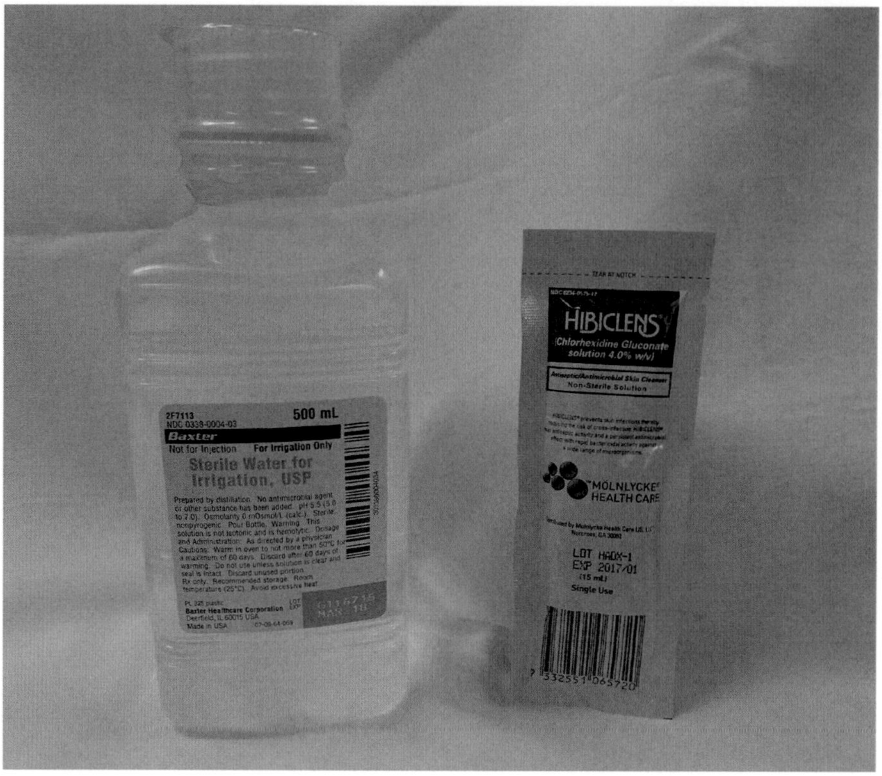

Sterile water and Hibiclens

4. *Drying Agents*

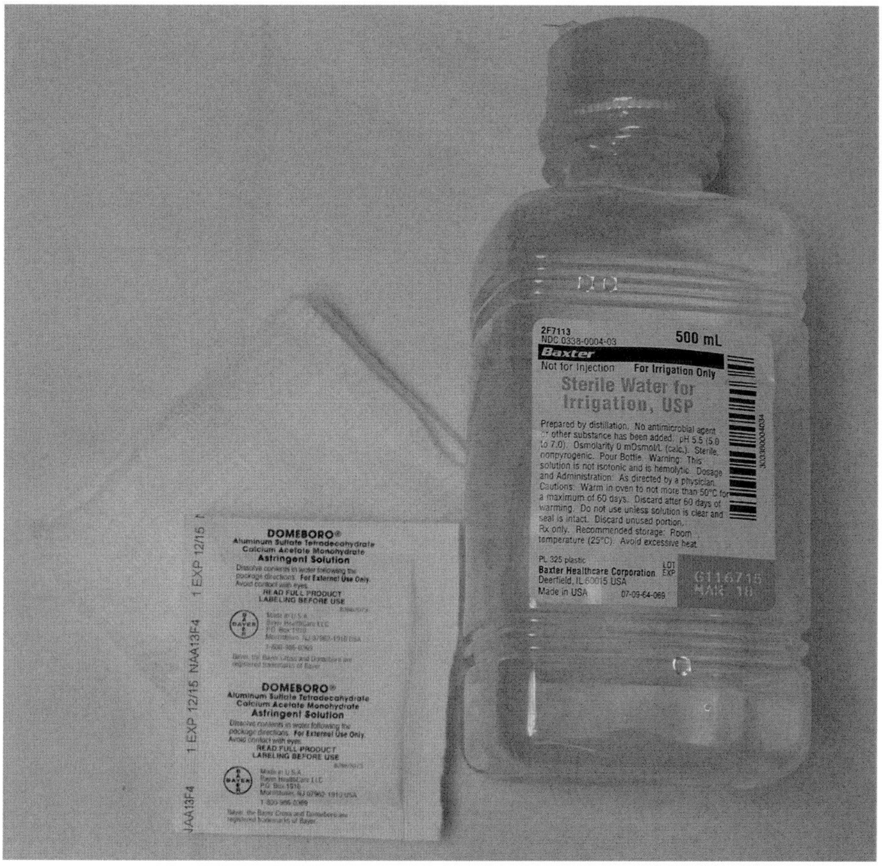

Domeboro (Burow's solution) with sterile water

5. *Anti-infective*

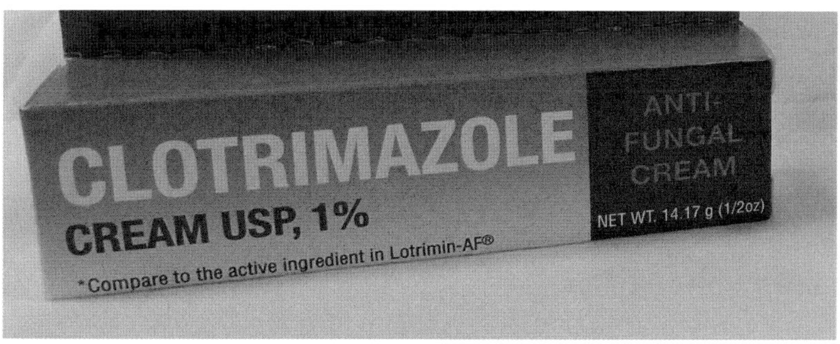

Clotrimazole cream

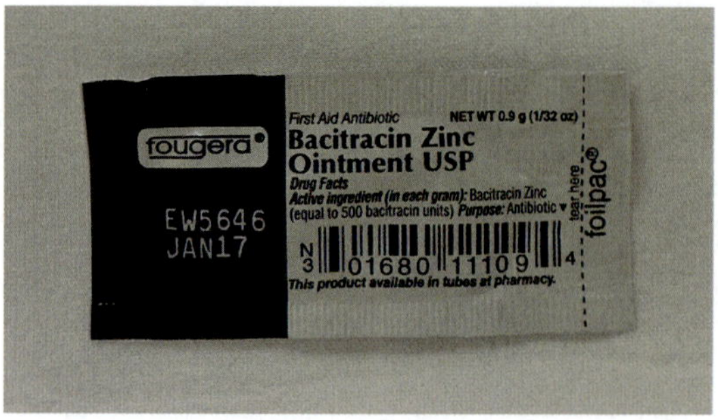

Bacitracin zinc ointment

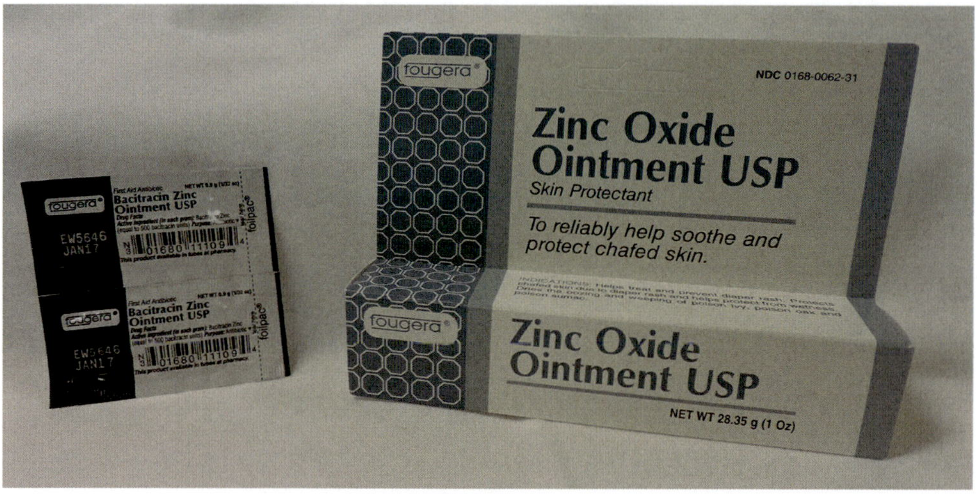

Bacitracin zinc ointment and zinc oxide ointment

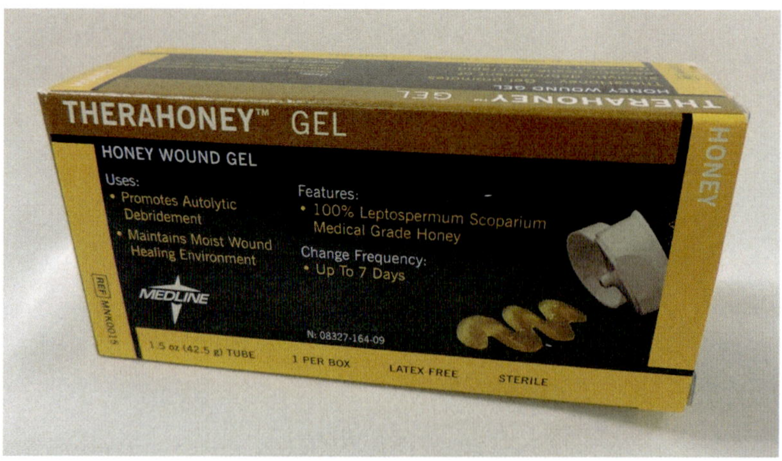

Therahoney gel

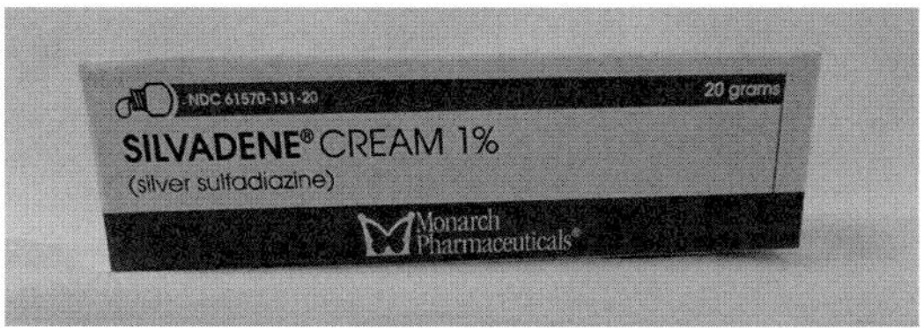

Silver sulfadiazine (not recommended)

6. *Skin Barriers*

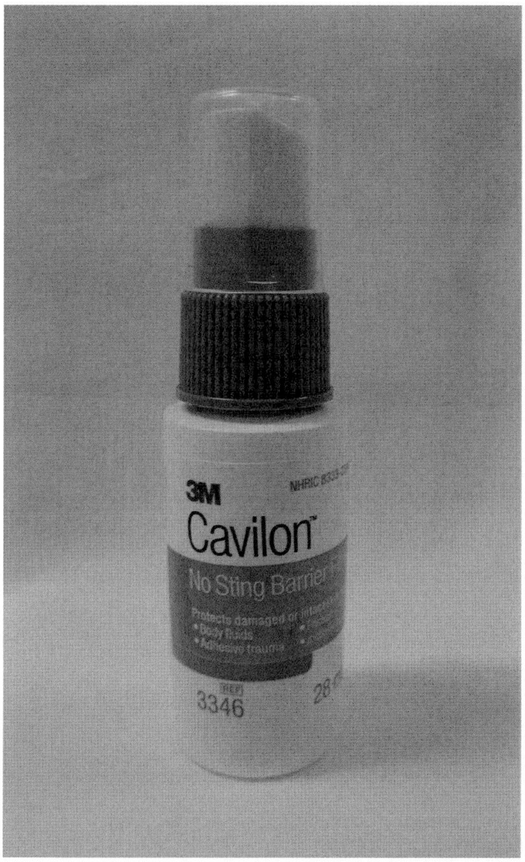

Cavilon

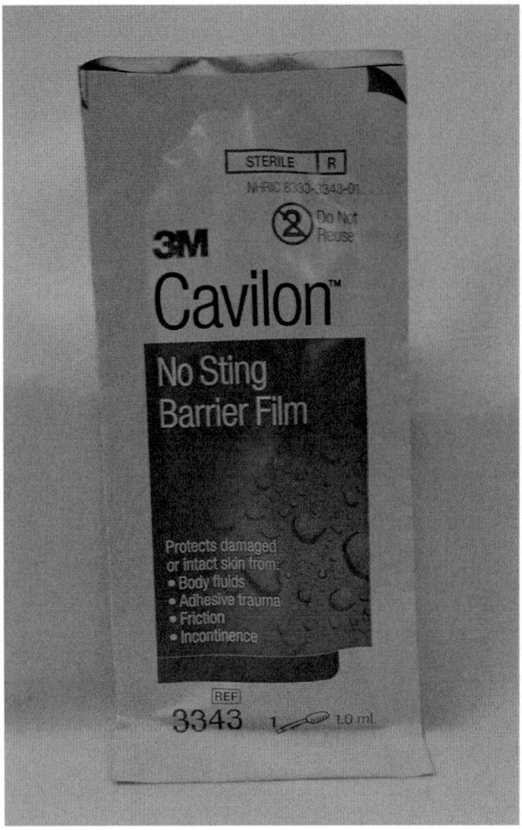
STERILE R
Do Not Reuse
3M
Cavilon™
No Sting Barrier Film
Protects damaged or intact skin from:
• Body fluids
• Adhesive trauma
• Friction
• Incontinence
REF
3343
1.0 ml

Cavilon

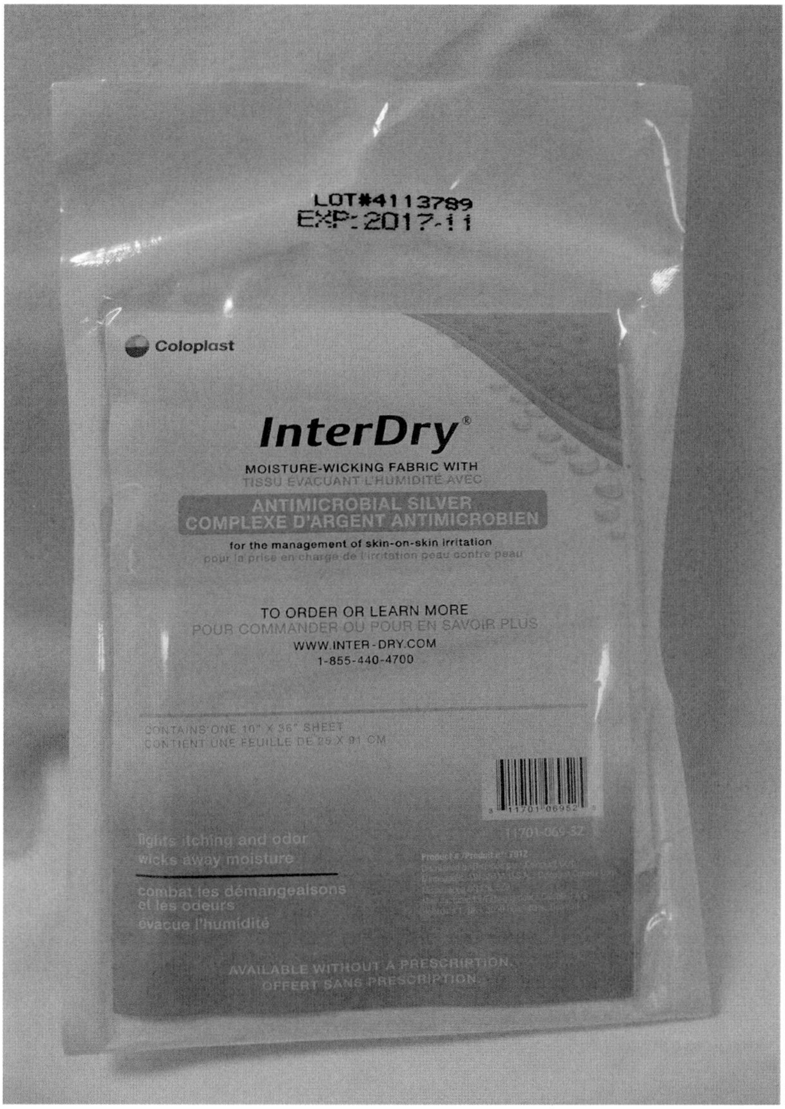
LOT#4113789
EXP:2017-11
Coloplast
InterDry®
MOISTURE-WICKING FABRIC WITH
TISSU ÉVACUANT L'HUMIDITÉ AVEC
ANTIMICROBIAL SILVER
COMPLEXE D'ARGENT ANTIMICROBIEN
for the management of skin-on-skin irritation
TO ORDER OR LEARN MORE
POUR COMMANDER OU POUR EN SAVOIR PLUS
WWW.INTER-DRY.COM
1-855-440-4700
fights itching and odor
wicks away moisture
combat les démangeaisons
et les odeurs
évacue l'humidité
AVAILABLE WITHOUT A PRESCRIPTION.
OFFERT SANS PRESCRIPTION.

InterDry

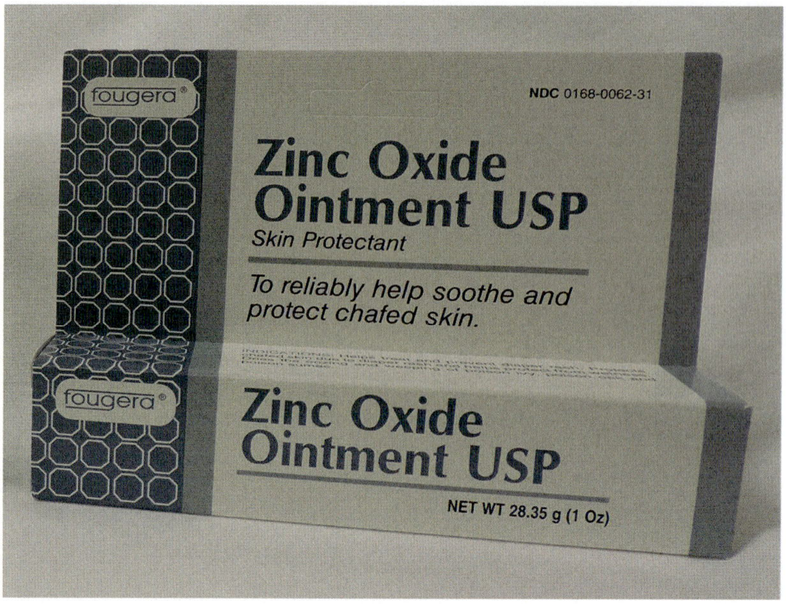

Zinc oxide

7. *Dressings*

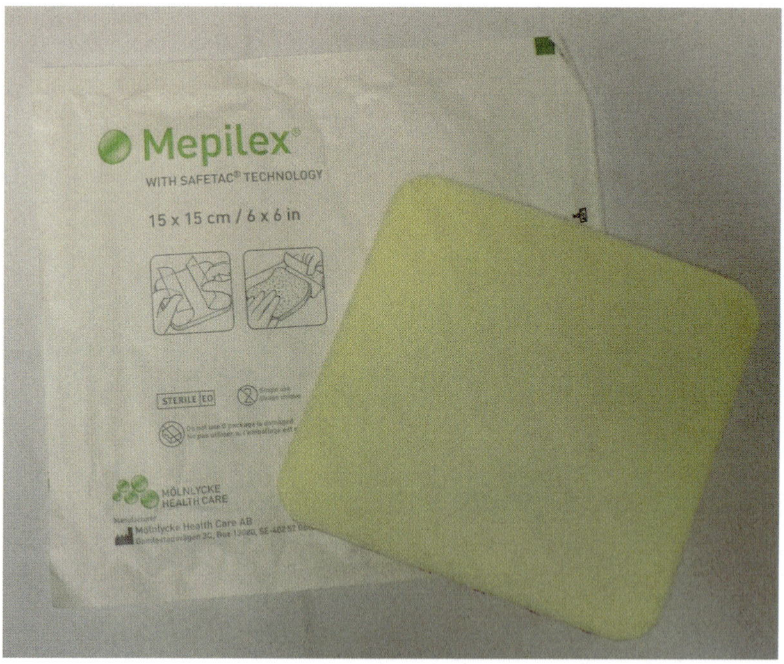

Mepilex

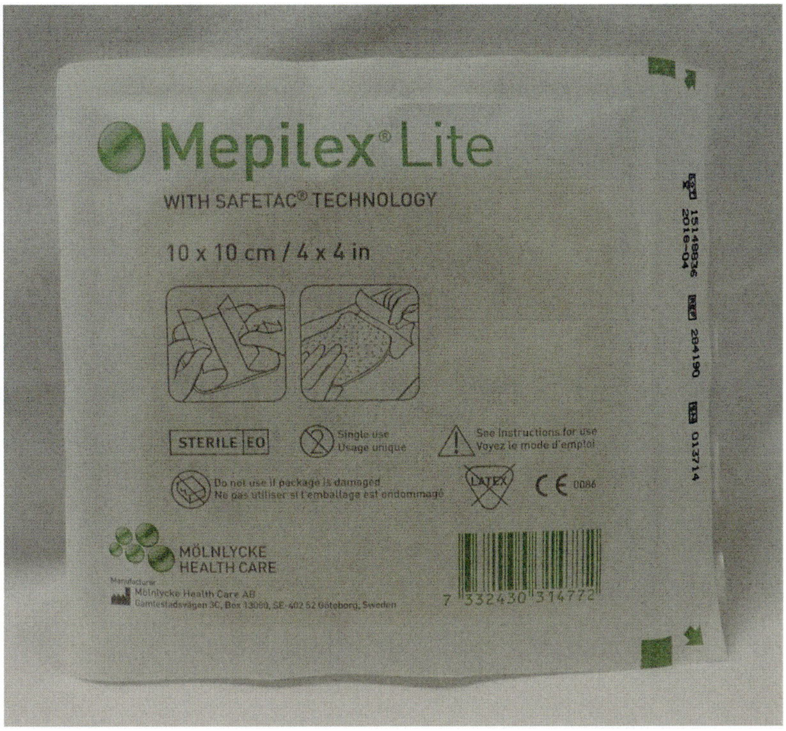

Mepilex Lite (small)

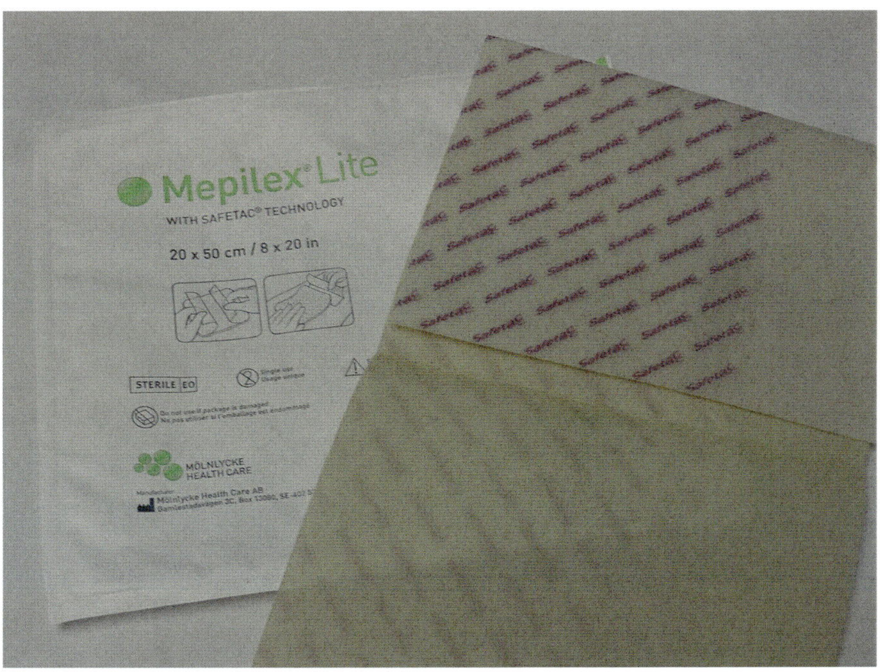

Mepilex Lite (large, cut to fit)

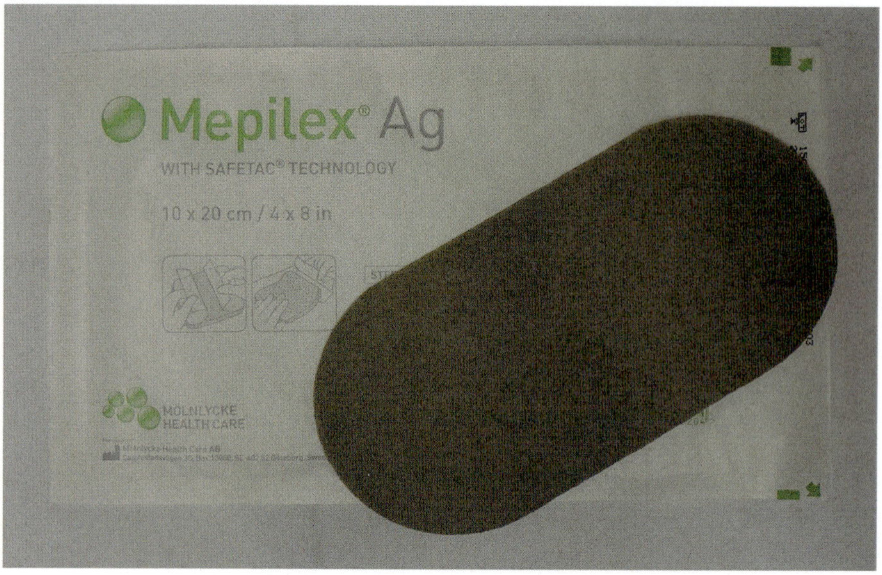

Mepilex Ag

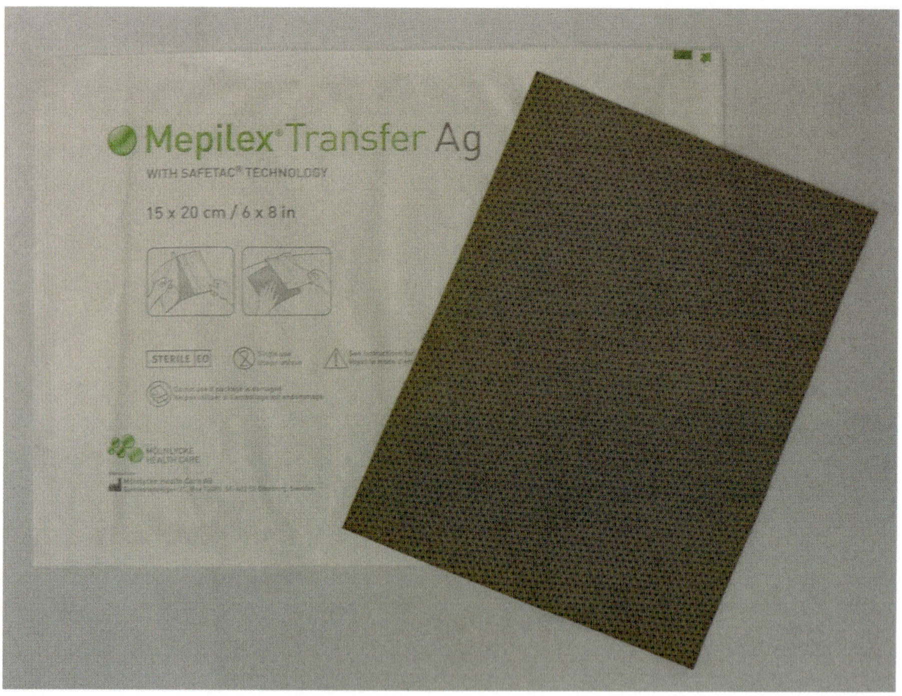

Mepilex Transfer Ag

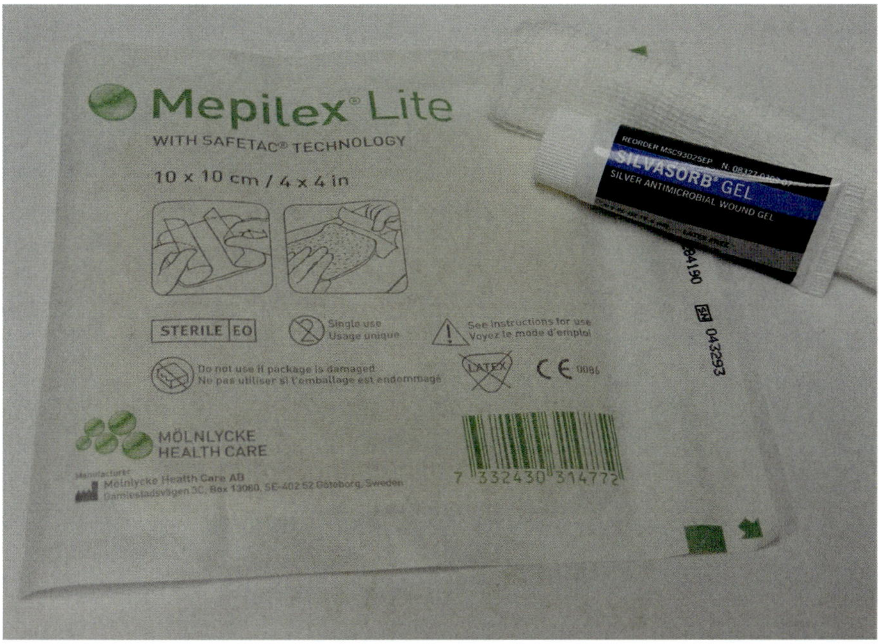

Mepilex Lite with Silvasorb Gel

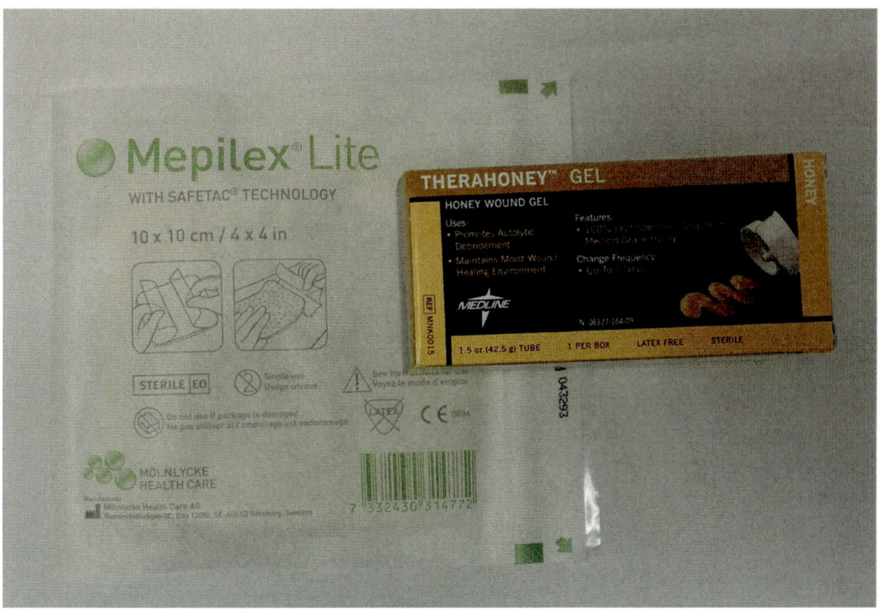

Mepilex Lite with Therahoney

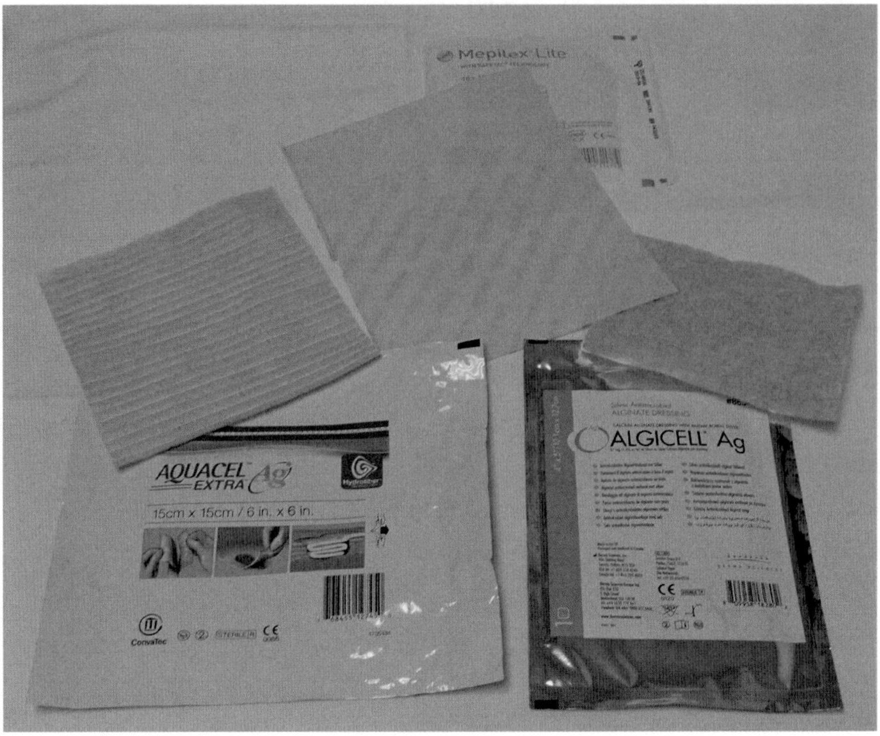

Aquacel Extra Ag and Algicell Ag with Mepilex Lite

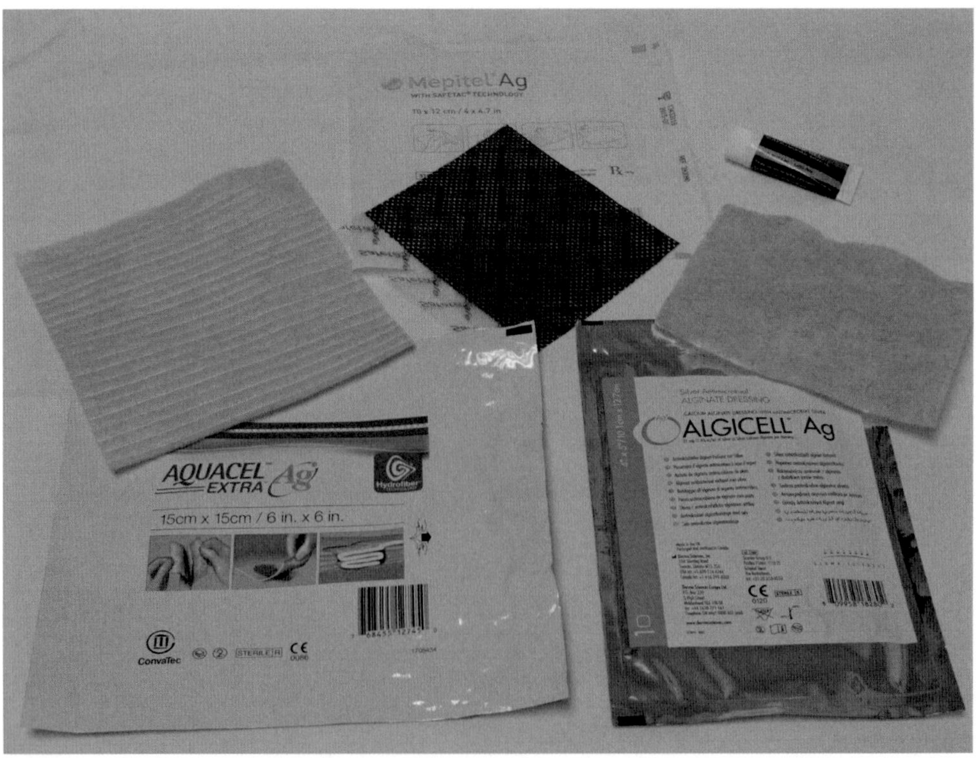

Aquacel Extra Ag, Algicell Ag, Mepitel Ag, and Silvasorb gel

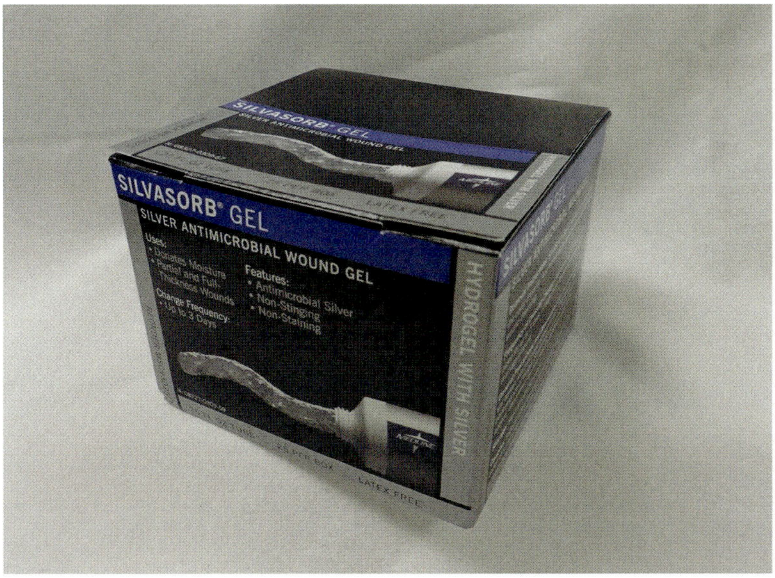

Silvasorb Gel

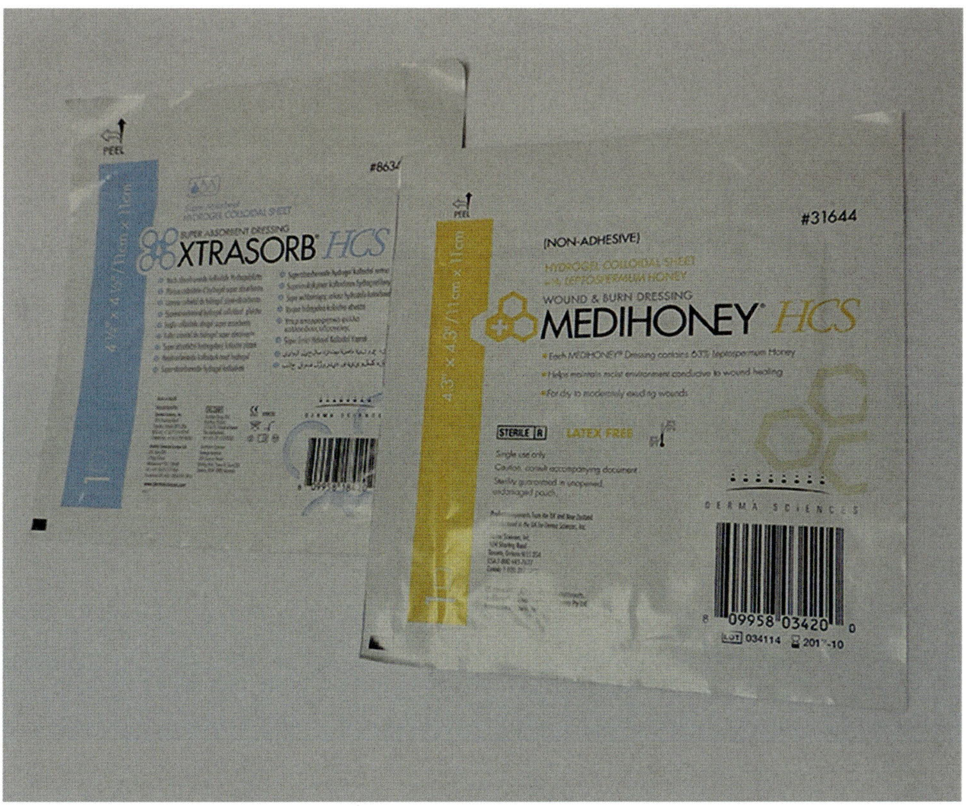

Hydrocolloidal Dressings with and without medical-grade honey

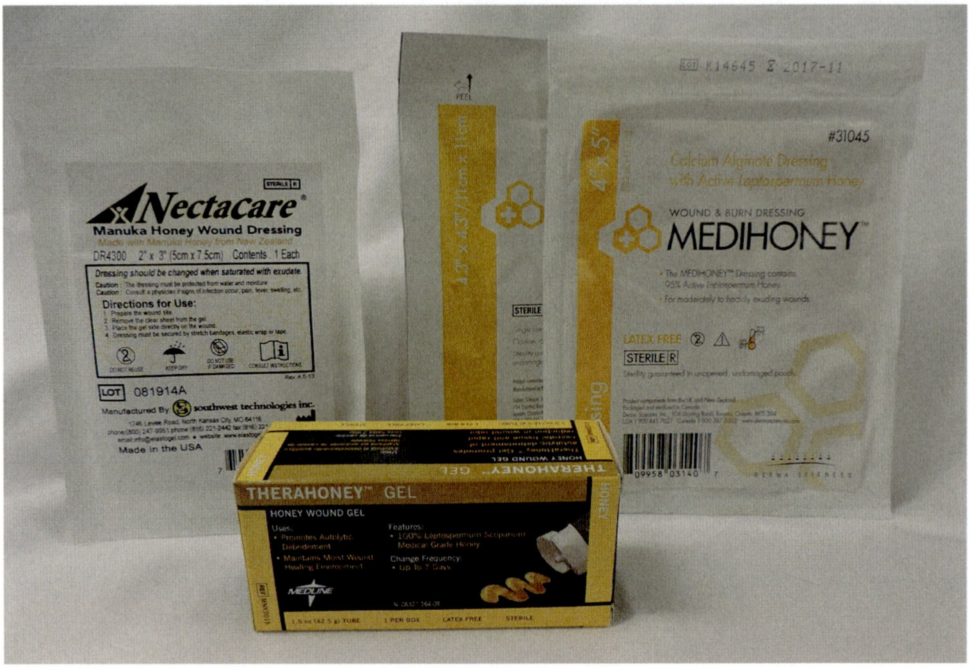

Medical-grade honey products

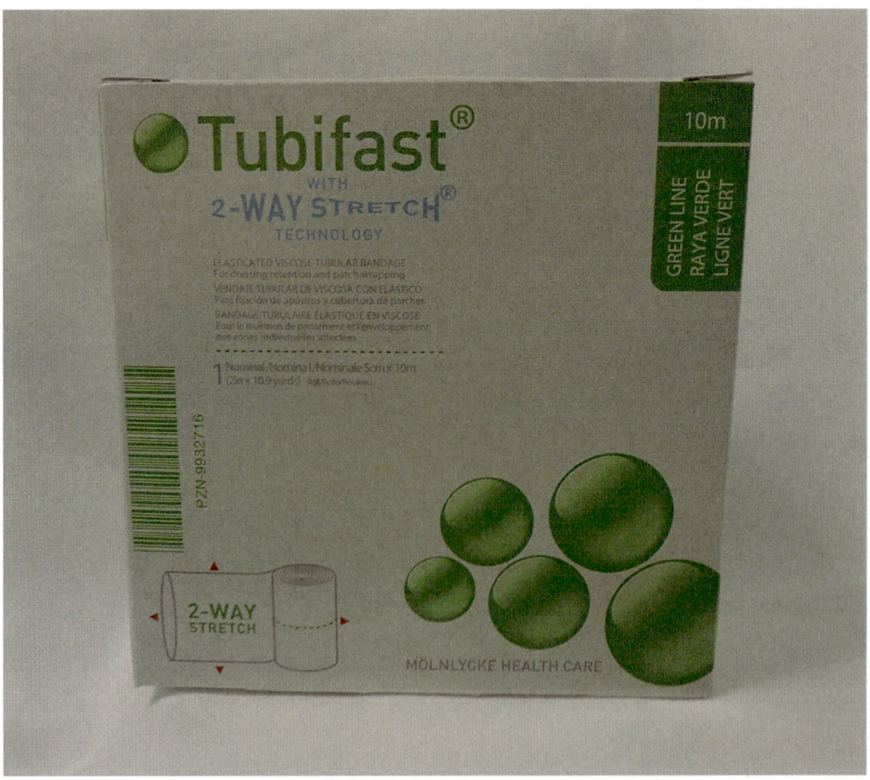

Tubifast

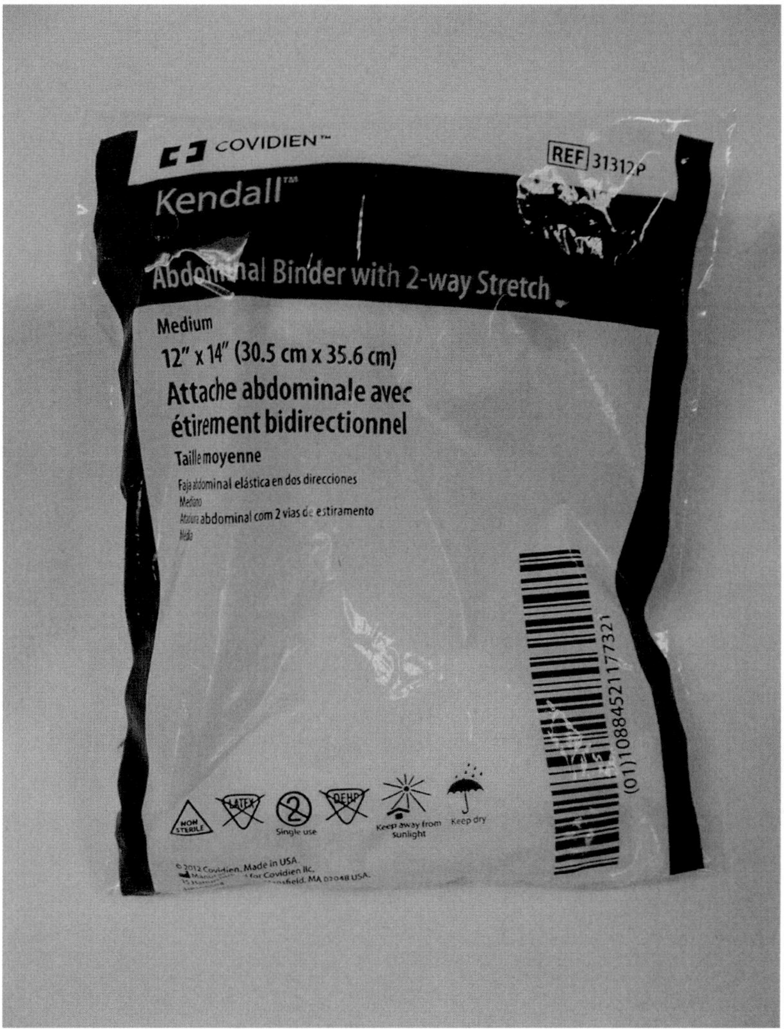

Kendall Abdominal Binder

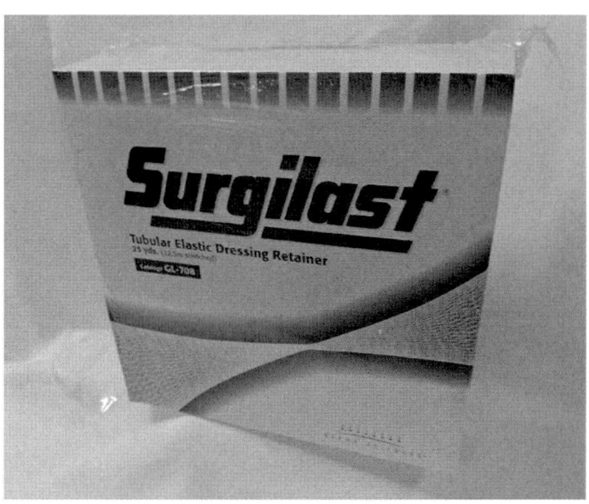

Surgilast

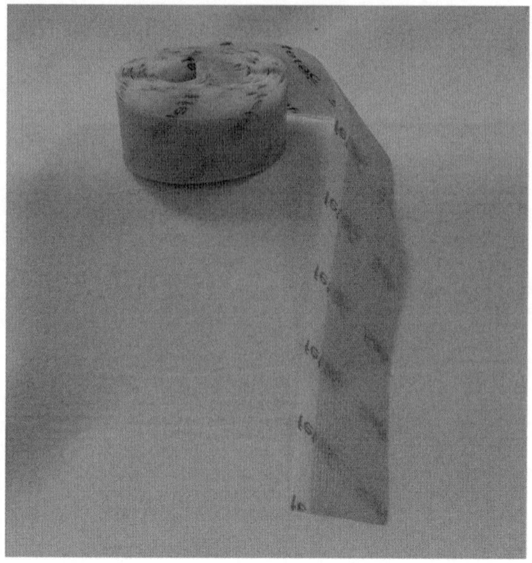

Silicone tape

8. *Miscellaneous*

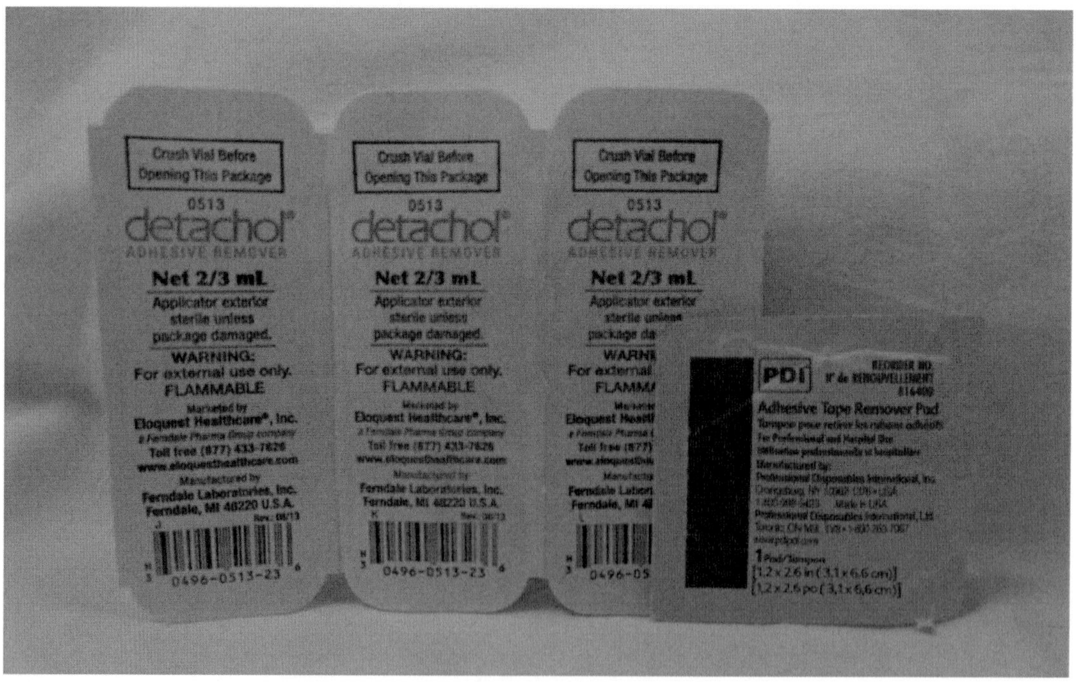

Detachol and Adhesive Tape Remover Pad

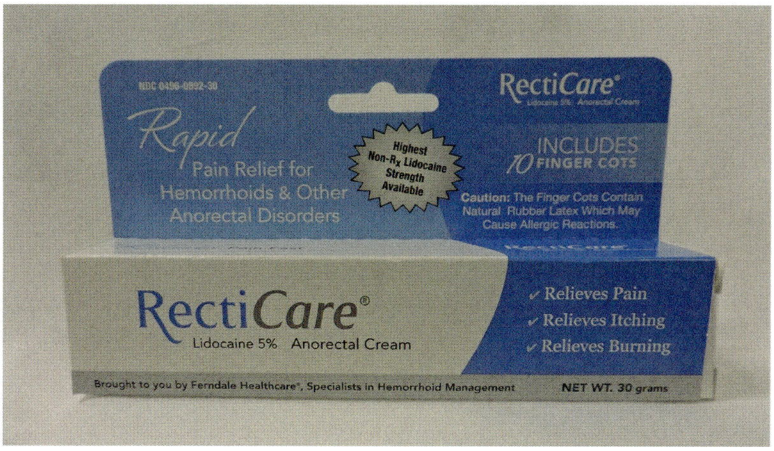

Lidocaine 5 % cream

Index

B. Fowble et al. (eds.), *Skin Care in Radiation Oncology*, DOI 10.1007/978-3-319-31460-0

Made in the USA
San Bernardino, CA
23 July 2020

75861759R00142